Günter Köhler, Matthias Evert, Katja Evert, Marek Zygmunt
Sarcoma of the female genitalia

Günter Köhler, Matthias Evert, Katja Evert,
Marek Zygmunt

Sarcoma of the female genitalia

Volume 2: Other rare sarcomas, mixed tumors, genital sarcomas and pregnancy

In collaboration with
Philipp-Andreas Hessler, Lars Kaderali,
Hanka Lehnhoff, Lisa Linke

DE GRUYTER

Authors
Prof. Dr. Günter Köhler
Department of Obstetrics and Gynecology, University Medicine Greifswald and German Clinical Center of Excellence for Genital Sarcomas and Mixed Tumors
Ferdinand-Sauerbruch-Straße
17475 Greifswald, Germany
e-mail: koehlerg@uni-greifswald.de

Prof. Dr. Marek Zygmunt
Department of Obstetrics and Gynecology, University Medicine Greifswald and German Clinical Center of Excellence for Genital Sarcomas and Mixed Tumors
Ferdinand-Sauerbruch-Straße
17475 Greifswald, Germany
e-mail: zygmunt@uni-greifswald.de

Prof. Dr. Matthias Evert
Institute of Pathology, University Hospital Regensburg and German Clinical Center of Excellence for Genital Sarcomas and Mixed Tumors, Greifswald
Franz-Josef-Strauß-Allee 11
93053 Regensburg, Deutschland
e-mail: matthias.evert@ukr.de

Dr. Katja Evert
Institute of Pathology, University Hospital Regensburg and German Clinical Center of Excellence for Genital Sarcomas and Mixed Tumors, Greifswald
Franz-Josef-Strauß-Allee 11
93053 Regensburg, Deutschland
e-mail: katja.evert@ukr.de

Collaborators
Dr. Philipp-Andreas Hessler
Department of Gynecologic Surgery, Center of Minimal-Invasive Surgery, Sachsenhausen, Frankfurt/Main/Germany

Prof. Dr. Lars Kaderali
Institute for Bioinformatics, University Medicine Greifswald/Germany

Hanka Lehnhoff
Department of Obstetrics and Gynecology University Medicine Greifswald and German Clinical Center of Excellence for Genital Sarcomas and Mixed Tumors, Greifswald/Germany

Lisa Linke
Department of Obstetrics and Gynecology University Medicine Greifswald and German Clinical Center of Excellence for Genital Sarcomas and Mixed Tumors, Greifswald/Germany

ISBN 978-3-11-045921-0
e-ISBN (PDF) 978-3-11-046002-5
e-ISBN (EPUB) 978-3-11-045925-8

Library of Congress Cataloging-in-Publication Data
A CIP catalog record for this book has been applied for at the Library of Congress.

Bibliographic information published by the Deutsche Nationalbibliothek
The Deutsche Nationalbibliothek lists this publication in the Deutsche Nationalbibliografie; detailed bibliographic data are available on the Internet at http://dnb.dnb.de.

Cover image: Dr. med. Peter Baier, Ketteler Hospital Offenbach, Gynecology and Obstetrics, Offenbach/Germany
Translation into English: Dr. jur. Philip Horsfield, Greifswald/Germany (translate@philiphorsfield.com)
Typesetting: PTP-Berlin, Protago-TEX-Production GmbH, Berlin
Printing and binding: Hubert & Co GmbH und Co KG, Göttingen
♾ Printed on acid-free paper
Printed in Germany

www.degruyter.com

Foreword

This monograph, comprising two volumes, discusses typical sarcomas of the female genitalia, including angiosarcoma, liposarcoma and rhabdomyosarcoma as well as the different types of mixed tumors. Other rare mesenchymal genital tumors are also comprehensively presented, such as the different variants of leiomyoma, smooth muscle tumors with uncertain malignant potential, endometrial stromal nodules, endometrial stromal tumors with sex cord-like elements (ESTSCLE), uterine tumor resembling ovarian sex-cord/stromal tumor (UTROCST) and PEComas. The behavior of the aforementioned neoplasms in relation to, and in the context of fertility and pregnancy is covered in a separate chapter. Another chapter is devoted to the prevention of subjecting sarcomas to inadequate surgical therapeutic measures under the assumed diagnosis of leiomyoma, and includes a diagnostic-therapeutic flowchart with a diagnostic score. The following subsections are provided for each of the tumor entities listed above: epidemiology, etiology, macroscopy and microscopy, clinical presentation, diagnostics, imaging, differential diagnostics, prognosis, surgical and radiation therapy for the primary tumor or recurrences and metastases including primary, adjuvant and palliative chemotherapy, hormone therapy, targeted therapy and aftercare.

The substantial basis for this monograph comprises 1,681 fully documented sarcoma consultation cases of the German Clinical Center of Excellence for Genital Sarcomas and Mixed Tumors ("Deutsches klinisches Kompetenzzentrum für genitale Sarkome und Mischtumoren", DKSM), University Medicine Greifswald/Germany, and the data kindly provided by our cooperation partners "Velener Working Group on Ambulatory Surgery" ("Velener Arbeitsgemeinschaft Ambulantes Operieren Deutschland", VAAO) and the Department Gynecologic Surgery, Center of Minimal-Invasive Surgery, Sachsenhausen/Frankfurt Main/Germany.

The overriding aim of this monograph is to identify and provide therapeutic guidance on the basis of evaluation of the DKSM data performed by the DKSM doctoral research group "uterine sarcomas", as well as on 2,025 literature sources, recommendations and studies published up to the end of May 2016. Particular attention has been devoted to determining, as far as possible, which measures can currently not be defined as standard practice. In total, 576 figures and illustrations have been incorporated and are comprehensively described.

The listed tumor entities also constitute a particular diagnostic challenge for pathologists that is beset with numerous pitfalls and difficulties. This monograph, therefore, addresses gynecologists and pathologists in both clinical and private practice, but also surgeons and hemato-oncologists.

Sincere thanks must be extended to a total of 112 gynecologists, pathologists, radiologists, hemato-oncologists and medical practitioners in clinical and private practice, but also affected patients, who kindly provided figures, images and data for use in this monograph.

Greifswald and Regensburg, June 2016

Prof. Dr. G. Köhler, Prof. Dr. M. Zygmunt,
Department of Obstetrics and Gynecology, University Medicine Greifswald
and German Clinical Center of Excellence for Sarcomas and Mixed Tumors,
Greifswald

Prof. Dr. M. Evert, Dr. Katja Evert
Institute of Pathology, University Hospital Regensburg
and German Clinical Center of Excellence for Genital Sarcomas and Mixed Tumors,
Greifswald

Sarcoma of the female genitalia
Volume 1: Smooth muscle and stromal tumors and the prevention of inadequate sarcoma surgery (ISBN: 978-3-11-035141-5)
Volume 2: Other rare sarcomas, mixed tumors, genital sarcomas and pregnancy (ISBN: 978-3-11-045921-0)

Contents

Volume 2

List of abbreviations

AAGL	American Association of Gynecologic Laparoscopists
AB	Antibody
AF	Adenofibroma
AI	Aromatase inhibitors
AJCC	American Joint Cancer Committee
ALM	Angioleiomyoma
ANS	Angiosarcoma
AR	Androgen receptor
ARMS	Alveolar rhabdomyosarcoma
AS	Adenosarcoma
AUB	Abnormal uterine bleeding(s)
BSO	Bilateral Salpingo-oophorectomy
BT	Brachytherapy
CBR	Clinical benefit rate (CR + PR + SD)
CECT	Contrast-enhanced CT
CHT	Chemotherapy
CHT-RT	Chemoradiotherapy
CLM	Cellular leiomyoma
CR	Complete response
CS	Carcinosarcoma
CT	Computed tomography
d	Day
DD	Differential diagnostics
DLM	Degenerated leiomyoma
DFS	Disease free survival
DKSM	Deutsches klinisches Kompetenzzentrum für genitale Sarkome und Mischtumoren Universitätsmedizin Greifswald (German Clinical Center of Excellence for Genital Sarcomas and Mixed Tumors, University Medicine Greifswald)
DNG	Dienogest
DPLM	Disseminated (diffuse) peritoneal leiomyomatosis
DSS	Disease specific survival
DW-MRI	Diffusion-weighted magnetic resonance imaging
EGF(R)	Epithelial growth factor (receptor)
EC	Endometrial carcinoma
ER	Estrogen receptor
ERMS	Embryonal rhabdomyosarcoma
ERT	External (percutaneous) radiotherapy
ESN	Endometrial stromal nodule
EST	Endometrial stromal tumor
ESTSCLE	Endometrial stromal tumor with sex cord-like elements

FDG-PET	F-FDG-PET (^{18}F-2-Fluor-2-deoxy-D-glucose-PET)
FES-PET	F-FES-PET (16α-^{18}F-fluoro-17β estradiol-PET)
FS	Fibrosarcoma
GCIG	Gynecologic Cancer InterGroup
GIST	Gastrointestinal stromal tumors
GnRH	Gonadotropin-releasing hormone
HE	Hysterectomy
HE-stain	Hematoxylin and eosin stain
HG-ESS	High-grade endometrial stromal sarcoma
HMB45	Human melanoma black 45
HPF	High power field (400× magnification)
HR	Hormone receptor
HRT	Hormone replacement therapy
HSC	Hysteroscopy
HT	Hormone therapy
HU	Hounsfield unit
IHC	Immunohistochemistry, immunohistochemical
IVLM	Intravenous leiomyomatosis
LAVH	Laparoscopically assisted vaginal hysterectomy
LDH	Lactate dehydrogenase
Lig.	Ligamentum, ligament
LG-ESS	Low-grade endometrial stromal sarcoma
LITT	Laser-induced thermotherapy
LLM	Lipoleiomyoma
LM	Leiomyoma
L/M-ratio	Lymphocyte-monocyte ratio
LMS	Leiomyosarcoma
LN	Lymph node
LNE	Lymphadenectomy
LS	Liposarcoma
LSC	Laparoscopy
LVI	Lymphovascular invasion
M/10 HPF	Counted mitoses per 10 HPF
max	Maximal
MGA	Megestrol acetate
ME	Myomectomy, myoma enucleation
MI	Mitotic index
min	Minimal
MLM	Benign metastasizing leiomyoma
mo	Months
MPA	Medroxyprogesterone acetate
MRI	Magnetic resonance imaging
MRT	Magnetic resonance tomography
mTOR	Mammalian target of rapamycin

N/L-ratio	Neutrophil/lymphocyte ratio
NOS	Not otherwise specified
NPV	Negative predictive value
PD	Progressive disease
PDGF(R)	Platelet-derived growth factor (receptors)
PEComa	Perivascular epithelioid cell tumor
PET-CT	Positron emission tomography
PFI	Progression free interval
PFS	Progression free survival
PGR	Progesterone receptor
PHH3	Phospho-histone H3
PPV	Positive predictive value
PR	Partial response
PRMS	Pleomorphic rhabdomyosarcoma
q	Time interval
RAH	Radical abdominal hysterectomy
RFA	Radiofrequency ablation
RFI	Relapse free interval
RFS	Relapse free survival
RI	Resistance index
RMS	Rhabdomyosarcoma
RR	Remission rate
RT	Radiation therapy, radiotherapy, ERT with and without VBT
RVH	Radical vaginal hysterectomy
SAH	Supracervical abdominal hysterectomy
SD	Stable disease
SEER	Surveillance, Epidemiology and End Results
SERM	Selective estrogen receptor modulator
SHE	Supracervical hysterectomy
SI	Signal intensity (in MRI)
SIRT	Selective internal radiation therapy
SLH	Supracervical laparoscopic hysterectomy
SLN	Sentinel lymph node
SMA	Smooth muscle actin
SO	Sarcomatous overgrowth
STS	Soft tissue sarcoma
STUMP	Smooth muscle tumor with uncertain malignant potential
SUV	Standardized uptake value
T1W, T2W	T1/T2 weighted MRI
T1WC	T1 weighted contrast MRI
T1W-FS	T1 or T2 weighted MRI with fat suppression, occasionally also T1/2W STIR
T2W-FS	see T1W-FS
TAH	Total abdominal hysterectomy
TAS	Transabdominal sonography

TCN	Tumor cell necrosis
THE	Total hysterectomy
TKI	Tyrosine kinase inhibitor
TCS	Tubal carcinosarcoma
TLH	Total laparoscopic hysterectomy
TVH	Total vaginal hysterectomy
TVS	Transvaginal sonography
UCS	Uterine carcinosarcoma
UES	Undifferentiated endometrial sarcoma
UPA	Ulipristal acetate
UTROSCT	Uterine tumor resembling ovarian sex-cord stromal tumor
UUS	Undifferentiated uterine sarcoma
VA	Vincristine plus actinomycin
VAC	Vincristine plus actinomycin D plus cyclophosphamide
VAI	Vincristine plus actinomycin D plus ifosfamide
VBT	Vaginal brachytherapy
VEGF(R)	Vascular endothelial growth factor (receptor)
VI	Vascular invasion
wk	Weeks
WOP	Week(s) of pregnancy
WT-1	Wilms tumor Gen 1

Definition of cytoreduction, NCCN-Guidelines

Cytoreduction (debulking)

- Maximal cytoreduction (debulking): no macroscopically visible residual disease, patient clinically tumor-free
- Optimal cytoreduction (debulking): only residual disease with a diameter or height of < 1 cm (< 2 cm according to some sources)
- Suboptimal cytoreduction (debulking): residual disease > 1 cm (> 2 cm according to some sources)

NCCN Clinical Practice Guidelines in Oncology (NCCN Recommendations)

- NCCN Clinical Practice Guidelines in Oncology – Uterine neoplasms 1.2016, Ovarian Cancer 2.2015, Soft tissue sarcoma 2.2015
- NCCN 1 Recommendation: Based upon high-level evidence, there is uniform NCCN consensus that the intervention is appropriate
- NCCN 2A Recommendation: Based upon lower-level evidence, there is uniform NCCN consensus that the intervention is appropriate
- NCCN 2B Recommendation: Based upon lower-level evidence, there is NCCN consensus that the intervention is appropriate
- NCCN 3 Recommendation: Based upon any level of evidence, there is major NCCN disagreement that the intervention is appropriate

Immunohistochemistry table

		Actin	SMA	Desmin	h-Caldesmon	ER	PGR	HMB 45	Melan A	S100	CD 10	Cytokeratin	Vimentin	Myogenin	Myo D1	Cyclin D1	CD34	CD31	ERG	Inhibin-alpha	CD99	Calretinin	WT1
ESN		(+)	+	–	–	++	++	–	–	–	++	–	++	–	–	–	–	–	–	(+)	–	(+)	
ESTSCLE		(+)	+	–	–	++	++	–	–	–	++	–/+	++	–	–	–	–	–	–	+	(+)	(+)	(+)
UTROSCT		(+)	+	–	–	++	++	–	+	–	++	+	++	–	–	–	–	–	–	++	+	+	+
LG-ESS		(+)	+	–	–	+	+	–	–	–	++	–	++	–	–	–	–	–	–	–	–	–	–
HG-ESS	LG-Comp.	(+)	+	–	–	+	+	–	–	–	++	–	++	–	–	–	–	–	–	–	–	–	–
	HG-Comp.	(+)	(+)	–	–	–	–	–	–	–	(+)	–	–	–	–	++	–	–	–	–	–	–	–
UUS		(+)	(+)	–	–	–	–	–	–	–	(+)	–	–	–	–	–	–	–	–	–	–	–	–
LM/Var.*		++	++	++	++	++	++	–	–	–	+	–	+	–	–	–	–	–	–	–	–	–	–
LMS		+	+	+	+	+	(+)	–	–	–	+	–	+	–	–	–	–	–	–	–	–	–	–
AF	epithelial	–	–	–	–	+	+	–	–	–	–	++	+	–	–	–	–	–	–	–	–	–	(+)
	mesench.	(+)	+	(+)	(+)	+	+	–	–	–	++	–	+	–	–	–	–	–	–	–	–	–	–
AS	epithelial	–	–	–	–	+	+	–	–	–	–	++	+	–	–	–	–	–	–	–	–	–	(+)
	mesench.	(+)	+	(+)	(+)	+	+	–	–	–	++	–	++	–	–	–	–	–	–	–	–	–	–
KS	epithelial	–	–	–	–	+	+	–	–	–	–	+	+	–	–	–	–	–		–	–	–	–
	mesench.	(+)	(+)	(+)	(+)	–/(+)	–/(+)	–	–	–	(+)	(+)	+	–	–	(+)	–	–	–	–	–	–	–
PECom	spindle cell	+	++	+	+	+	+	+	+	(+)	(+)	–	+	–	–	–	–	–	–	–	–	–	–
	epitheloid	(+)	+	+	+	+	+	++	++	(+)	(+)	–	+	–	–	–	–	–	–	–	–	–	–
RMS		(+)	(+)	+	–	–	–	–	–	–	(+)	(+)	++	+	+	(+)	–	–	–	–	–	–	–
ANS		–	(+)	–	–	–	–	–	–	–	–	(+)	++	–	–	–	++	+	++	–	–	–	+
LS		–	–	–	–	–	–	–	–	+	–	–	+	–	–	–	–	–	–	–	–	–	–

Smooth muscle markers: SMA, desmin, h-caldesmon; steroid receptors: ER, PGR; Melanocytic markers: HMB45, melan A, S100; Skeletal/striated muscle markers: myogenin, myo D1; gene fusion markers: cyclin D1; vessel markers: CD 31, CD 34, ERG; Epithelial markers: cytokeratins; sex cord markers: inhibin, CD99

++ normally strongly positive; **+** normally positive, sometimes weak; **(+)** sometimes positive, usually weak; **–** negative

* the different LM variants show barely any differences in terms of the IHC-profile

Günter Köhler, Katja Evert, Marek Zygmunt and Matthias Evert

1 Angiosarcoma

1.1 Uterine angiosarcoma

1.1.1 General, epidemiology, etiology, pathogenesis, staging

The term angiosarcoma (ANS) nowadays comprises lymphangiosarcomas and hemangiosarcomas (94). ANS only account for approximately 1 % of all STS, with a respective incidence of 0.1/100,000 (men and women) (89). The term hemangioendothelioma, previously used synonymously for ANS, is now used for a vascular tumor of borderline malignancy (94). Fifty percent of ANS are located in the skin and are closely associated with radiation exposure when so localized. What all ANS have in common is the presence of malignant endothelial cells. ANS are currently categorized into four clinical groups: primarily cutaneous ANS not associated with lymphedema or subjection to radiation; ANS associated with lymphedema (Stewart–Treves syndrome); ANS following subjection to radiation; ANS of the deep soft tissue/ANS of parenchymal organs (liver, spleen, breast) (94). Uterine ANS falls within the latter category and constitutes a purely homologous uterine sarcoma. The uterine variety is rare among all ANS. From 1902 to 2010, only 30 cases were described in the literature (22). ANS occurs in women aged between 17 and 81 years. A further overview (22) reports 14 cases since 1987 in women aged between 35 and 86 years (mean: 62 years).

Only deficient data are available pertaining to a connection between uterine ANS and prior RT. One case of uterine ANS in a patient with tuberous sclerosis complex has been reported (35), in which the patient also had accompanying lymphangioleiomyomatosis. The ANS showed mutations of the tumor suppressor genes p53 and TSC2. It is assumed that these genetic dysfunctions contributed to the pathogenesis of the ANS. However, the ANS differed significantly from the lymphangioleiomyomatosis in that it did not express HMB45. A very recent study of an ANS revealed breakages at three loci, YWHAE (17pl3), FAM22A (10q23) and FAM22B (10q22) (84). Abnormalities/fusions of these genes also play an important role in the genesis of LG-ESS (cf. Vol. 1, Chapter 4). A further study has reported on the association between ANS and retained foreign body materials (39). In some cases, uterine ANS develop within or in direct connection with an LM (19, 76, 86).

No phase III and only very few phase II studies have focused on either general ANS or on uterine ANS in particular. Therapeutic recommendations are based almost solely on retrospective accumulative statistics that cover ANS with different localizations.

Staging for STS applies for uterine ANS (cf. Vol. 1, Chapter 2). Uterine ANS are thus always classified as deep tumors. Accordingly, disease stages T1a and T2a are not possible according to the AJCC. ANS are not included in UICC classification (95).

Uterine angiosarcomas are extremely rare. There is apparently no association with prior subjection to radiation. Gene breakages can play a role in pathogenesis. Staging for soft tissue sarcomas applies, according to which angiosarcomas are deep tumors.

1.1.2 Macroscopic and microscopic features

At the time of initial presentation, ANS usually appear as large, fleshy, often polypous tumors that can involve the endometrium and the myometrium (14), with a mean size of 13 cm (5–29 cm) (76). These relatively soft tumors usually have a brown to bright red color on the cut surface (44). The macroscopic appearance of ANS can also bear resemblance to an LM, with whorled structures and central necroses or cysts. It is common for such tumors to exhibit extensive necrosis with numerous hemorrhages (44, 100). Polypoid ANS originating in the endometrium or tumors that occupy the entire uterine wall have also been reported (76). ANS diffusely infiltrate the uterus, causing it to expand and grow rapidly. Extensive destructive invasion of the myometrium is a typical finding (100). ANS have no capsule and lack clear margins.

At the microscopic level, most ANS have a lobulated structure with infiltrating margins. The presence of numerous open, slit-like blood-carrying vascular spaces that are irregularly anastomosed with each other, and that are also connected to the regular vessels, is particularly characteristic. The vascular sinusoids are lined with atypical cuboidal or polygonal endothelial cells (100). The cells show numerous atypical, pleomorphic hyperchromatic nuclei with ample mitoses. The number of cells lining the vascular spaces is significantly higher than usual. They can be multilayered compared to normal endothelial tissue and can exhibit papillary growth into the vascular spaces (98) (Fig. 1.1.1 (A)). Some ANS also have solid sections that can be associated with smooth muscle proliferations. These proliferations are characterized by clearly defined margins, unsuspicious cytological characteristics and a lack of mitotic activity. In these cases, the highly vascularized tumor spreads outside of the smooth muscle proliferate. Interestingly, in particular in combination with the presence of smooth muscle shares, the endothelial cells also exhibit an epithelioid morphology, with round cells, eosinophilic cytoplasm, a high nucleus-cytoplasm ratio, and prominent nucleons (19). The epithelioid cells can also form nests. Epithelioid ANS consist almost exclusively of layered epithelioid cells. The vascular spaces lined with pleomorphic cells, as described above, are mostly not so dominant in such tumors and can sometimes be difficult to recognize. They can occasionally bear resemblance to primitive glands. Taken together with the aberrant expression of cytokeratins that can be observed in virtually all epithelioid ANS, these factors pose the significant risk of misdiagnosing the tumor as poorly differentiated adenocarcinoma. Notwithstanding, the focal presence of slit-like spaces with erythrocytes is a factor suggestive of an ANS, a suspicion that can be immunohistochemically verified (51).

Some ANS have been described as small solid nodules with a predominant presence of spindle cells lining the vascular spaces. In ANS, the endometrial glands and their surrounding vicinity are often strongly infiltrated, which in turn can cause cavernous spaces to develop within the tumor. The benign glands are, however, confined to the remaining or previously endometrial tissue – no glandular differentiation can be found in the remainder of the ANS. In terms of their grading, uterine ANS are generally regarded as high-grade sarcomas, so that no other grading need be provided.

The endothelial tumor cells in the vascular spaces usually express CD31, CD34, and Factor VIII. Vascular marker CD31, in particular, shows diffuse and intensive staining (Fig. 1.1.1 (B)). Fli1 (Friend leukemia integration 1 transcription factor) and, more recently, ERG (erythroblast transformation specific related gene) are regarded as further promising nuclear markers for endothelial cells (55, 83). ERG is a proto-oncogene and a member of the erythroblast transformation specific transcription factor family, and is apparently involved in the regulation of angiogenesis. In 25 ANS diagnosed on fine needle aspirates, ERG, CD31, and CD34 had sensitivities of 100 %, 100 %, and only 60 %, respectively (83). Positive CD31 and ERG staining usually allows for a reliable diagnosis of ANS as such, even on the basis of cytological material gathered via aspirates (83). These positive findings notwithstanding, these markers are not monospecific! However, combining the two is by far more conclusive than measuring CD31 plus CD34, not least since the latter is expressed in only around 50 % of all vascular tumors (55). ERG can also sometimes be found in epithelioid sarcomas and in variants of myxoid LS, and is also expressed in carcinoma of the prostate. The smooth muscle markers SMA and desmin as well as ER and PGR test positive in potential accompanying smooth muscle proliferations, however not in the actual tumor cells themselves. Present residual endometrial glands also stain with cytokeratins and likewise express ER and PGR (76). P53 mutations are regarded as a typical characteristic of ANS (59). The Ki-67 index is usually clearly elevated in epithelioid ANS in particular, an expression of their strong proliferative activity (Fig. 1.1.1 (C)). ANS also express VEGFR1/2 and 3 (6, 38, 67), but show no reaction to S100, HMB45, and CD99.

Uterine angiosarcoma is a bluish-red, usually relatively soft tumor with necroses, hemorrhages, and cystic areas. Histological examination reveals ample vascular blood-carrying spaces that are lined with pleomorphic malignant cells and that communicate with each other. Epithelioid ANS can also grow as purely solid tumors. Smooth muscle differentiations can occur within the tumor, in some cases there are larger sections with epithelioid cells. Trapped endometrial glands can be present on the fringes of the tumor. Angiosarcomas are immunoreactive to CD31, CD34, and Factor VIII. Combining CD31 and ERG allows for a relatively reliable and secure diagnosis to be reached. The fact that epithelioid ANS show an aberrant expression of epithelial markers (e.g. cytokeratins) must be borne in mind.

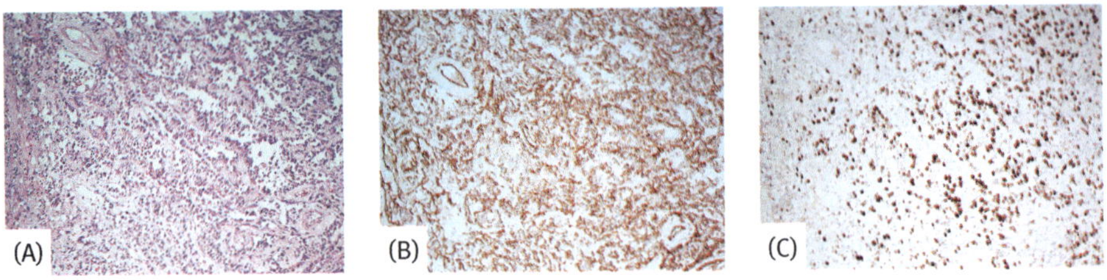

Fig. 1.1.1: Histological image of an angiosarcoma. (A) typical appearance of a high-grade angiosarcoma with pathological (in this case relatively wide) vascular lumina lined with highly atypical, in part epithelioid neoplastic endothelial cells. This produces a pseudoglandular morphological appearance that should not be confused with adenosarcoma; (B) immunohistochemical testing using a typical, albeit nonspecific endothelial marker (CD31 in this case) will serve to avoid such confusion in most cases; (C) the tumor cells exhibit a high degree of proliferative activity (Ki-67 index) that matches the tumors' generally high level of malignancy. Small non-neoplastic arteries (top left and lower right of the image) are recognizable in (A) and in the serial sections (B and C), the flat, non-atypical endothelia of which tested positive for CD31 (B), but negative for Ki-67 (C).

1.1.3 Clinical presentation, diagnostics, screening

AUB as well as postmenopausal bleeding are the most important symptoms. The bleeding is often so severe that it results in anemia (76). Clinically, ANS present as large palpable unclear uterine tumors that are rather soft to touch. Patients often complain of lower abdominal pains due to the size of the tumor and/or the rapidity of its growth (22). Roughly 50 % of ANS have already spread beyond the uterus at the time of primary diagnosis. The diagnostic approach does not differ from that applied for LMS or UUS. According to the NCCN Guidelines for soft tissue sarcomas, CT or MRI should be performed on the abdomen, the pelvis, and the brain whenever an ANS has been identified as such (60). To date, no specific screening approaches have been established or "taken root" in practice.

Abnormal bleeding and lower abdominal pains are the key symptoms of uterine angiosarcomas.

1.1.4 Imaging

Barely any data are available pertaining to the sonographic appearance of ANS.

CT is not suitable for securely identifying this specific tumor. CECT reveals tumor masses within the uterus that show a heterogeneous enhancement (36). The frequent presence of central necroses has the effect that the visible enhancement is limited to the periphery of the tumor in many cases (80). While such findings are indeed typical, they are by no means exclusive of other types of sarcoma.

A noticeable degree of heterogeneity in T2W-MRI – with overall low SI and focal pockets of very high SI – is the most important diagnostic characteristic, and gives the ANS its typical cauliflower-like appearance. ANS show a strong enhancement in T1WC (36, 43). In terms of differential diagnosis, neither CT nor MRI allow for ANS to be reliably and securely discerned from LMS (43).

F-18 FDG PET/CT images show mild to moderate metabolic activity with an SUV max of 6.5. Extensive hemorrhagic and necrotic areas are low in metabolic activity, so that the resulting image can be a rather heterogeneous one. In terms of differential diagnosis, an LMS or an LM must be considered as possible alternatives when interpreting PET-CT images (36).

PET-CT is thus inadequate for reaching a primary diagnosis, but can be helpful when searching for metastases.

Barely any ultrasound images of angiosarcomas are known to exist. In contrast-CECT, due to ample central necroses, enhancement is usually limited to the periphery. T2W-MRI images are characterized by a noticeable degree of heterogeneity, with low overall SI as well as focal pockets of very high SI, which gives the ANS a typical cauliflower-like appearance. PET-CT is rather not suitable for primary diagnostics.

1.1.5 Differential diagnostics

From a clinical and macroscopical perspective, all other uterine sarcomas as well as AS and CS need to be included in any DD considerations. Particularly severe bleeding, often connected to anemia, is one important clinical factor suggestive of an ANS. In terms of the clinical aspect of ANS, their consistency, their color on the cut surface, and the presence of strong bleeding, an ALM should also be considered as a potential DD.

At the microscopic level, spindle cell or epithelioid LMS need to be drawn into consideration whenever spindle or epithelioid cells are present. Differentiation should best be made on the basis of the vascular marker CD31 and ERG (55, 65) (Fig. 1.1.1 (B)). However, it is worthy of note that epithelioid sarcomas, too, can be ERG positive (55). Despite the fact that epithelioid ANS generally show positive cytokeratin expression, they must not be mistaken for carcinomas, a major diagnostic challenge for this subtype. Differentiating an ANS from an AS with SO can be extremely difficult when trapped endometrial glands are present, not least because there are known cases of AS with SO with histologically pure angiosarcomatous components (45). While in ANS the trapped glands can only be found in the regions affected by endometrial infiltration, in AS they are spread across the whole lesion, except when the AS has SO. Misdiagnoses are, therefore, inevitable when only small tissue samples have been taken/are available. A definitive diagnosis can thus often only be reached on the basis of the primary surgical specimen. Since uterine ANS are even rarer than the already seldom AS, the entire tumor should be meticulously checked for glands, for instance using cytokeratin markers. The same applies to CS with SO consisting of an ANS component. If cytokeratins are found, it must be borne in mind that the epithelioid cells in ANS can also express cytokeratins. Such expression is, however, weak and only focal in the majority of cases (27, 31, 76).

Hemangiopericytoma must also be considered as a potential DD. The presence of diffuse and strong immunoreactivity to vascular marker CD31 and to Factor VIII, however, would serve to exclude this tumor type from diagnostic consideration (27).

Uterine angiosarcoma can bear gross resemblance to angioleiomyoma as well as to the other histologically pure types of sarcoma. Adenosarcoma should be taken into consideration when endometrial glands are present. A hemangiopericytoma can be relatively easily ruled out via immunohistochemical examination.

1.1.6 Course, prognosis

Uterine ANS are highly malignant and are classed as high-risk tumors per se. The following criteria are regarded as unfavorable factors for all ANS: size > 5 cm, deep and retroperitoneal localization, ANS of body cavities, epithelioid tumors, necroses, and positive resection margins (70, 94, 98). Low or no VEGFR2 expression is reported to be associated with a significantly unfavorable prognosis (38).

Sixty-two percent of patients suffering from ANS (all sites, men and women) present with metastasis at the time of primary diagnosis (70). More than 50 % of patients with uterine ANS succumb to their disease within one year of initial diagnosis (9, 22). A further study measured a 1-year OS of 43 % (54). Median OS is said to be at 13.5 mo (18). In one case, metastases developed in the vagina, the lung, and the brain within six weeks of primary therapy (54). One case study suggests that polypoid intramural tumors might have a more promising prognosis (76). Improved survival is observed in particular in cases in which smaller lesions are subjected to clear R0 resection (54). Notwithstanding, the prognosis for uterine (!) ANS does not appear to necessarily depend on tumor size (22, 44).

Disregarding the small number of observed cases, the available data nonetheless allow the conclusion to be drawn that adjuvant RT and/or CHT will have no influence on the generally poor prognosis with which uterine ANS are associated (22, 76).

Overall, angiosarcomas localized in body cavities have a poorer prognosis than those at other sites. Uterine angiosarcomas are highly malignant tumors. Median overall survival is at roughly one year.

1.1.7 Primary surgery

While the different STS guidelines do indeed also include ANS, there is as of yet no "evidence-based therapy" specific to the different sites at which the disease can be localized (21, 78, 98).

The therapeutic method of choice for all ANS regardless of their localization is performing and securely achieving R0 resection (21, 60, 98). For uterine ANS, performing THE without injuring the uterus is thus the therapeutic approach that is to be opted for. In practically all cases referred to in the literature, patients underwent TAH in combination with a BSO (18, 22, 54, 76). There are no data pertaining to the potential benefits of performing a BSO – ANS do not express ER and PGR, and for uterine ANS, it remains questionable whether or not there is a pathogenetic connection to hormone exposure. Similarly, there are no data suggesting that undergoing a BSO has any influence or effect on the further course of the disease. What is noteworthy, though, is that, in the cases described, all women who underwent a BSO were postmenopausal. For premenopausal women, therefore, the adnexa can be left in situ so long as the results from clinical examination and/or imaging diagnostics are not suggestive of adnexal involvement.

No data are currently available concerning the performance of systematic LNE on uterine ANS, nor have there been any accounts of metastasis to the LN in the literature. Analogous to the other homologous and heterologous uterine sarcoma types, there is no indication for performing an LNE, i.e. it has yet to be scientifically proven that doing so can be beneficial for DFS and OS (54, 74, 86). The same applies to sentinel LN biopsies (98).

Overall, THE without injury to the uterus and the tumor must be regarded as the most adequate surgical option. Due to the very unfavorable prognosis, the absence of a capsule, and the typical presence of extensive myometrial infiltrations with unclear margins, organ preserving surgical procedures must be refrained from, regardless of the indication under which they would otherwise have been performed.

Analogous to the other types of uterine sarcoma and STS, maximal cytoreductive surgery (debulking) is recommended in cases of extrauterine peritoneal dissemination (60, 64). Reference should be made to the chapter on LMS (Vol. 1, Chapter 2) for more detailed particularities to this end. Since invasion into neighboring tissues and organs is predominantly diffuse, achieving R0 resection margins can be very difficult or even technically and practically impossible. Consequently, it is imperative that patients undergo detailed, precise imaging diagnostic procedures prior to surgery.

Total hysterectomy without injuring the uterus and/or the tumor is the therapeutic method of choice for patients with uterine angiosarcoma. Performing an adnexectomy has yet to be scientifically proven as a beneficial course of action. There is no indication for performing a lymphonodectomy. Maximal cytoreductive surgery (debulking) is recommended when there is extrauterine dissemination.

1.1.8 Adjuvant and additive radio-, chemo- and hormone therapy

No formal studies have yet been devoted to the effects of performing postoperative RT on ANS patients. Recommendations (98) for postoperative RT following surgery on an ANS are based only on retrospective studies. More specifically, they are primarily based on two studies that covered all types of ANS. The first study only considered cutaneous ANS (68), while the second study (50) covered a sample of 67 ANS of different sites, including only 1 cervical, 1 ovarian, and 1 retroperitoneal ANS. However, the analyses only revealed a nonsignificant effect on DFS and OS. In actual fact, the data are not simply transferable or applicable to uterine ANS, as they are based almost entirely on cutaneous and breast ANS. They also include cases in which only R1/2 resection margins were achieved, while uterine ANS are generally subjected to R0 resection or the compartment "uterus" is removed completely. Likewise, the available case studies with and without meta-analyses (22, 44, 54, 76) do not suggest that undergoing adjuvant RT following R0 resection yields any benefits. Overall, there is no indication for subjecting uterine ANS patients who have undergone an R0 resection to postoperative RT. Nor is such course of action supported in the NCCN Guidelines (60, 61). Further retrospective analyses yielded no findings suggestive of effects on DFS and OS, including CHT (1, 25).

To date, scientific studies, including some larger-scale analyses (87, 96), have yet to prove that adjuvant CHT bears any benefits for STS patients, including those with ANS. The same applies to uterine ANS in particular. Meta-analyses (22, 44, 54, 76) have reported on cases in which subjection to adjuvant CHT was following by survival periods beyond one year, but also extremely short DFS. Overall, there appears to be no difference in this context to the other pure uterine sarcomas, like LMS, HG-ESS, UUS, and LS (cf. Vol. 1, Chapters 2, 4, 5 and LS next chapter). In one reported case, a patient survived disease-free for 4 years following adjuvant CHT with cisplatin and doxorubicin (74). There is also a report of a patient who was started on an adjuvant CHT regimen of albumin-bound paclitaxel and the VEGF-AB bevacizumab. She remained recurrence-free over a follow-up period of 12 mo (64). The aforementioned individual cases do not, however, suffice to justify administering adjuvant CHT or VEGF antibodies as standard procedure. ANS are not covered in the NCCN Guidelines for uterine sarcomas (61). There is no indication for adjuvant HT for ANS.

Uterine ANS exhibiting extrauterine spread should not be routinely subjected to RT following R0 resection. Operated cases with recurrences that could result in significant morbidity due to their critically close proximity to neighboring structures constitute an exception in this regard (60). The same essentially also applies to cases in which R1 resection margins have been achieved. Targeted postoperative RT can, however, be considered as an option (60).

Uterine ANS that have spread beyond the uterus and for which R2 resection margins have been achieved should be subjected to follow-up resection. Should such course of action not be possible, "downstaging" should be resorted to via combination

CHT, CHT-RT or standalone RT. Where downstaging fails or cannot be achieved, the principles of palliative therapy or best supportive care should apply (60).

The NCCN Guidelines do not envisage that R0 and R1 resections in cases of advanced disease be followed up by postoperative CHT (60). In actual fact, there are no data to suggest that doing so would have any beneficial effects on PFI and OS.

Likewise, there have been no studies to date that suggest that immediately subjecting patients in whom R2 resections have been achieved to postoperative CHT yields more promising results than can be achieved by adhering to a more observant, reserved strategy. Accordingly, CHT can only then be administered to symptomatic patients or when recurrences/metastases occur in critical locations. In general, the approach envisaged for and applied to LMS and UUS can be followed.

There is no indication for routinely subjecting patients with uterine angiosarcomas in whom R0 resection has been achieved to postoperative radiotherapy. This is true also in cases that have spread beyond the uterus. The same applies to R1 resections. In both instances, however, targeted radiotherapy can be considered if recurrences could result in significant morbidity due to their critical proximity to neighboring structures. Patients with uterine ANS that have spread beyond the uterus and in whom R2 resection margins have been achieved should be subjected to follow-up resection. If this is not possible, downstaging should be sought via combination chemotherapy, radiochemotherapy or standalone radiotherapy. Palliative therapeutic strategies should be resorted to when downstaging cannot be achieved.

There is currently no indication for the administration of adjuvant or postoperative chemotherapy, except in the context of downstaging cases of R2 resections.

1.1.9 Primary radio-, chemo- and hormone therapy, approach in cases of general inoperability

Subjecting operable ANS to standalone RT is deemed an inadequate therapeutic approach that lacks any indication (50). No data are available pertaining to primary RT in uterine ANS patients. In cases of local and general inoperability, administering a CHT regimen with ANS-effective cytostatic agents would be a conceivable option. Where neoadjuvant therapy with the option for surgery is planned, combination CHT (see palliative CHT), sequential CHT-RT, but also standalone RT can be considered as means for achieving swift remission. All three of these options are supported in the current NCCN Guidelines (60).

There is a known case in which remission of an inoperable extragenital cutaneous ANS was achieved using RT plus VEGF-AB bevacizumab (17). For localized tumors that are generally inoperable, targeted RT in combination with bevacizumab would be a justifiable therapeutic approach. Whether or not this combination is in fact superior to CHT or CHT-RT remains questionable. According to a further study, CR of an ANS was achieved in one case using a combination of docetaxel (50 mg/m^2), gemcitabine

(1500 mg/m^2 every 2 weeks), and bevacizumab 5 mg/kg (91). There is no indication for primary HT for ANS patients.

There is no indication for subjecting operable uterine angiosarcomas to primary radiotherapy. Inoperable angiosarcomas can be treated with chemotherapy and/or targeted radiotherapy, potentially in combination with a VEGF antibody, in order to achieve operability.

1.1.10 Aftercare, recurrences, metastases

Aftercare should be approached in the same fashion as described for LMS and UUS (Vol. 1, Chapters 2, 5). There are no suitable or adequate tumor markers. However, it is recommended that imaging diagnostics be expanded to include a brain CT scan (21). This should be done relatively early on when the present symptoms justify it. It is, however, questionable whether doing so offers any benefits in terms of OS. There are also no data which would suggest that subjecting ANS patients who have undergone surgery to HRT has any influence on prognosis.

According to a meta-analysis and some individual publications, the metastatic spread of uterine ANS predominantly occurs to the abdominal cavity, the lung, the vagina, the bones, and the brain (51, 54). Cases of cardiac and gingival metastasis have also been reported (18, 53). Untreated metastases are associated with a median OS of 2.2 mo (70). Independent of the individual treatment methods, performance status is regarded as the most important prognostic factor at the metastatic stage (70). Local recurrence and distant metastases had 5-year OS of 42 % and 10 %, respectively. The difference was statistically significant (46).

Follow-up and aftercare for uterine angiosarcomas should be designed in accordance with the approach adopted for the other types of uterine sarcoma. Metastases occur in the abdominal cavity and in the lungs in particular. Brain metastases are relatively common. Performing imaging procedures on the brain can thus be included in aftercare strategies for uterine ANS.

1.1.11 Surgery and postoperative additive therapy for recurrences and metastases

Barely any data are available that pertain to uterine ANS in this context. The meta-analysis stated above (54) only mentions in passing that recurrences and metastases should rather be subjected to resection. Recourse must thus be had to the literature on ANS of all localizations and sites, which states that recurrences and operable metastases should first be subjected to R0 resection, a course of action that is also supported by the NCCN Guidelines for soft tissue sarcomas (60) in the form of a 2A recommendation. Seventy-six percent of ANS-distant metastases are solitary tumors. Surgery seems to be possible in 20 % of cases, and can be performed either with curative intent or as a means of palliative symptom treatment (46). More recent data pertaining to ANS of all sites suggest that performing a metastasectomy is associated with improved survival (70). According to another study, however, there is no correlation between resecting distant metastases and improvements in OS. In contrast, administration of paclitaxel-based CHT regimens (paclitaxel mono-CHT or paclitaxel plus gemcitabine) is predictive of longer OS, albeit only just beyond the threshold of statistical significance (46). Prognosis for patients who underwent resection of LN metastases was no better than for those who were treated with CHT. Overall, though, patients with LN metastases had a clearly favorable prognosis over patients with distant metastasization. Median PFI for distant metastatic disease is only 10 mo from the onset of treatment (46).

No remaining tumor material can be found under the microscope in 70 % of cases in which complete gross clinical resection of local recurrences has been achieved. Resection is associated with improved OS in particular in cases in which tumor size is < 5 cm (50). Incomplete resection or a lack of resectability, by contrast, are associated with a less favorable prognosis and an increased rate of distant metastasis (46). Overall, the size of local tumor recurrences (< or > 5 cm) is the only independent predictor for survival.

According to an NCCN 2A recommendation, R0 resections of local recurrences should not routinely be followed up with CHT and/or RT (60). In actual fact, it has yet to be sufficiently and adequately examined or verified in scientific studies that any form of postoperative intervention bears any benefits for PFI and OS. Even the larger-scale retrospective studies (70) do not allow the conclusion to be drawn that postoperative CHT and/or RT have any beneficial effects on PFI or OS in patients who have undergone R0 resections of local recurrences and/or metastases. According to the current NCCN Guidelines for soft tissue sarcomas, RT can be considered if further recurrences in potentially critical locations would cause significant morbidity (60). An identical approach is recommended for R1 resections, however RT can also be applied optionally. For R2 resections, the guidelines recommend follow-up resection or "downstaging" via combination CHT, CHT-RT or RT with subsequent surgery. Should this be unsuccessful or if such surgery is technically impossible (i.e. progressive disease or unresectability), palliative therapy or best supportive care are indicated (46, 60). Ultimately, there are no data to suggest that assuming a more reserved, observant postoperative approach is associated with detrimental effects on PFI and OS in this situation. Accordingly, all measures can be held back and only applied once strong symptoms occur or when recurrences/metastases are in critical locations.

Embolization or other minimally invasive therapeutic methods constitute a further option.

First and foremost, operable local recurrences and metastases should be subjected to R0 resection. There is no evidence to suggest that following up R0 resections with radiotherapy or chemotherapy bears any benefits. Radiotherapy can be administered if potential recurrences in critical locations could cause significant morbidity. The same rules apply in principle to R1 resections. For R2 resections, follow-up resection should be considered, possibly following downstaging via chemotherapy, radiochemotherapy or standalone radiotherapy. There is no clear indication for applying chemotherapy in cases of asymptomatic residual masses in noncritical locations. Primarily inoperable recurrences/metastases can be subjected to radiotherapy, chemotherapy or radiochemotherapy in order to achieve operability.

1.1.12 Palliative radio-, chemo- and hormone therapy, small molecule therapy, supportive therapy

Adopting an observant approach or providing best supportive care are acceptable options for asymptomatic patients with disseminated metastasis to noncritical locations (64). Primary RT is most likely suitable for patients with bone metastases (46). CHT is indicated when patients with inoperable recurrent and/or metastatic disease are symptomatic or when said recurrences/metastases are in critical locations.

First and foremost, a monotherapy is indicated in the palliative context. Paclitaxel appears to be the most effective agent according to more recent data. In a small cohort of 8 ANS localized at various different sites, monotherapy with paclitaxel effected CR in 2 and PR in 3 cases (81). An RR of 89 % and a median PFI of 5 mo were measured in a further small cohort (24). In a study covering 60 cutaneous and non-cutaneous ANS, paclitaxel monotherapy administered with palliative intent achieved an RR of 56 % with a median OS of 11.2 mo. The disparities between the two tumor groups (cutaneous and non-cutaneous) in terms of survival were not statistically significant (23). In an extensive retrospective study of STS including ANS, ANS of primary sites other than the scalp showed an RR of 58 % (14 of 24 cases). Median PFI for all ANS was 7.6 mo (77). Weekly administration of paclitaxel is said to be superior to regimens in which the agent is applied every three weeks (69, 70). Paclitaxel is also among the substances recommended in current guidelines (21, 60, 78).

The efficacy of doxorubicin for treating ANS has been known for quite some time. In a small sample of 9 patients, administering doxorubicin effected an RR of 67 %, and median PFI was 9.5 mo (58). In one study, 3 of 6 ANS patients who were started on liposomal doxorubicin showed PR for between 6 and > 20 mo, while 2 patients had SD for 7 and 11 mo, respectively (81). For unresectable ANS, doxorubicin-based CHT regimens achieved PFI of 3.7–5.4 mo; a PFI of 6.8 mo was achieved using paclitaxel. Subclavicular ANS were associated with a shorter PFI (28). Paclitaxel and doxorubicin have also been proven to be effective in in vitro experiments using cutaneous ANS cell lines (99). In case of resistance or secondary progression under doxorubicin or paclitaxel, a switch to the respective alternate agent is possible (78). Where ineffectiveness persists, subsequent administration of gemcitabine or ifosfamide regimens is a viable possibility (21, 60, 78).

An extensive randomized phase II study of STS including ANS compared the efficacy of doxorubicin monotherapy (75 mg/m^2 d 1, q 3 weeks) with a dose-intensified combination CHT regimen of doxorubicin 25 mg/m^2 d 1–3 plus ifosfamide (2–5 g/m^2 d 1–4, q 3 weeks) (41). While the study revealed no significant differences between the two groups in terms of OS (12 vs. 14.3 mo doxorubicin vs. combination), median PFI was significantly longer following intensified therapy (7.4 vs. 4.6 mo). Furthermore, the combination group showed a higher RR than the monotherapy group (26 % vs. 14 %), albeit with clearly higher toxic effects among the former. Referring in particular to the virtually identical survival-related data, the research group agrees that intensified combination CHT should only be administered when there is significant urgency for achieving disease remission, i.e. when symptoms are severe or when the critical location of recurrent or metastatic lesions makes effecting tumor shrinkage necessary (41).

In one case of a uterine ANS that had metastasized to the lungs and the bones, CR of the target lesion could be achieved using a CHT regimen of ifosfamide plus doxorubicin. However, a new metastasis developed in the upper jaw during ongoing treatment that had to be surgically removed. The patient remained disease-free for 1½ years following surgery and completion of CHT, and subsequently developed a metastasis to the heart. In total, bearing in mind the fact that she was primarily metastatic, the patient survived for an uncommonly long time, a fact that the authors suspect was a lasting effect of the administered CHT combination.

Paclitaxel and gemcitabine are occasionally administered in second-line therapy (46). According to the current NCCN Guidelines for soft tissue sarcomas, the combinations epirubicin plus ifosfamide and paclitaxel plus gemcitabine can also be used (60).

Remissions of inoperable vaginal ANS have been observed in two cases in which the patients underwent a combination of poly-CHT (CYVADIC-protocol) plus intravenous interleukin (IL-2, 40IE p.d.), with a PFI of up to 9 mo (57). Where tumors are localized, a palliative combination of RT plus administration of interleukin could be recommendable in individual cases (85).

There is no indication for palliative HT for ANS patients.

It is generally conceivable that VEGF antibodies like bevacizumab will have an effect on vascular tumors. The same equally applies to multi-TKI like sunitinib and sorafenib, which direct their activity against VEGFR. In vitro experiments with cutaneous ANS cell lines have revealed the VEGF-AB bevacizumab to be practically ineffective (99). In a phase II trial, among 23 ANS patients who underwent bevacizumab monotherapy (15 mg/kg, q 3 weeks), 2 showed PR and 11 showed SD, a CBR of 52 %. Median PFI and OS were 12 and 53 weeks, respectively (2). In a study investigating the efficacy of sorafenib in sarcoma patients, among them 37 ANS, 1 patient showed CR, 4 had PR (RR 14 %), and 21 had SD. Median PFI was 3.8 mo (48). By contrast, sunitinib appears to have no activity against ANS (29). These findings notwithstanding, according to the current NCCN Guidelines for soft tissue sarcomas, in addition to bevacizumab, both sorafenib and sunitinib can be administered in a palliative context

(60). The German guidelines state that sorafenib can be administered to STS patients when CHT has failed (78).

There is also a report of an ANS patient showing CR to a combination of docetaxel, gemcitabine, and bevacizumab administered with palliative intent (91).

Overall, an effective cytostatic agent plus bevacizumab appears to be the most suitable combination for palliative contexts. In any case, doing so must be regarded as merely a "therapy attempt".

Good supportive therapy is also an acceptable option when metastatic disease is widespread and diffuse (60, 61).

Chemotherapy is indicated for inoperable and/or diffuse recurrences/metastases in symptomatic patients or when recurrences/metastases are in critical locations. Monochemotherapy should generally be given priority. Combination chemotherapy should only be administered when symptoms are severe and the need to achieve tumor remission is great. Paclitaxel and doxorubicin are regarded as the agents of choice. Combination chemotherapy should be a regimen of doxorubicin and ifosfamide. Administering antibodies or tyrosine kinase inhibitors like bevacizumab and sorafinib is possible, either as monotherapy or in combination with a cytostatic agent.

1.2 Extrauterine angiosarcomas

1.2.1 Angiosarcomas of the vulva and the vagina

General, pathogenesis, pathologico-anatomical features

ANS occasionally also occur in the vulva. Depending on their pathogenesis, vulvar ANS can be categorized as primary cutaneous ANS not associated with lymphedema or irradiation, as lymphedema-associated ANS, or as ANS associated with irradiation. In actual fact, vulvar ANS occur in connection with lymphedemas (12) and following exposure of vulvar sarcomas and other lower genital sarcomas or carcinomas to radiation (30, 33). The timeframe following exposure is stated as being between 4 and 29 years. Such cases thus primarily involve women aged 70 and above (44).

Vulvar ANS does not constitute a specific gynecological tumor type, but is rather the result of coincidental localization at that site that is not discussed as an independent tumor type in the NCCN and other guidelines. Vulvar ANS must thus be categorized under STS of the extremities/trunk, and respective staging must be applied (cf. Vol. 1, Chapter 2). The majority of vulvar ANS are superficial tumors in stage Ia (≤ 5 cm) or IIa (> 5 cm). If the fascia or the levator muscle have been invaded or penetrated, the tumor must be classified as a deep tumor in either stage Ib (≤ 5 cm) or IIb (> 5 cm) (60). The challenges faced in staging cutaneous ANS are addressed in the NCCN Guidelines (60).

Only very few cases of vaginal ANS have been described in the literature to date (51, 72, 75, 88). Like its vulvar equivalent, vaginal ANS, too, is not a tumor type specific to the genitalia. Vaginal ANS are located above the pelvic floor and should thus, unlike their vulvar counterparts, be classified as retroperitoneal STS. Vaginal ANS seem to be much more frequently associated with previous exposure to RT than their uterine, vulvar, and ovarian equivalents (13, 56, 63, 72, 85). In the described cases, the interval from previous RT to diagnosis was 9–21 years (57). One study has found a connection between ANS with the long-term presence of foreign objects, for example vaginal pessaries (51). In terms of staging, vaginal angiosarcomas are classified as deep tumors (stage Ib or IIb) in accordance with the criteria for retroperitoneal soft tissue sarcomas provided in the AJCC Classification.

Angiosarcomas of the vagina and the vulva do occur. They do not constitute independent genital tumor types. There is often a correlation to previous radiotherapy. Vulvar angiosarcomas are staged in accordance with the criteria for soft tissue sarcomas of the trunk, while staging of vaginal angiosarcomas is in accordance with the criteria for retroperitoneal soft tissue sarcomas provided in the AJCC Classification. Vulvar angiosarcomas can be classified either as superficial or as deep tumors (irruption or penetration of the pelvic musculature).

Clinical presentation, diagnostics, differential diagnostics

Vulvar and vaginal angiosarcomas typically appear as purplish-red to red lesions in skin that has usually sustained prior radiogenic damage. They can grossly present as bruise-like blotches, plaques or (most commonly) nodules, occasionally with ulcerations (26, 63). The characteristic bluish-red color becomes particularly noticeable on the cut surface of the specimen. The resulting gross image strongly resembles that of ANS of the breast (Fig. 1.2.1).

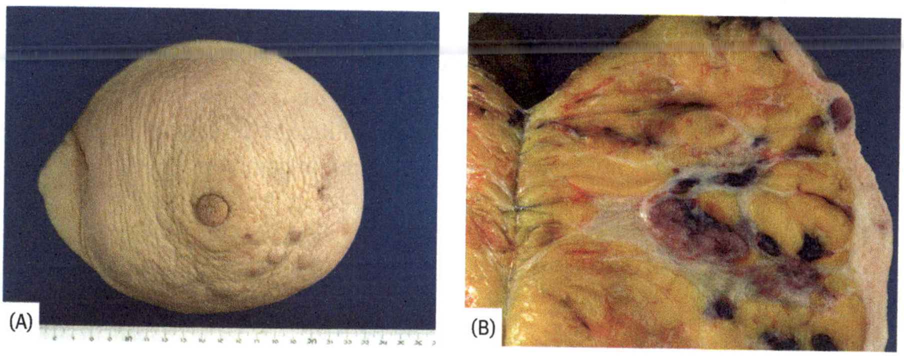

Fig. 1.2.1: Typical angiosarcoma of the breast, the clinical appearance of vulvar angiosarcoma is largely identical in terms of macroscopic and cut surface appearance.

Vaginal ANS have numerous purplish nodules and vesicles that can be accompanied by ulcerous tumor segments with conspicuous hemorrhaging. It is possible for such tumors to rupture and invade the bladder and to cause hematuria (51, 56, 57).

Microscopic appearance is described in the subchapter on uterine ANS. Vulvar ANS are often already clinically diagnosed on the basis of gross appearance and patients' medical history. In such cases, the tumors should already be resected with wide clear margins at the time of clinical diagnosis. The extremely rare epithelioid ANS of the vagina can be mistaken for an epithelial tumor if an immunohistochemical examination is not conducted. The strong expression of CD31, CD34, Factor VIII, and focally positive staining with vimentin, SMA, WT-1, and keratin 8/18 serve to secure a correct diagnosis as ANS (75). ANS of the vagina can also clinically resemble malignant melanoma. The lack of HMB-45, Melan A and S100 expression serves to largely exclude melanocytic tumors (51). The tumors reportedly have high density in CT (57).

From a clinical standpoint, vulvar and vaginal angiosarcomas usually present as reddish, sometimes ulcerated nodules. Histologically they correspond to uterine angiosarcoma. Vulvar and vaginal angiosarcomas can be clinically mistaken for melanoma.

Course, prognosis, primary surgery, primary and adjuvant radio-, chemo- and hormone therapy

According to SEER data, ANS of the skin, the trunk, the lower extremities, the hips, and the vulva have a 10-year OS of 75.3 %. In general, cutaneous ANS of the trunk, patients aged < 50 years, and localized tumors are factors associated with having the most promising prognoses (4). As of yet, there is no evidence to suggest that there is a correlation between tumor size and prognosis for patients with cutaneous ANS, not least because their growth pattern often makes precise measurements impossible. The few cases of vaginal ANS that have been described to date have been consistently associated with a poor prognosis (51).

For sarcomas of the trunk (as which vulvar ANS must be classified), a therapeutic approach will be deemed adequate if the tumor is removed leaving wide, clear resection margins (21, 60). Since ANS have often widely infiltrated the surrounding tissues and are often multifocal, R1/2 resection margins are not uncommon. Reresection with a resection margin of at least 1 cm is generally called for in these cases (21, 60).

The same conditions essentially also apply for vaginal ANS. However, in the majority of such cases, the conditions for adequate surgical therapy cannot be fulfilled (51).

Postoperative treatment of vulvar and vaginal ANS can be managed in accordance with the current NCCN Guidelines on soft tissue sarcomas extremity/trunk and retroperitoneal/intra-abdominal (60). Bar some marginal deviations, the recommendations made in the ESMO Guidelines conform to those provided in the NCCN Guidelines (21, 61).

For retroperitoneal STS, the general rule is that postoperative RT is not necessary when R0 resection margins have been achieved, unless potential recurrences would be associated with a high degree of morbidity, for example severely disturbing the functionality of neighboring organs, or would be difficult to resect (60). Due to the close proximity of both bladder and rectum, such a situation can practically be assumed to exist for all vaginal ANS. From this perspective, postoperative RT is indicated for vaginal ANS. The same recommendation applies to R1 resections (60).

Regarding vulvar ANS, too, it must be borne in mind that they are high-grade tumors. Accordingly, the NCCN Guidelines indicate that virtually all patients with such tumors must be subjected to postoperative RT (60). For small tumors resected with wide clear margins, surgery with subsequent observation alone may be sufficient. For more details, reference should be made to the chapter on vulvar LMS (Vol. 1, Chapter 2) as well as the respective table. However, the NCCN Guidelines do not clearly specify a specific tumor size above or below which RT should be performed in stage pT1a cases. RT should always be considered when there is any doubt as to the true dimensions and reach of the tumor.

In cases in which ANS of the vagina and the vulva are primarily inoperable or in which only an R2 resection could be achieved, combination CHT, CHT-RT or RT can be considered as means for achieving tumor shrinkage to allow subsequent (re)resection (cf. uterine ANS) (21, 32, 60, 78). Combining a CHT regimen with regional hypothermia (± radiotherapy) is also a conceivable option. According to the results of a phase III trial, the aforementioned combination can improve local tumor control and result in a longer PFS in patients with locally advanced STS, and can thus be sensible in individual cases (21, 37, 78).

RT is indicated if R0 resection margins cannot be achieved despite reresection, i.e. when resection margins are positive (21). There is consensus that postoperative RT cannot replace reresection. Local control cannot be achieved via RT when gross tumor residuals remain (5). The patient must be assigned to palliative or supportive therapy in such cases (cf. uterine ANS). In one case, a patient was subjected to incomplete resection and subsequent postoperative RT. The patient had a PFI of over 3 years, at which point follow-ups ceased (72).

RT should be applied with a sufficiently high dose (> 50 Gy) over a wide field (50). According to the NCCN Guidelines, for vaginal ANS, standalone VBT is also a possibility depending on the size of the tumor bed. In general, postoperative RT is only associated with an improved DFS, without effects on OS (21). Patients must be informed to this end. For patients with vaginal ANS who are generally inoperable, symptoms can be temporarily controlled by subjecting them to ERT or VBT (51).

Patients whose ANS are associated with prior radiation therapy should not be subjected to further RT (98).

It remains unsubstantiated that adjuvant CHT offers any benefits. Accordingly, such course of action is generally not recommended except for select individual cases (21, 32, 60, 78). There is no indication for adjuvant HT for vulvar and vaginal ANS.

Vulvar angiosarcomas have a better prognosis than their vaginal and uterine equivalents. Resection leaving wide clear resection margins is the therapeutic method of choice for angiosarcomas primarily originating in the vulva and the vagina. Cases in which such margins cannot be achieved must be subjected to reresection. Since vulvar and vaginal angiosarcomas are high-grade tumors, postoperative radiotherapy is indicated. Since vaginal angiosarcomas are retroperitoneal tumors, postoperative radiotherapy can be abstained from in cases in which the resection margins are clearly negative. However, postoperative irradiation is nonetheless recommended, since potential recurrences of vaginal angiosarcomas can be associated with high rates of morbidity (e.g. significant negative impacts on the functionality of adjacent organs, or problematic resection/questionable resectability). Small vulvar angiosarcomas resected with wide margins can also be merely subjected to observation. Adjuvant chemotherapy has not been proven to be beneficial. Tumor shrinkage can be pursued via chemotherapy, radio-chemotherapy or radiotherapy when tumors are primarily inoperable or when reresection is not possible. Patients with inoperable/unresectable tumors are subjected to palliative or supportive therapy.

Aftercare, recurrences, metastases and their therapeutic management

Aftercare and follow-up care should be organized in accordance with the rules and recommendations for uterine ANS. Local imaging of vulvar ANS using CT and/or MRI is not necessary so long as they can be subject to good clinical control (60). Regarding the therapeutic management of recurrences and metastases, reference can be made to the measures and strategies described for uterine ANS.

Aftercare and follow-up care for vulvar and vaginal angiosarcomas as well as the strategy for therapeutically managing recurrences and metastases thereof should be designed in accordance to what has been stated for uterine angiosarcomas.

1.2.2 Angiosarcoma of the ovary and the tuba uterina

General, pathogenesis, pathologico-anatomical features

Only very few primary ANS of the ovary have been described in the literature. ANS of the fallopian tube are practically unknown. Ovarian ANS receive no mention in the NCCN Guidelines. Ovarian ANS fall with the group of ovarian STS according to the new WHO Classification (52). According to one review (44), affected women are aged between 7 and 77 years (mean: 37 years); postmenopausal occurrence is rather rare, and an absolute exception in women aged 81 (8). Little is known about these tumors in terms of etiology and pathogenesis. A Finnish study investigated the association between the exposure of mamma and genital carcinoma patients to RT and the occurrence of ANS (92). Development from ovarian vessels is possible. Another plausible pathogenetic option could be that the tumor has developed from ovarian carcinosarcoma with a sarcomatous ANS component. There are also accounts of ovarian angiosarcoma developing from or within mature teratomas or other sex-cord tumors (3, 15, 47, 49). In some cases, residuals of dermoid cysts can be found within ovarian

ANS (62). It is known that other pure sarcomas like LMS, FS, RMS, osteosarcomas, chondrosarcomas, and carcinosarcomas can arise in teratomas (97). There are no reports of associations between ovarian ANS and previous radiation exposure. ANS occasionally also occur as mixed tumors, together with or within cystadenocarcinoma, borderline carcinoma, mucinous cystadenoma or ovarian fibroma (7, 8, 10, 42, 66, 71).

ANS can also occur as a metastatic tumor in the ovary. ANS of the breast appear to be the most common primary tumors in such cases (93). What is noticeable is that the ovarian metastases only occur unilaterally, which gives rise to the assumption that such lesions might well in fact be independent tumors (93).

Whether staging should occur in accordance with the rules for ovarian carcinoma or those for STS is unclear, while the former does, however, appear to be the more sensible option from a clinical perspective. The STS criteria only allow for stages Ib and IIb. The pathologist should always note which staging criteria are being drawn on.

Ovarian angiosarcomas do occur. Affected women are predominantly premenopausal. Development from a dermoid is not unusual. The possibility that an ovarian angiosarcoma could in fact be metastasis from an angiosarcoma of another site must be considered. Staging for ovarian carcinomas is applied in most cases.

Analogous to other pure ovarian sarcomas, only one ovary appears to be primarily affected in the majority of cases (44, 73, 90). Tumor size ranges from 3.5 to 25 cm (90). Macroscopic appearance is characterized by cystic structures, often with visible necroses and hemorrhages, with a puce or bluish-red color on the cut surface.

As evidenced by the described and reported cases, ovarian ANS, independent of their pathogenesis, do not histologically or immunohistochemically differ from uterine ANS (3, 26, 73).

Clinical presentation, diagnostics, imaging, differential diagnostics

Ovarian ANS can have a clinical appearance that resembles both benign and malignant ovarian tumors. Rapid growth attended by increased abdominal girth is a common finding (73). Furthermore, abdominal pains, uriesthesis, and nausea are the most common symptoms; ascites or a hematoperitoneum are not unusual (44, 73, 90). Fatal bleeding can occasionally occur in cases of advanced disease, sometimes within only a few weeks of cytoreductive surgery (34).

Both solid and cystic components are visible in sonography (90). CT reveals a solid tumor that is isodense to the soft tissues and that can contain larger cystic areas (11, 73), that in turn can increase in size during the course of observation (82). In MRI, the solid components have been reported to have a high SI in T2W, a low SI in T1W images, and show enhancement in T1WC images (82). Ultimately, imaging via CT and MRI is unspecific.

In the context of DD, it must be borne in mind that ovarian ANS can also be the result of metastatic spread of ANS from other sites, in particular the breast but also the subcutis (11, 82, 93). In contrast to the spread of metastatic carcinomas, ANS metastases in such cases are virtually always unilaterally localized. One case report describes a well circumscribed solid tumor that exhibited no cystic structures, neither macroscopically nor in MRI (93). The discussed possibility of ANS independently developing simultaneously at various sites thus requires that lungs, abdomen, and pelvis be subjected to imaging whenever an ANS has been identified as such.

Hemangioma, embryonic and poorly differentiated carcinomas, other pure sarcomas like FS, RMS, LMS, chondrosarcoma, and osteosarcoma as well as malignant peripheral nerve sheath tumors are further differential diagnostic options. In this context, verifying the presence or absence of endothelial immunohistochemical markers serves as the most important factor pertaining to DD.

There are no known usable tumor markers.

Angiosarcomas usually give the impression of ovarian carcinoma, both clinically and in terms of their imaging characteristics. Tumors are usually bluish-red, often with cystic structures, necroses, and hemorrhages. Verifying the presence of endothelial markers serves as the most reliable means for histologically excluding undifferentiated carcinomas and other pure sarcoma types.

Course, prognosis, primary surgery, primary and adjuvant radio-, chemo- and hormone therapy

About 30 to 50 % of cases are in stage I at the time of primary diagnosis, while the remainder are already in stages III and IV (44, 73). Almost without exception, patients with stage III and IV succumb to their disease within one year. Median survival for all deceased patients of all stages is only 10.2 mo (44).

Ovarectomy is the therapeutic option of choice. In the majority of cases only a unilateral or bilateral adnexectomy was performed (44). There is no evidence to suggest that expanding surgical therapy to include a THE or an omentectomy is beneficial in cases in which the tumor is confined to the ovary. As for uterine ANS, maximal cytoreductive surgery (debulking) is indicated for ovarian tumors that have spread beyond the ovaries, and is line with current NCCN Guidelines for soft tissue sarcomas (60).

As is also the case for uterine, vulvar, and vaginal ANS, subjecting patients with R0 resected ovarian ANS to adjuvant CHT has yet to be proven a beneficial strategy (73). Cases are known in which patients have deceased while still under adjuvant CHT (90). There is no indication for adjuvant HT for ovarian and tubal ANS.

In light of the fact that practically no patients with primary advanced disease (stage III and IV) survive for longer than one year, subjecting them to postoperative CHT would be a highly palliative strategy to adopt. Moreover, there are no data that suggest that immediate subjection to postoperative CHT yields better results than initially adopting a more cautious or observant approach. Accordingly, CHT can only be applied when there are strong or severe symptoms or when further tumor growth would endanger or restrict the proper functioning of organs.

Ovarian angiosarcomas have an extremely poor prognosis. Ovarectomy is the therapeutic option of choice. There is no indication for expanding surgical measures to include total hysterectomy, lymphonodectomy or omentectomy. Maximal cytoreductive surgery (debulking) should be performed in cases of extrauterine spread. Postoperative chemotherapy and/or radiotherapy have not yet been proven as beneficial, neither for R0 resections nor for R1/2 resections. It is generally acceptable to adhere to the approach recommended for uterine ANS.

Aftercare, recurrences and metastases and their therapeutic management

Aftercare should be rendered in a fashion analogous to the approach described for uterine ANS. Metastasis to the lungs appears to be most common. Omental, peritoneal, and retroperitoneal metastasis occurs in up to 20 % of cases.

The criteria for the surgical management of recurrences and metastases as well as for potential subsequent follow-up treatment correspond to those for uterine and other genital ANS.

There is one account of recurrent ovarian ANS in which the local recurrence was subjected to R1 resection followed by a CHT regimen of doxorubicin plus ifosfamide. The patient became pregnant after two years without disease and subsequently delivered a healthy child (40).

There are only few reports pertaining to palliative therapy of ovarian ANS. In one case, complete radiologic response was achieved by administering epirubicin 60 mg/m^2 d 1 and 2 plus ifosfamide 1.8 g/m^2 d 1–5. The patient was alive without evidence of disease for 12 mo (end of control period) after the onset of treatment (79). In a further case, 3 mo of doxorubicin and ifosfamide effected a clinical CR and complete disappearance of symptoms. After a total of 5 mo there was an onset of rapid growth that could not even be halted by a regimen of cisplatin plus etoposide (16). Overall, palliative therapy of ovarian ANS as well as the substances/agents to be administered can be guided by the approach applied for uterine ANS.

Aftercare as well as the therapeutic approach to recurrent and metastatic ovarian angiosarcomas correspond to the approaches adhered to for uterine angiosarcomas.

References

(1) Abraham JA, Hornicek FJ, Kaufman AM, Harmon DC, Springfield DS, Raskin KA, Mankin HJ, Kirsch DG, Rosenberg AE, Nielsen GP, Desphpande V, Suit HD, DeLaney TF, Yoon SS. Treatment and outcome of 78 patients with angiosarcoma. Ann Surg Oncol. 2007; 14: 1953–1967

(2) Agulnik M, Yarber JL, Okuno SH, von Mehren M, Jovanovic BD, Brockstein BE, Evens AM, Benjamin RS. An open-label, multicenter, phase II study of bevacizumab for the treatment of angiosarcoma and epithelioid hemangioendotheliomas. Ann Oncol. 2013; 24: 257–263

(3) Albertin C, Johnson KA, Connor JP, Al-Niaimi AN. Angiosarcoma originating from an ovarian mature teratoma, a rare disease with complex treatment modalities. Gynecol Oncol Case Rep 2013; 5: 31–33

(4) Albores-Saavedra J, Schwartz AM, Henson DE, Kostun L, Hart A, Angeles-Albores D, Chablé-Montero F. Cutaneous angiosarcoma. Analysis of 434 cases from the Surveillance, Epidemiology, and End Results Program, 1973–2007. Ann Diagn Pathol 2011; 15: 93–97

(5) Alektiar KM, Velasco J, Zelefsky MJ, Woodruff JM, Lewis JJ, Brennan MF. Adjuvant radiotherapy for margin-positive high-grade soft tissue sarcoma of the extremity. Int J Radiat Oncol Biol Phys 2000; 48: 1051–1058

(6) Antonescu CR, Yoshida A, Guo T, Chang NE, Zhang L, Agaram NP, Qin LX, Brennan MF, Singer S, Maki RG. KDR activating mutations in human angiosarcomas are sensitive to specific kinase inhibitors. Cancer Res 2009; 69: 7171–7179

(7) Aragon L, Terreros D, Ho H, Greenberg H, Kupesic Plavsic S. Angiosarcoma of the ovary arising in a mucinous cystadenoma. J Clin Ultrasound 2011; 39: 351–355

(8) Bösmüller H, Gruber C, Haitchi-Petnehazy S, Wagner D, Webersinke G, Hauptmann S. Primary angiosarcoma of the ovary with prominent fibrosis of the ovarian stroma. Case report of an 81-year-old patient. Diagn Pathol 2011; 6: 65

(9) Brooks SE, Zhan M, Cote T, Baquet CR. Surveillance, epidemiology, and end results analysis of 2677 cases of uterine sarcoma 1989–1999. Gynecol Oncol 2004; 93: 204–208

(10) Cambruzzi E, Pegas KL, Milani DM, Cruz RP, Guerra EH, Ferrari MB. Angiosarcoma arising in an ovarian fibroma: A case report. Patholog Res Int 2010; Article ID: 842592. DOI: 10.4061/2010/842592

(11) Cantú De León D, Pérez Montiel D, Chanona Vilchis J. Unusual case of subcutaneous angiosarcoma metastatic to the ovary. Pathol Oncol Res 2007; 13: 379–381

(12) Cerri A, Gianni C, Corbellino M, Pizzuto M, Moneghini L, Crosti C. Lymphangiosarcoma of the pubic region: A rare complication arising in congenital non-hereditary lymphedema. Eur J Dermatol 1998; 8: 511–514

(13) Chan WW, SenGupta SK. Postirradiation angiosarcoma of the vaginal vault. Arch Pathol Lab Med 1991; 115: 527–528

(14) Clement PB, Young, RH. Atlas of gynaecologic surgical pathology. Elsevier Saunders 3rd ed. 2014

(15) Contreras AL, Mapca A. Angiosarcoma arising in mature cystic teratoma of the ovary: A case report and review of the literature. Int J Gynecol Pathol 2009; 28: 453–457

(16) Cunningham MJ, Brooks JS, Noumoff JS. Treatment of primary ovarian angiosarcoma with ifosfamide and doxorubicin. Gynecol Oncol 1994; 53: 265–268

(17) De Yao JT, Sun D, Powell AT, Rehmus EH. Scalp angiosarcoma remission with bevacizumab and radiotherapy without surgery: A case report and review of the literature. Sarcoma 2011; 2011: 160369 DOI: 10.1155/2011/160369

(18) Donnez O, Marbaux E, Van Ruyssevelt P, Mitri S, Donnez J. Cardiac and gingival metastasis after total abdominal hysterectomy with bilateral salpingo-oophorectomy for primary epithelioid angiosarcoma: Case report and review of the literature. Gynecol Surg 2001; 8: 207–212

(19) Drachenberg CB, Faust FJ, Borkowski A, Papadimitriuo JC. Epithelioid angiosarcoma of the uterus arising in a leiomyoma with associated ovarian and tubal angiomatosis. Am J Clin Pathol 1994; 102: 388–389

(20) Ehrmann RL, Griffiths CT. Malignant hemangioendothelioma of the uterus. Gynecol Oncol 1979; 8: 376–383

(21) ESMO – European Sarcoma Network Working Group. Soft tissue and visceral sarcomas: ESMO Clinical Practice Guidelines for diagnosis, treatment and follow-up. Ann Oncol 2012 Oct; 23 Suppl 7: vii 92–9

(22) Fadare O. Heterologous and rare homologous sarcomas of the uterine corpus: A clinicopathologic review. Adv Anat Pathol 2011; 18: 60–74

(23) Farid M, Ong WS, Lee MJ, Jeevan R, Ho ZC, Sairi AN, Soh LT, Poon D, Teh J, Chin F, Teo M, Quek R. Cutaneous versus non-cutaneous angiosarcoma: clinicopathologic features and treatment outcomes in 60 patients at a single Asian cancer centre. Oncology 2013; 85: 182–190

(24) Fata F, O'Reilly E, Ilson D, Pfister D, Leffel D, Kelsen DP, Schwartz GK, Casper ES. Paclitaxel in the treatment of patients with angiosarcoma of the scalp or face. Cancer 1999; 86: 2034–2037

(25) Fayette J, Martin E, Piperno-Neumann S, Le Cesne A, Robert C, Bonvalot S, Ranchère D, Pouillart P, Coindre JM, Blay JY. Angiosarcomas, a heterogeneous group of sarcomas with specific behavior depending on primary site: A retrospective study of 161 cases. Ann Oncol 2007; 18: 2030–36

(26) Fetsch JF, Laskin WB. soft tissue lesions involving female reproductive organs. In: Kurman RJ, Ellenson LH, Ronnett BM (eds). Blaustein's Pathology of the Female Tract. 6th ed. Springer 2011; pp. 1159–1203

(27) Fletcher CDM, Beham A, Bekir S, Clarke AMT, Marley NJE. Epithelioid angiosarcoma of deep soft tissue: A distinctive tumor readily mistaken for an epithelial neoplasm. Am J Surg Pathol 1991; 15: 915–924

(28) Fury MG, Antonescu CR, Van Zee KJ, Brennan MF, Maki RG. A 14-year retrospective review of angiosarcoma: Clinical characteristics, prognostic factors, and treatment outcomes with surgery and chemotherapy. Cancer J 2005; 11: 241–247

(29) George S, Merriam P, Maki RG, Van den Abbeele AD, Yap JT, Akhurst T, Harmon DC, Bhuchar G, O'Mara MM, D'Adamo DR, Morgan J, Schwartz GK, Wagner AJ, Butrynski JE, Demetri GD, Keohan ML. Multicenter phase II trial of sunitinib in the treatment of nongastrointestinal stromal tumor sarcomas. J Clin Oncol 2009; 27: 3154–3160

(30) Goette DK, Detlefs RL. Postirradiation angiosarcoma. J Am Acad Dermatol. 1985; 12: 922–926

(31) Gray MH, Rosenberg AE, Dickersin GR, Bhan AK. Cytokeratin expression in epithelioid vascular neoplasms. Hum Pathol 1990; 21: 212–217

(32) Grimer R, Judson I, Peake D, Seddon B. Guidelines for the management of soft tissue sarcomas. Sarcoma. 2010; 2010: 506182. DOI: 10.1155/2010/506182

(33) Guirguis A, Kanbour-Shakir A, Kelley J. Epithelioid angiosarcoma of the mons after chemoradiation for vulvar cancer. Int J Gynecol Pathol 2007; 26: 265–268

(34) Guseh SH, Bradford LS, Hariri LP, Schorge JO. Ovarian angiosarcoma: Extended survival following optimal cytoreductive surgery and adjuvant chemotherapy. Gynecol Oncol Case Rep. 2012; 4: 23–25

(35) Hayashi T, Koike K, Kumasaka T, Saito T, Mitani K, Terao Y, Ogishima D, Yao T, Takeda S, Takahashi K, Seyama K. Uterine angiosarcoma associated with lymphangioleiomyomatosis in a patient with tuberous sclerosis complex: An autopsy case report with immunohistochemical and genetic analysis. Hum Pathol 2012; 43: 1777–1784

(36) Hwang JP, Lim SM. Uterine epithelioid angiosarcoma on F-18 FDG PET/CT. Nucl Med Mol Imag 2013; 47: 134–137

(37) Issels RD, Lindner LH, Verweij J, Wust P, Reichardt P, Schem BC, Abdel-Rahman S, Daugaard S, Salat C, Wendtner CM, Vujaskovic Z, Wessalowski R, Jauch KW, Dürr HR, Ploner F, Baur-Melnyk A, Mansmann U, Hiddemann W, Blay JY, Hohenberger P. Neo-adjuvant chemotherapy alone or with regional hyperthermia for localised high-risk soft-tissue sarcoma: A randomised phase 3 multicentre study. Lancet Oncol 2010; 11: 61–70

(38) Itakura E, Yamamoto H, Oda Y, Tsuneyoshi M. Detection and characterization of vascular endothelial growth factors and their receptors in a series of angiosarcomas. J Surg Oncol 2008; 97: 74–81

(39) Jennings TA, Peterson L, Axiotis CA, Friedlaender GE, Cooke RA, Rosai J. Angiosarcoma associated with foreign body material. A report of three cases. Cancer 1988; 62: 2436–2444

(40) Jha S, Chan KK, Poole CJ, Rollason TP. Pregnancy following recurrent angiosarcoma of the ovary – A case report and review of literature. Gynecol Oncol 2005; 97: 935–937

(41) Judson I, Verweij J, Gelderblom H, Hartmann JT, Schöffski P, Blay JY, Kerst JM, Sufliarsky J, Whelan J, Hohenberger P, Krarup-Hansen A, Alcindor T, Marreaud S, Litière S, Hermans C, Fisher C, Hogendoorn PC, dei Tos AP, van der Graaf WT. European Organisation and Treatment of Cancer Soft Tissue and Bone Sarcoma Group Doxorubicin alone versus intensified doxorubicin plus ifosfamide for first-line treatment of advanced or metastatic soft-tissue sarcoma: A randomised controlled phase 3 trial. Lancet Oncol 2014; 15: 415–423

(42) Jylling AM, Jørgensen L, Hølund B. Mucinous cystadenocarcinoma in combination with hemangiosarcoma in the ovary. Pathol Oncol Res 1999; 5: 318–319

(43) Konishi Y, Sato H, Fujinioto T, Tanaka H, Takahashi O, Tanaka T. A case of primary uterine angiosarcoma: magnetic resonance imaging and computed tomography findings. Int J Gynecol Cancer 2007; 17: 280–284

(44) Kruse AJ, Sep S, Slangen BF, Vandevijver NM, Van Gorp T, Kruitwagen RF, Van de Vijver KK. Angiosarcomas of primary gynecologic origin: A clinicopathologic review and quantitative analysis of survival. Int J Gynecol Cancer 2014; 24: 4–12

(45) Lack EE, Bitterman P, Sundeen JT. Müllerian angiosarcoma of the uterus with pure angiosarcoma: A case report. Hum Pathol 1991; 22: 1289–1291

(46) Lahat G, Dhuka AR, Lahat S, Smith KD, Pollock RE, Hunt KK, Ravi V, Lazar AJ, Lev D. Outcome of locally recurrent and metastatic angiosarcoma. Ann Surg Oncol 2009; 16: 2502–2509.

(47) Lifschitz-Mercer B, Leider-Trejo L, Messer G, Peyser MR, Czernobilsky B. Primary angiosarcoma of the ovary: a clinicopathologic, immunohistochemical and electronmicroscopic study. Pathol Res Pract 1998; 194: 183–187

(48) Maki RG, D'Adamo DR, Keohan ML, Saulle M, Schuetze SM, Undevia SD, Livingston MB, Cooney MM, Hensley ML, Mita MM, Takimoto CH, Kraft AS, Elias AD, Brockstein B, Blachère NE, Edgar MA, Schwartz LH, Qin LX, Antonescu CR, Schwartz GK. Phase II study of sorafenib in patients with metastatic or recurrent sarcomas. J Clin Oncol 2009; 27: 3133–3140.

(49) Malagon HD, Valdez AM, Moran CA, Suster S. Germ cell tumors with sarcomatous components: clinicopathologic and immunohistochemical study of 46 cases. Am J Surg Pathol 2007; 31: 1356–1362

(50) Mark RJ, Poen JC, Tran LM, Fu YS, Juillard GF. Angiosarcoma. A report of 67 patients and a review of the literature. Cancer 1996; 77: 2400–2406

(51) McAdam JA, Stewart F, Reid R. Vaginal epithelioid angiosarcoma. J Clin Pathol 1998; 51: 928–930

(52) McCluggae WG, Daya D, Ip P, Malpica A, Nielsen GP, Oliva E, Young RH. Soft tissue tumors. In: Kurman RJ, Carcangiu ML, Herrington CS, Young RH (eds.): WHO classification of tumors of female reproductive organs. 4th ed. IARC: Lyon 2014, p. 74

(53) Medina BR, Barba EM, Torres AV, Trujillo SM. Gingival metastases as first sign of a primary uterine angiosarcoma. J Oral Maxillofac Surg 2001; 59: 467–471

(54) Mendez LE, Joy S, Angioli R, Estape R, Penalver M. Primary uterine angiosarcoma. Gynecol Oncol 1999; 75: 272–276

(55) Miettinen M. Immunohistochemistry of soft tissue tumours – review with emphasis on 10 markers. Histopathology 2014; 64: 101–118

(56) Morgan MA, Moutos DM, Pippitt CH Jr, Suda RR, Smith JJ, Thurnau GR. Vaginal and bladder angiosarcoma after therapeutic irradiation. South Med J 1989; 82: 1434–1436

(57) Morimura Y1, Hashimoto T, Soeda S, Fujimori K, Yamada H, Yanagida K, Sato A. Angiosarcoma of vagina successfully treated with interleukin-2 therapy and chemotherapy: A case report. J Obstet Gynaecol Res 2001; 27: 231–235

(58) Nagano T, Yamada Y, Ikeda T, Kanki H, Kamo T, Nishigori C. Docetaxel: a therapeutic option in the treatment of cutaneous angiosarcoma: report of 9 patients. Cancer 2007; 110: 648–651

(59) Naka N, Tomita Y, Nakanishi H, et al. Mutations of p53 tumor suppressor gene in angiosarcoma. Int J Cancer 1997; 71: 952–955

(60) National Comprehensive Cancer Network: NCCN Practice Guidelines in Oncology – Soft Tissue Sarcoma – Version 2.2016 www.nccn.org

(61) National Comprehensive Cancer Network: NCCN Practice Guidelines in Oncology – Uterine Tumors – Version 2.2016 www.nccn.org

(62) Nielsen GP, Young RH, Prat J, Scully RE. Primary angiosarcoma of the ovary: A report of seven cases and review of the literature. Int J Gynecol Pathol 1997; 16: 378–382

(63) Nirenberg A, Ostor AG, Slavin J, Riley CB, Rome RM. Primary vulvar sarcomas. Int J Gynecol Pathol 1995; 14: 55–62

(64) Olawaiye AB, Morgan JA, Goodman A, Fuller AF Jr, Penson RT. Epithelioid angiosarcoma of the uterus: A review of management. Arch Gynecol Obstet 2008; 278: 401–404

(65) Oliva E. Leiomyoma and variants. In: Nucci MR, Oliva E (eds.). Diagnostic Pathology Gynaecological. Amirsys 2014; 3-180–191

(66) Ongkasuwan C, Taylor JE, Tang CK, Prempree T. Angiosarcomas of the uterus and ovary: clinicopathologic report. Cancer 1982; 49: 1469–1475

(67) Park MS, Ravi V, Araujo DM. Inhibiting the VEGF-VEGFR pathway in angiosarcoma, epithelioid hemangioendothelioma, and hemangiopericytoma/solitary fibrous tumor. Curr Opin Oncol 2010; 22: 351–355

(68) Pawlik TM, Paulino AF, McGinn CJ, Baker LH, Cohen DS, Morris JS, Rees R, Sondak VK. Cutaneous angiosarcoma of the scalp: A multidisciplinary approach. Cancer 2003; 98: 1716–1726

(69) Penel N, Bui Nguyen B, Bay JO, Cupissol D, Ray-Coquard I, Piperno-Neumann S, Kerbrat P, Fournier C, Mahier C, Blay JY. Weekly paclitaxel in metastatic angiosarcoma. A FNCLCC French Sarcoma Group (6SF-GETO) phase II trial (ASCO Annual Meeting Proceedings). J Clin Oncol 2007; 25: (Abstr 10002).

(70) Penel N, Italiano A, Ray-Coquard I, Chaigneau L, Delcambre C, Robin YM, Bui B, Bertucci F, Isambert N, Cupissol D, Bompas E, Bay JO, Duffaud F, Guillemet C, Blay JY. French Sarcoma Group (GSF/GETO). Metastatic angiosarcomas: doxorubicin-based regimens, weekly paclitaxel and metastasectomy significantly improve the outcome. Ann Oncol 2012; 23: 517–23

(71) Pillay K, Essa AS, Chetty FT. Borderline serous cystadenocarcinoma with coexistent angiosarcoma: An unusual form of ovarian carcinosarcoma. Int J Surg Pathol 2001; 9: 317–321

(72) Prempree T, Tang CK, Hatef A, Forster S. Angiosarcoma of the vagina: A clinicopathologic report. A reappraisal of the radiation treatment of angiosarcomas of the female genital tract. Cancer 1983; 15: 618–622
(73) Quesenberry CD, Li C, Chen AH, Zweizig SL, Ball HG. Primary angiosarcoma of the ovary: A case report of Stage I disease. Gynecol Oncol 2005; 99: 218–221
(74) Quinonez GE. Paraskevas MP. Diocee MS. Lorimer SM. Angiosarcoma of the uterus: A case report. Am J Obstet Gynecol 1991; 164: 90–92
(75) Richer M, Barkati M, Meunier C, Fortin S, Provencher D, Rahimi K. Vaginal epithelioid angiosarcoma: A potential pitfall in gynecologic pathology. J Low Genit Tract Dis 2014; 18: E38–42
(76) Schammel DP, Tavassoli FA. Uterine angiosarcomas: A morphologic and immunohistochemical study of four cases. Am J Surg Pathol 1998; 22: 246–250
(77) Schlemmer M, Reichardt P, Verweij J, Hartmann JT, Judson I, Thyss A, Hogendoorn PC, Marreaud S, Van Glabbeke M, Blay JY. Paclitaxel in patients with advanced angiosarcomas of soft tissue: A retrospective study of the EORTC soft tissue and bone sarcoma group. Eur J Cancer 2008; 44: 2433–2436
(78) Schütte J, Hartmann JH, Reichardt P, Issels RD, Tunn PU, Budach V. Weichteilsarkome – Onkopedia Leitlinie 2011. www.dgho-onkopedia.de/de/onkopedia/leitlinien/weichteilsarkome
(79) Serrano C, García Á, Brana I, Pérez-Benavente A, Oaknin A. Angiosarcoma of the ovary: Is it always a lethal disease? J Clin Oncol. 2010; 28: e675–677
(80) Shin YR, Rha SE. Miscellaneous tumors of the uterus. In: Kim SH. (ed) Radiology Illustrated Gynecologic Imaging. 2nd. edn, Springer 2012; pp. 249–297
(81) Skubitz KM, Haddad PA. Paditaxel and pegylated-liposomal doxorubicin are both active in angiosarcoma. Cancer 2005; 104: 361–366
(82) Souza FF, Katkar A, den Abbeele AD, Dipiro PJ. Breast angiosarcoma metastatic to the ovary. Case Rep Med 2009; 2009:381015. DOI: 10.1155/2009/381015
(83) Sullivan HC, Edgar MA, Cohen C, Kovach CK, HooKim K, Reid MD. The utility of ERG, CD31 and CD34 in the cytological diagnosis of angiosarcoma: An analysis of 25 cases. J Clin Pathol 2015; 68: 44–50
(84) Suzuki S, Tanioka F, Minato H, Ayhan A, Kasami M, Sugimura H. Breakages at YWHAE, FAM22A, and FAM22B loci in uterine angiosarcoma: A case report with immunohistochemical and genetic analysis. Pathol Res Pract 2014; 210: 130–134.
(85) Takeuchi K1, Deguchi M, Hamana S, Motoyama S, Kitazawa S, Maruo T. A case of postirradiation vaginal angiosarcoma treated with recombinant interleukin-2 therapy. Int J Gynecol Cancer 2005; 15: 1163–1165
(86) Tallini G, Price FV, Carcangiu ML. Epithelioid angiosarcoma arising in uterine leiomyomas. Am J Clin Pathol 1993; 100: 514–518
(87) Tierney JF, Stewart LA, Parmar MKB (Writing Committee). Sarcoma Meta-analysis Collaboration. Adjuvant chemotherapy for localised resectable soft-tissue sarcoma of adults: meta-analysis of individual data. Lancet 1997; 350: 1647–1654
(88) Tohya T, Katabuchi H, Fukuma K, Fujisaki S, Okamura H. Angiosarcoma of the vagina. A light and electron microscopy study. Acta Obstet Gynecol Scand 1991; 70: 169–172
(89) Toro JR, Travis LB, Wu HJ, Zhu K, Fletcher CD, Devesa SS. Incidence patterns of soft tissue sarcomas, regardless of primary site, in the surveillance, epidemiology and end results program, 1978–2001: An analysis of 26,758 cases. Int J Cancer 2006; 119: 2922–2930
(90) Vavilis D, Papadopoulos N, Agorastos T, Efstratiou I, Kommoss F, Bontis IN. Primary ovarian angiosarcoma – review of the literature and report of a case with coexisting chylothorax. Eur J Gynaecol Oncol 2007; 28: 287–289
(91) Verschraegen CF, Arias-Pulido H, Lee SJ, Movva S, Cerilli LA, Eberhardt S, Schmit B, Quinn R, Muller CY, Rabinowitz I, Purdy M, Snyder D, Bocklage T. Phase IB study of the combination of

docetaxel, gemcitabine, and bevacizumab in patients with advanced or recurrent soft tissue sarcoma: The Axtell regimen. Ann Oncol 2012; 23: 785–790
(92) Virtanen A, Pukkala E, Auvinen A. Angiosarcoma after radiotherapy: A cohort study of 332,163 Finnish cancer patients. Br J Cancer 2007; 97: 115–117
(93) Wang J, Fisher C, Thway K. Angiosarcoma of the breast with solitary metastasis to the ovary during pregnancy: An uncommon pattern of metastatic disease. Case Rep Oncol Med. 2013; 2013: 209610 DOI: 10.1155/2013/209610
(94) Weiss SW, Goldblum JR, Folpe AL, Weiss SW. Malignant vasular tumors. In: Weiss SW, Goldblum JR Folpe AL, Weiss SW (eds). Enzinger and Weiss's Soft Tissue Tumors. 6th edn, Elsevier Saunders 2014, pp. 703–732
(95) Wittekind C, Comptom CC, Brierley J, Sobin LH. TNM-Supplement – A commentary on uniform use. 4th ed. UICC and John Wiley & Sons, 2012
(96) Woll PJ, van Glabbeke M, Hohenberger P, et al. Adjuvant chemotherapy (CT) with doxorubicin and ifosfamide in resected soft tissue sarcoma (STS): Interim analysis of a randomised phase III trial. Proc Am Soc Clin Oncol 2007; 25: abstr 10008
(97) Yaqoob N, Nemenqani D, Khoja H, Hafez M, Tulbah A, Al-Dayel F. Ovarian angiosarcoma: a case report and review of the literature. J Med Case Rep 2014; 8: 47
(98) Young RJ, Brown NJ, Reed MW, et al. Angiosarcoma. Lancet Oncol 2010; 11: 983–991
(99) Young RJ, Woll PJ, Staton CA, Reed MW, Brown NJ. Vascular-targeted agents for the treatment of angiosarcoma. Cancer Chemother Pharmacol 2014; 73: 259–270
(100) Zaloudek, C, Hendrickson MR. Soslow RA. Mesenchymal tumors of the uterus. In: Kurman, RJ. Ellenson LH, Ronnett BM. Blaustein's Pathology of the Female Tract. 6th edn. Springer 2011; 452–527

Image references

Evert M, Evert K. Universitätsmedizin Greifswald, Institut für Pathologie, Greifswald.
Figs. 1.1.1 (A)–(C); 1.2.1 (A), (B)

Günter Köhler, Katja Evert, Marek Zygmunt and Matthias Evert

2 Liposarcoma

Generally speaking, liposarcomas (LS) are among the most common sarcomas in adults, without a clear preference for gender (52). They account for 17–20 % of all STS, third only behind LMS and malignant fibrous histiocytoma (13, 77). The extremities and retroperitoneal localizations are the most common sites. LS of the female reproductive organs are so rare that only individual case studies or small retrospective studies exist. There is currently no evidence to suggest that genital LS significantly differ from their extrauterine equivalents, either clinically, pathologico-anatomically or in terms of prognosis. Due to the limited number of cases of LS of female reproductive organs that have been published, any characterization thereof must be widely based on what is known about their extragenital counterparts.

According to the current WHO Classification, uterine LS are categorized as "other mesenchymal tumors" (61). WHO Classification (18) differentiates adipogenic tumors into intermediate (locally aggressive) tumors and malignant adipocytic tumors. The former group essentially covers well-differentiated LS. These neoplasms are termed atypical lipomatous tumors (atypical lipoma) when located at superficial sites, while deep, retroperitoneally localized tumors are termed well-differentiated LS (2, 3). The group of malignant adipocytic tumors, on the other hand, covers dedifferentiated LS, myxoid round cell LS, and pleomorphic LS. According to WHO Classification, this group also includes mixed-type LS and LS not otherwise specified (NOS) (18).

Liposarcomas only exceptionally occur in the female reproductive organs.

2.1 Uterine liposarcoma

2.1.1 General, epidemiology, etiology, pathogenesis, staging

LS in the uterus are to be classified as heterologous sarcomas. To date, fewer than 20 cases of uterine LS have been described in the literature. The true incidence rate is, however, likely to be markedly higher. LS account for 0.4 % of all pure uterine sarcomas covered in the DKSM database (42). Among uterine sarcomas that are encountered only occasionally, only alveolar soft tissue sarcomas and malignant extrarenal rhabdoid tumors are even rarer than LS (16). It has yet to be reported that a well-differentiated LS has arisen in the uterus. Instead, the LS types that are most frequently known to be encountered at this site are the myxoid round cell and pleomorphic types. By contrast, with a share of 40–50 %, well-differentiated LS is the most common lipoma in extrauterine sites, followed by pleomorphic LS (about 30 %), and myxoid round cell LS (about 10 %). Well-differentiated, dedifferentiated, and pleomorphic LS of all sites predominantly occur in patients older than 50, but are also known to arise in patients under the age of 20. Myxoid round cell LS are usually observed in patients who are slightly younger on average (25 to 45 years old). The average age of women with all forms of LS is 59 years (16).

Only little is known about uterine LS in terms of etiology and pathogenesis. As is also the case for most other uterine and also extrauterine STS, previous RT is assumed to be an etiological factor in LS as well. Different genetic factors have been identified for the different individual types of LS. In well-differentiated and dedifferentiated LS, structural anomalies can be found, for instance chromosome 12-derived ring and giant chromosomes that subsequently lead to the amplification of defined genes (MDM2, CDK4). t(12;16) (q13;p11) or t(12;22) (q13;q12) chromosomal translocations are known oncogenic factors for myxoid round cell LS, and complex chromosomal alterations can be found in pleomorphic LS (1, 5). The aforementioned translocations in myxoid round cell LS result in a subsequent gene fusion and thus to an expression of FUS-DDIT3 or EWS-DDIT3 fusion genes and their proteins (67). Myxoid round cell LS, therefore, belong to the group of translocation-associated sarcomas, which also encompasses LG-ESS, alveolar RMS, alveolar STS, and ANS. Among other effects, the stated fusion genes and fusion proteins disturb adipocytic differentiation.

Well-differentiated and dedifferentiated LS are closely pathogenetically related. The dedifferentiation of LS is probably a temporally contingent consequence of a tumor being present yet undetected for a longer period of time. Dedifferentiated LS virtually never arise from well-differentiated subcutaneous LS, while the opposite applies for larger and thus usually older retroperitoneal neoplasms. It occasionally so happens that the dedifferentiation only becomes evident upon disease recurrence.

In contrast to well-differentiated LS, the p53 protein is mutated in up to 30 % of myxoid round cell LS. More than half of all uterine adipocytic tumors are in some way or another associated with smooth muscle neoplasia and/or can contain elements or components of an LM. Such observations have not been made for extrauterine lipogenous tumors. It is thus assumed that uterine LS can also arise from an LM or an LLM (cf. Vol. 1, Chapter 1) (17, 31, 49). There are also (albeit rare) known cases of LLM in the uterus. The adipocytic component usually has the morphology of myxoid LS in such cases (45). Otherwise, lipoleiomyosarcomas in the pelvic region are usually only encountered retroperitoneally (20).

Uterine LS have no separate staging. Staging for STS (cf. Vol. 1, Chapter 2) applies unless otherwise stated. According to STS classification, uterine LS are always deep tumors. Consequently, there are no stages T1a and T2a for this type of neoplasm. In theory, pathologists could also refer to staging for uterine LMS or stromal sarcomas. They should always clearly note which staging they are applying in the individual case.

Well-differentiated liposarcomas are not known to arise in the uterus. Dedifferentiated, myxoid round cell and pleomorphic liposarcomas do occur in the uterus, albeit rarely. Uterine liposarcomas predominantly occur in postmenopausal women. Genetic aberrations are present in all types of liposarcoma. Myxoid round cell liposarcoma belong to the group of translocation-associated sarcomas. No separate staging exists for uterine liposarcoma. Reference should be made to staging for soft tissue sarcomas, according to which such neoplasms are always deep tumors.

2.1.2 Macroscopic and microscopic features

Uterine LS are usually even larger than LMS at the time of primary diagnosis. They have a mean diameter of around 16 cm. Their size exceeds 10 cm in the majority of cases and is only exceptionally under 5 cm (16, 17, 49). LS are usually well-circumscribed masses located within the myometrium. Due to their large size, there is very often also cervical infiltration/involvement. Almost one third are primarily located in the cervix or in the lower uterine segment (47). Despite their size, LS usually remain confined to the uterus.

To date, there are no accounts of well-differentiated LS in the uterus without signs of dedifferentiation. They can, however, occur in immediate proximity to the uterus, for example in the ligamentum latum. The well-circumscribed nodules usually have an intense yellow color (Fig. 2.1.1 (A)).

Dedifferentiated LS usually have a multinodus macroscopic appearance; cohesion between the individual nodes is only loose or weak in most cases. They are almost always free of necrosis, but sometimes hemorrhaging can be observed. Depending on the share of fat or dedifferentiated tissue in the nodes, they can be either soft or rather solid, with a lipoid or greyish-brown appearance.

Myxoid round cell LS are characterized either by a more gelatinous or a more solid whitish or yellowish cut surface, depending on the present shares of myxoid, round, and/or fat cells. The round-celled histological sections macroscopically present as opaque-whitish, fleshy nodules.

Pleomorphic LS are usually not macroscopically recognizable as such. Such tumors are most commonly solid, are occasionally knotty/nodular, and the cut surface presents a fleshy grayish-yellow to grayish-white, sometimes even brownish-yellow to brownish-white appearance. It is common for signs of necrosis and degeneration to be visible on macroscopic inspection. The different components of which mixed myxoid-pleomorphic LS consist provide these neoplasms with a polymorphic macroscopic appearance.

Well-differentiated LS are characterized by abundant adipocytes of varying size with minor nuclear atypia as well as by the ample presence of fibrous septa. The latter also contain cells with atypical nuclei. Lipoblasts are present, but that presence is not decisive. The atypical adipocytes almost always express S100, as do non-neoplastic fat cells (50).

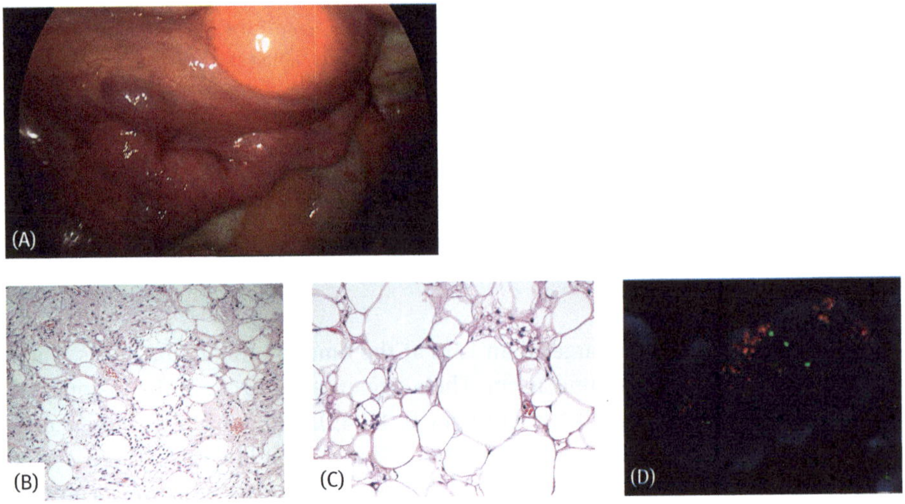

Fig. 2.1.1: Macroscopic and microscopic appearance of a well-differentiated liposarcoma. (A) laparoscopic aspect of a well-differentiated liposarcoma located within the ligamentum latum; (B) typical appearance of a well-differentiated liposarcoma with usually well-differentiated univacuolar fat cells that are barely or not at all discernible from normal cells, with interjacent fusicellular connective tissue that is typically found in the majority of such tumors, but also in variants of benign lipoma; (C) using strong magnification and searching for a considerable amount of time reveals the morphologically important multivacuolar lipoblasts (two cells in this image) that do not occur in mature cell lipomas; (D) the verification of MDM2 amplification (multiplicity of red signals) in the tumor cell nuclei via fluorescence in situ hybridization (FISH) constitutes a major diagnostic advance.

Microscopically speaking, dedifferentiated LS are well-differentiated LS in which an additional non-adipocytic sarcomatous component has developed or in which progression to a non-lipogenic tumor is recognizable (3, 39) (Fig. 2.1.2 (A), (B)). An LS should only be classified as a dedifferentiated LS when dedifferentiation is also macroscopically visible (> 1 cm). Masses with a size of 1–2 cm should be termed minimal or early dedifferentiation (25). The boundary between the two components is abruptly clear in all but exceptional cases. The dedifferentiated component usually consists of high-grade, sometimes (albeit rarely) of low-grade non-lipogenous sarcoma. Providing a more detailed description of the dedifferentiated sections – that can consist of homologous and/or heterologous components – would go too far for the context at hand, and should be read up in the specialist pathologico-anatomical literature (25). In order to secure and verify the diagnosis, at least 5 M/10 HPF should be measured in the dedifferentiated area. Unlike their pleomorphic counterparts, dedifferentiated LS always have a well-differentiated adipocytic component. They are also classified as dedifferentiated LS if the dedifferentiated component is an undifferentiated pleomorphic sarcoma. Dedifferentiated LS show a positive reaction to CD34, though the strength of the reaction varies from case to case (50).

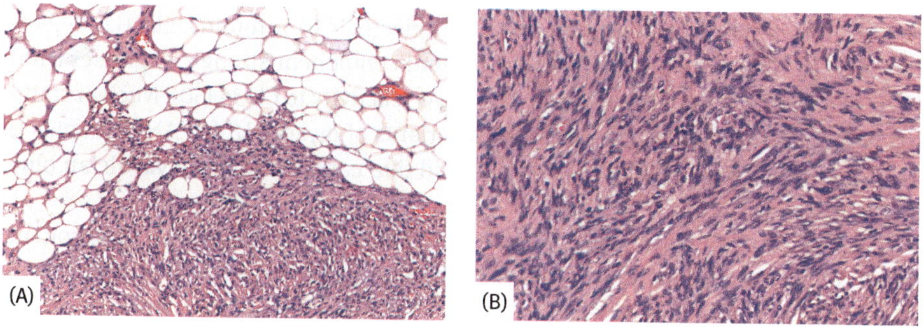

Fig. 2.1.2: Microscopic image of a dedifferentiated liposarcoma. (A) typical aspect of a dedifferentiated liposarcoma with abrupt transition from a well-differentiated liposarcoma to a spindle cell sarcoma, the most common morphological type of the dedifferentiated component; (B) recurrences can consist only of the dedifferentiated component. Verification of MDM2 amplification, e.g. via FISH (see Fig. 2.1.1 (D)), is usually decisive for reaching the proper diagnosis, since this typical gene modification remains detectable in the dedifferentiated component of the tumor.

Molecular verification of the presence of MDM2 amplification using FISH is a helpful option when only the dedifferentiated tumor component remains (as is often the case in recurrent tumors); not doing so will inevitably result in the tumor being misdiagnosed (e.g. as pleomorphic sarcoma, NOS) on the basis of the dedifferentiated sarcoma. In this regard, it is of vital importance that any prior knowledge of the presence of a well-differentiated sarcoma is shared during anamnesis. Otherwise, the attending physicians are unlikely to have any clues suggesting a necessity for molecular analyses!

Myxoid round cell LS typically consist of ample extracellular myxoid material with few mature adipocytes, as well as immature lipoblasts and round cells. Myxoid round cell LS with large myxoid shares can also exhibit cysts that form in extracellular mucin. A prominently myxoid background inevitably results in hypocellularity, in turn effecting that an MI of 7 M/10 HPF is only rarely reached (49). The tumor is usually pervaded by a striking vascular network (25). There are purely myxoid LS without round cells (myxoid LS), and LS with round cells that are poorly differentiated almost without exception. Essentially, however, both constitute variants of the same tumor (20). The term "round cell LM" has been dropped in the new WHO Classification and replaced with the term "high-grade myxoid LS" (19). The stronger the degree to which the adipocytic cells lose their differentiation, the more they assume round cell or spindle cell character. Generally, these cells are tightly grouped in a decreasing myxoid matrix. In cases in which no lipoblasts are distinguishable, the correct diagnosis can be securely confirmed by verifying the presence of chromosome translocation t(12;16)(q13;p11). Doing so is also necessary in view of the spectrum of "small round blue cell" tumors. Myxoid round cell LS can occasionally also exhibit chondroid, osseous or leiomyomatous differentiations. Malignancy and grading of myxoid round cell LS are determined by the share of round cells (G1 < 10 % round cells, G2 10–25 % round cells, G3 > 25 % round cells). The myxoid component strongly expresses S100 (49). The spindle cell component can also show reactivity to CD 34 (50). Nuclear staining with ERG is occasionally successful in variants of myxoid LS (cf. ANS, Chapter 1) (50). The stroma also contains hyaluronic acid that can be visualized via alcian blue staining.

Uterine lipoleiomyosarcomas consist of a predominantly myxoid LS component and an LMS component that are focally intermingled, however without invading each other (45).

Pleomorphic LS consist of uncharacteristic high-grade mesenchymal tissue with intercalated pleomorphic and multivacuolar lipoblasts. The extremely high degree of cellular pleomorphism also encompasses bizarre giant cells. Histologically, tumors of this type are strongly reminiscent of pleomorphic sarcomas NOS (previously: malignant fibrous histiocytoma). However, large lipoblasts with bizarre hyperchromatic nuclei cannot be traced in the latter. The diagnosis "pleomorphic LS" thus has its footing in the verification of the presence of lipoblasts. Should lipoblasts be absent or overlooked, the tumor will inevitably be identified as a pleomorphic sarcoma, NOS (24). Pleomorphic LS with focal leiomyosarcomatous components have also been reported. There have also been (albeit few) known cases of pleomorphic LS occurring as malignant mesenchymoma with lipo-, leio- and osteosarcomatous components (16). Pleomorphic LS are occasionally positive for CD34 expression.

In one case, a uterine pleomorphic LS was positively immunoreactive for ER and negative for PGR. Smooth muscle elements in this tumor were positive for both ER and PGR (47).

Liposarcomas can reach a considerable size in the uterus. They usually have a yellowish-brownish appearance if they contain ample adipocytes. Myxoid round cell liposarcomas often have a gelatinous appearance, while their pleomorphic counterparts are usually unspecifically fleshy.

There are to date no accounts of well-differentiated liposarcomas arising in the uterus. Well-differentiated liposarcomas are characterized by the presence of adipocytes of varying size with nuclear atypia as well as by fibrous septa that likewise contain cells with atypical nuclei. Histologically, dedifferentiated liposarcomas are well-differentiated liposarcomas in which an additional non-adipocytic sarcomatous component has developed, or in which progression to a non-lipogenic tumor is recognizable. An MI of at least 5 M/HPF should be measurable in the dedifferentiated component. Myxoid round cell liposarcomas typically consist of ample extracellular myxoid matrix with few mature adipocytes as well as of immature lipoblasts and round cells. Purely myxoid liposarcomas do not contain round cells. Grading is determined by the relative share of round cells. Pleomorphic liposarcomas contain uncharacteristic high-grade mesenchymal tissue with intercalated pleomorphic and multivacuolar lipoblasts.

2.1.3 Clinical presentation, diagnostics, screening

Uterine LS are often incidental findings. Uterine LS essentially exhibit the same clinical behavior as LM or LMS. AUB and dysmenorrhea are key symptoms. Uterine LS often exhibit rapid growth. The presence of rapid growth in combination with symptoms is suggestive of sarcoma (cf. Vol. 1, Chapter 6), but is not monospecific to adipocytic malignancies. Analogous to the other uterine sarcomas, the pelvic pains that LS patient frequently present with are to be understood as a consequence of said rapid growth. Depending on the size of the lesion, increases in girth as well as dysuria and obstipation are also known to occur.

LS are mostly softer than LM on palpation due to their higher share of fat tissue. The suspicion of a lipomatous tumor is at least partially granted in particular in cases of younger women with relatively soft nodules in the vicinity of the cervix or the isthmus. It is thus imperative that LM that are clinically suspicious in any way be subjected to imaging diagnostic procedures, not least because lipogenous tumors can be easily identified as such via sonography, CT, and MRI. Particularities to this end and a respective flow chart can be found in Chapter 6 (Vol. 1). An LS will only be recognizable as such in hysteroscopy in exceptional cases, and fractional curettage, analogous to LMS, will regularly yield negative results. If patients are not subjected to sonographic examination, the different forms and variants of LS will only be incidentally diagnosed as such following an HE or uterus preserving surgery performed under the assumption of a uterine myomatosis. Suspicious results from sonographic examination (see below) should be followed up by further imaging diagnostic procedures, as doing so is the best means for avoiding incidental intraoperative or postoperative findings. LLM is the most important clinical DD (cf. Vol. 1, Chapter 1), as it is barely discernible from LS in imaging. LLM are benign tumors that predominantly occur in the uterus, but also in the cervix. The localizations in which uterine LS arise largely correspond to those of uterine LM. Patients with LLM are either asymptomatic or their symptoms correspond to those with which LM are associated (10). No particular screening strategy for LS has taken root in practice.

Symptoms, clinical findings, and hysteroscopic findings pertaining to uterine liposarcomas largely correspond to those of leiomyoma. The tumors are noticeably soft and often exhibit rapid growth. No specific screening methods have been established in practice.

2.1.4 Imaging

The following imaging characteristics primarily refer to the uterine variants of LS, but also apply to LS of other genital sites and retroperitoneal LS.

Lipomatous uterine and extrauterine tumors stand out in sonography because they typically have a visibly discernible high level of echogenicity (Figs. 2.1.3 (A),

2.2.2) that clearly delineates them from the surrounding myometrium. That high echogenicity, however, corresponds to the presence of lipogenous cells and can thus also be largely absent. Therefore, the generally hyperechoic tumors can contain, to varying extents, sections that are isoechoic and/or hypoechoic to normal myometrium (Fig. 2.1.3 (A)). The borders to the myometrium can be more or less sharply/clearly delineated, depending on the infiltrative behavior of the tumor. The septa (that are so typical for well-differentiated LS) can usually also be nicely visualized in sonography. Those septa are not found in the uterus, however, but are abundant in the vulva. Lipogenous tumors are occasionally surrounded by a hypoechoic "capsule" that likely corresponds to compressed myometrium. LLM appear much more frequently in the uterus than LS do, and likewise appear as well-defined, predominantly hyperechoic lesions in ultrasound (10, 72). Reliable discrimination from the other adipocytic tumor types is barely possible.

At -120 to -10 HU, LS have a very low density in CT that is below that of water yet above that of air. Depending on the number of adipocytes, lipogenous tumors can be isodense to subcutaneous fat tissue. In CT, the tumor margins or resection margins of lesions that are particularly rich in fat can be difficult to precisely discern against the backdrop of the retroperitoneal area that itself exhibits significant fat levels (73). Infiltrations of adjacent organs are, however, easy to recognize and can be helpful in making decisions pertaining to neoadjuvant therapy.

As the degree of dedifferentiation increases, so, too, does the density of the soft tissue, making the tumors noticeably lighter than water in CT. The density of the dedifferentiated sections of the tumor becomes increasingly unspecific (43). The remaining adipocytic areas remain as visible masses isodense to water. The solid sections as well as the septa of well-differentiated LS show a clear and strong enhancement in CECT, while the lipogenous components show none at all (10, 72).

Myxoid LS show attenuation comparable to that of muscle tissue (43, 73). Hemorrhages, myxoid areas, and necroses exhibit lower density or attenuation and thus appear dark in the image.

When an LS has been diagnosed, staging requires at the very least that the patient undergoes pulmonary CT. As is also the case for sonographic examination, in CT, too, accurately and reliably discerning an LS from an LLM is virtually impossible. The attenuation that the recurrences of well-differentiated LS show in CT is stronger than that of the present retroperitoneal fat (43). Remissions of advanced tumors and metastases are visualized in CT insofar as they cause a decrease in density (27). CT can thus be a helpful and useful tool for assessing disease remission.

MRI has the highest sensitivity and specificity for identifying the presence of fat tissue, and is thus regarded as the diagnostic method of choice for lipogenous tumors (55). However, benign neoplasms like lipoma, atypical lipomatous tumors, and well-differentiated LS cannot always be distinguished from each other.

The adipose tissue sections of all lipogenous tumors share identical characteristics in MRI (Tab. 2.1.1). The presence or extent of the high SI (a typical characteristic of

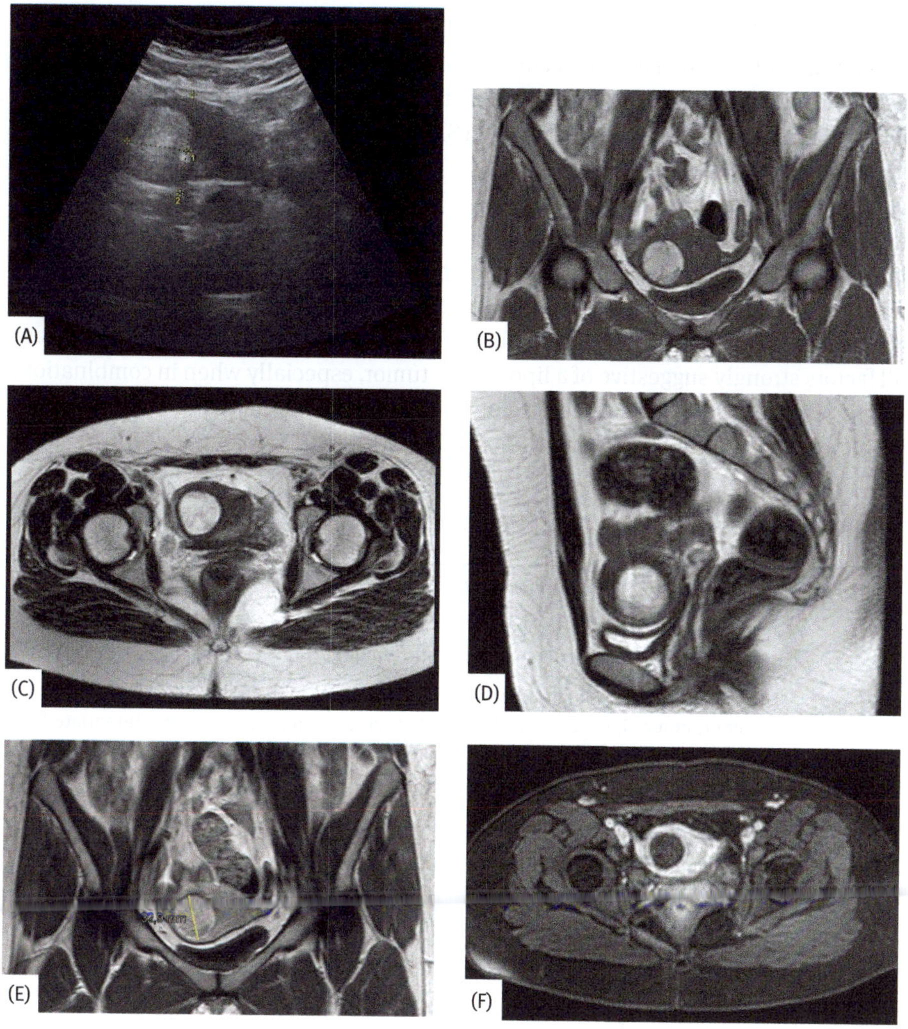

Fig. 2.1.3: Results from imaging diagnostics performed on a 23-year-old woman with dedifferentiated uterine liposarcoma; (A) the tumor's heterogeneous hyperechoicity to normal myometrium is clearly recognizable in abdominal sonography; (B) coronal T1-weighted MRI reveals a hyperintense tumor with a clearly distinguishable (also from normal myometrium) hypointense margin as well as hypointense bands, or seams, that correspond to the dedifferentiated sections of the tumor; (C), (D) axial and sagittal T2-weighted MRI likewise reveals a tumor with high signal intensity and a hypointense border margin; (E) in T1WC, the tumor does not enhance compared to normal myometrium, the hypointense margin remains; (F) T1WC with fat suppression serves to verify the diagnosis of adipocytic tumors as the fat suppression agent causes such tumors to lose all signal intensity.

fat tissue in MRI) is thus dependent on the share of adipocytes within the tumor. Well-differentiated LS (which do not occur in the uterus) thus exclusively exhibit the characteristics of adipocytic tumors. Analogous to subcutaneous fat tissue, the sections of adipose tissue within the tumor show high SI in T1 and T2W images and are isointense to fat (Fig. 2.1.3 (B)–(D)). These sections do not enhance in T1WC (Fig. 2.1.3 (E)), but show signal drop-out in T1/2-FS (Fig. 2.1.3 (F)). In contrast, the septa and solid tissues (hypointense in T1W) do enhance (75), as is particularly visible in the fat-suppressed images. Compared to lipomas, the aforementioned septa are thicker, more irregular, and more nodular (43). Isointensity to subcutaneous fat tissue in T1/2W images, an absence of SI in T1WC with FS, and visibly enhancing septa and solid components are all factors strongly suggestive of a lipogenous tumor, especially when in combination. In T1/2W and T1WC images, there is a noticeable edge or margin that is hypointense to both the tumor and to the myometrium (Fig. 2.1.3 (B)–(F)).

Tab. 2.1.1: Sonographic and MRI characteristics of liposarcomas.

Sonography	Tumors hyperechoic, commensurate to their share of adipose tissue
T1W	High SI isointense to subcutaneous fat, hypointense margin, hypointense bands/seams reflecting non-adipocytic tumor portions
T2W	High SI corresponding to that of subcutaneous fat in the adipocytic parts of the tumor; non-adipocytic areas have an SI that is isointense to the dedifferentiated sarcomatous component of the tumor; hypointense margin
T1WC	No enhancement in the adipocytic portions; enhancement in the non-adipocytic portions of the tumor; hypointense margin
T1WC with FS	Lack of SI in the adipocytic tumor components

Myxoid LS exhibit high SI in T1W, except in the non-adipocytic areas. In T2-weighted images, the myxoid components or myxoid cysts also have a high SI (43). Islands or pockets of fat tissue are shown as areas of high SI in T1W images. The solid tumor tissues and septa enhance in T1WC, while the adipocytic components do not.

Beyond their typically high levels of SI in the dedifferentiated components in T1- and T2-weighted images, dedifferentiated LS also exhibit the MRI characteristics of the soft tissue of other STS (15). Fully dedifferentiated LS are then no longer discernible from other uterine sarcomas and STS in MRI.

Just like STS, round cell and pleomorphic LS are hypointense in T1W and slightly hyperintense in T2W images, and generally show a strong enhancement in T1WC. Focally high SI in T1W will usually correspond to hemorrhages that do not enhance in T1WC, and that do not change their SI in T1W-FS (75). Pleomorphic LS can generally not be differentiated from other STS in MRI.

In T2W, adipocytic tumors bear close similarity to LG-ESS as the latter, too, is hyperintense with a typical visible border margin with low SI (cf. Vol. 1, Chapter 4).

However, LG-ESS have a lower SI than that exhibited by adipocytic tumors and normal fat tissue. Furthermore, LG-ESS do not lose all signal intensity in fat-suppressed images and do not have high SI in T1W.

T1W-FS images should always be recorded in order to exclude hemorrhagic cysts, mucinous cysts, and degenerated LM – all of which also exhibit high SI – as possible alternative diagnoses. While in FS images SI will substantially decrease in the sections of the LS that are rich in fat, it will remain high in the aforementioned potential differential diagnostic alternatives.

Differentiating LS from pedunculated mature ovarian teratomas with fatty content can be very challenging. Metastases appear hypointense compared to the primary tumor in T1W images, and show heterogeneous enhancement in T1WC images. In T2W, both metastases and the primary tumor are hyperintense. (71).

RT- or CHT-induced remissions of advanced tumors or metastases are visualized in T1WC as decreases in enhancement (28). Administering an MRI can thus be helpful in assessing remissions.

LLM, which occur in the uterus more frequently than LS do, are also the most important DD for LS in MRI (72).

There is currently no clearly recognizable indication for administering FDG-PET-CT. However, if neither sonography nor MRI can provide sufficient clarification as to whether a lesion is potentially malignant, and the patient insists on conservative surgery, undergoing FDG-PET-CT can be indicated for further clarification. PET-CT is said to be an effective means for differentiating between atypical lipomas/well-differentiated LS and clearly more aggressive lipogenic tumors. However, FDG-PET-CT appears to be inadequate for detecting metastases due to the frequency of false-negative findings (71).

The most fundamental sonographic feature of adipocytic tumors is their hyperechoicity. Depending on the adipocyte levels in the dedifferentiated, round cell, and pleomorphic components, sections that are isoechoic and/or hyperechoic to the myometrium can also be visible.

In CT, lipogenic tumors, depending on the share of fat tissue in their makeup, are isodense to subcutaneous fat tissue. Density decreases as the degree of dedifferentiation increases, so that the respective sections of the tumor appear lighter than water, while the adipocytic masses remain darker than water. CT is a very adequate method for evaluating and assessing disease remission.

In MRI, adipocytic tissue is characterized by high signal intensity in T1- and T2-weighted images, and shows little to no enhancement in contrast MRI. In order to delineate the tumor from neighboring structures with high SI, both in T1- and T2-weighted images, visualization should be improved by using fat suppression which causes the adipocytic tissue to lose its high signal intensity. Dedifferentiation or decreasing numbers of fat cells cause the high level of signal intensity to drop off, leaving a signal image that closely resembles that emitted by non-adipocytic STS. Contrast MRI can be helpful in assessing and evaluating disease remission.

In exceptional cases, FDG-PET-CT can be useful for assessing whether a lipogenic tumor is benign or malignant. In contrast, it is rather inadequate for detecting and assessing metastasis.

2.1.5 Differential diagnostics

Histologically differentiating between undifferentiated pleomorphic sarcomas, pleomorphic RMS, and highly malignant myxofibrosarcomas can be very challenging. Telling dedifferentiated LS from pleomorphic sarcomas that have infiltrated adipose tissue is equally difficult.

LS sometimes constitutes the mesenchymal component of a CS or an AS. Therefore, whenever an LS is encountered in the uterus, it must always be borne in mind that a CS or an AS could also be present. Overall, heterologous CS with an adipocytic sarcomatous component appear to be much more common and frequent than purely heterologous uterine LS. Thus, every LS should be carefully scrutinized as to whether it contains epithelial components, if need be via immunohistochemical testing. Uterine LMS with lipomatous differentiation is another possible DD.

Lipoleiomyosarcoma can be wrongfully diagnosed as LMS or merely LS when diagnosis is based on curettage or smaller biopsy specimens. The metastatic masses that this entity can develop often lack any sign of the leiomyomatous component (44).

If myxoid round cell LS only contain round cells, i.e. if the presence of lipoblasts cannot be verified within the tumor, one must also consider other "small round blue cell" sarcomas and lymphomas as possible differential diagnoses. Myxoid round cell LS with high counts of myxoid cells can also be primarily mistaken to be myxoid sarcoma. The typical capillary network and the presence of lipoblasts are important characteristics suggestive of a lipogenous origin. Where the histological diagnosis remains unclear, searching for chromosome translocation t(12;16)(q13;p11) can be helpful. If the lipoblasts are either missing or overlooked in pleomorphic LS, the tumor will inevitably be mistaken for a malignant fibrous histiocytoma. Malignant fibrous histiocytoma constitutes the more important DD for pleomorphic LS.

> Liposarcoma can constitute the sarcomatous component of carcinosarcoma and adenosarcoma. Epithelial components must thus be concertedly sought after. Liposarcoma can also be a constituent element of a lipoleiomyosarcoma. Pleomorphic liposarcoma can be mistaken for other types of pleomorphic sarcoma. Predominantly round celled liposarcoma can be confused with other round cell sarcomas and lymphomas.

2.1.6 Course, prognosis

Since LS are only very rarely genitally localized, providing an accurate prognostic forecast for the uterine variants is extremely difficult. It is thus both reasonable and expedient to orient oneself along the prognostic lines adopted for lipogenous STS. The information provided largely applies and refers to intraabdominal and retroperitoneal LS. Unlike for other uterine sarcomas, for uterine LS, prognosis does not appear to be associated with tumor size (49). Overall, it is widely assumed that well-differentiated LS and atypical lipomatous tumors never metastasize, but that they do have a tendency to recur (13). Five year survival is at around 90 % and is exclusively determined by local recurrence, and thus by their complete surgical excision. Up to now, however, this tumor type has not yet been encountered within a uterus.

Prognosis for dedifferentiated LS is clearly worse than for its well-differentiated counterpart. As dedifferentiation increases, so, too, do the recurrence rate and metastatic potential. The rate of local recurrence is at 41 %, while 15–20 % of cases developed metastatic disease (13, 24). Most patients die from expansive, uncontrollable locally recurrent disease before metastatic spread can even occur. The 5-year survival rate is between 30–70 %. The non-lipogenous sarcoma component apparently has no influence on prognosis, regardless of whether it originates from a high-grade or a low-grade sarcoma (30, 39). The risk of metastasis is said to be elevated when a myxofibrosarcomatous component is present.

The prognosis for myxoid round cell tumors can and does vary. It primarily depends on cell density, proliferative activity, and the share of round cells. Thirty-five percent of patients with myxoid round cell LS develop metastases and 31 % die of this tumor. Presence or absence of necroses is associated with significantly different 5-year OS (25 vs. 90 %) (41). In myxoid round cell LS, the degree of round cell differentiation determines whether the tumor is benign or malignant, as the latter is a morphological correlate of dedifferentiation. Five year survival is at around 25 % for almost exclusively round celled tumors, at 90 % for low-grade myxoid tumors, and between 40 and 50 % for mixed myxoid-round cell sarcomas. A further study has likewise revealed that round cell LS have clearly poorer 5- and 10-year DFS compared to their purely myxoid equivalents (51). In principle, metastasis should be expected in any case in which round cells account for 10 % or more of the total tumor volume (3). In one study, 23 % of patients whose tumors contained 0–5 % round cell differentiation developed metastases (41). For tumors with 5–25 % round cell differentiation, the rate of developing metastatic disease was 35 %, while the rate of metastasis was 58 % in patients with tumors with > 25 % round cells (41). This prognostic assessment applies to myxoid round cell LS of all sites (39, 51). Furthermore, patient age (> 45 years) and large tumor size (> 10 cm) are associated with poorer prognosis for patients with myxoid round cell LS (51).

Pleomorphic LS are generally regarded as highly malignant high-grade tumors with a recurrence and metastasization rate of 30 to 50 % and a 5-year OS of 50–65 % (3, 23, 32, 39).

Among patients aged < 22 years, myxoid, well-differentiated, and pleomorphic LS had 5-year OS of 83, 67, and 25 %, respectively. Patients with low-grade myxoid and well-differentiated LS had a median survival of 7.3 years versus only 1.9 years in patients with pleomorphic LS (76).

The metastatic spread of myxoid round cell LS is much more frequently to other soft tissues than to the lungs or the bones.

Positive margins post-surgery are associated with having a dramatically detrimental impact on OS. Disease recurs in 67 % of patients with R1/2 resection margins, compared to 14 % when R0 margins have been achieved. Peripherally located LS statistically had a significantly better prognosis than central (i.e. intraabdominal, retroperitoneal) tumors (76).

As is also the case for other STS, and analogous to uterine LMS, metastasis to the locoregional lymph nodes is rare. The prognostic relevance of LN positivity and the benefits of performing LNE are currently unclear. Nodal status is also not considered in current prognostic nomograms for retroperitoneal LS and STS (4, 12).

Women with dedifferentiated liposarcomas who die predominantly do so as a consequence of expansive recurring disease. Prognosis for myxoid round cell liposarcomas depends on the number of tumor cell necroses and the share of round cell differentiation. Pleomorphic liposarcomas generally have a poorer prognosis. Resection margin status is a decisive prognostic factor in all cases. Locoregional lymph nodes are usually not affected in liposarcoma patients.

2.1.7 Primary surgery

Surgical excision with wide margins is the therapeutic method of choice for all STS, including LS. All uterine LS described in the literature to date were removed via THE. THE can thus be regarded as the optimal surgical method. The adnexa can be left in situ as a matter of principle. Performing a BSO would currently not be justifiable. There is no indication for performing RAH or BSO, unless the structures affected by such surgery are afflicted by the tumor. Analogous to LS located in extragenital sites, performing an LNE is generally not indicated, nor is doing so recommended in any publication pertaining to LS of all sites. Moreover, studies have shown that performing an LNE has no impact on prognosis (29). The current NCCN Guidelines on uterine sarcomas and soft tissue sarcomas do not envisage subjecting LS patients to an LNE.

There is no literature pertaining to uterus-preserving surgery and LS. A conservative approach would most likely be conceivable for well-differentiated LS. Since such tumors do not develop metastatic disease and only recur locally, TE could be a feasible option in cases in which the patient urgently desires to preserve fertility, not least because well-differentiated LS do not recur at all when R0 resection margins are achieved in primary surgery (3). Accounts of uterine well-differentiated LS have, however, yet to be scientifically described in the literature. Excision with wide clear resection margins seems to be the most conceivable option for dedifferentiated LS. The key problems in all cases are that the tumor could potentially be damaged during surgery and that the resection margins are drawn too narrowly. The reason why this risk is so great is because LS have no capsule – instead, the compressed myometrium or the compressed edge of the tumor forms a pseudo-capsule. In the case depicted in Fig. 2.1.3 (A)–(F), the patient underwent a conservative TE with clear margins – there was no recurrence of disease over a four-year follow-up period.

The absence of reliable data pertaining to uterine LS notwithstanding, it can nonetheless be assumed that predominantly round celled LS and pleomorphic LS present the same state of affairs as uterine LMS do in this context – tumor injury, RX or R1/2 resection margins are very likely to have a significant negative impact on prognosis (cf. Vol. 1, Chapter 2). Accordingly, as is the case for LMS, morcellating or clamping the uterus with sharp hooks should be refrained from. Patients who insist on uterus preserving surgery must be unequivocally informed of these circumstances. Generally speaking, performing conservative surgery on patients with adipocytic tumors can be planned rather well. Since conservative LM surgery always requires imaging diagnostics to be performed prior, at the very least sonography (cf. Vol. 1, Chapter 6), uterine LS should in fact only rarely arise as incidental findings during or following organ-sparing operations. Sonographic findings that suggest the presence of a lipogenous tumor can be reliably verified and widely substantiated via subsequent MRT, as can the margins of the tumor in particular (see imaging).

Overall, it would be sensible to base decisions for or against organ-sparing surgery on the sarcomatous component at hand, which is indeed a relevant prognostic factor as has already been stated previously (17). Referring to a diagnostic flowchart can also be helpful in this context (cf. flowchart Vol. 1, Chapter 6).

Patients in whom only an R2 resection could be achieved must at the very least be subjected to reresection. As is also the case for the other types of uterine sarcoma, the THE should be performed once the desire to preserve fertility has ceased to exist.

Total hysterectomy without injuring the uterus is the therapy of choice for uterine liposarcomas. There is no indication for further reaching surgical measures or lymphonodectomy. Uterus-preserving surgery can be considered in extremely rare cases without any damage to the tumor. This would most likely be a conceivable option for dedifferentiated liposarcomas. In this regard, the same criteria apply as for leiomyosarcoma.

2.1.8 Adjuvant and additive radio-, chemo- and hormone therapy

There are no data pertaining to adjuvant RT that refer specifically to uterine LS. A larger study on extrauterine myxoid round cell LS revealed no effect of adjuvant RT on survival. Postoperative RT on patients subjected to R1/2 resections served to significantly reduce the rate of local recurrence albeit with no effects on OS. In contrast, no benefits were observed for R0 resections (51). RT was shown to have had no effect in a further study covering patients aged < 22 with LS at various sites (76). In general, this also applies to other retroperitoneal STS (24). The results from some studies (the samples of which consisted largely of patients with LS) suggest that postoperative RT has a prolonging effect on DFS. Numerous biases, not entirely clear resection margin conditions, and the use of varying surgical methods, however, do not allow any final conclusions to be drawn (65). In two large SEER analyses, independent of resection margin status, no effects of postoperative RT on OS could be measured in retroperitoneal sarcomas the majority of which contained LS (9, 79). The current NCCN Guidelines for uterine sarcomas do not envisage adjuvant RT for cases in which R0 resection margins have been achieved, although it needs to be noted that this recommendation primarily refers to LMS, HG-ESS and UUS (53). The current NCCN recommendations for retroperitoneal and abdominal STS make a very weak 2B recommendation to consider RT in cases of high-grade or extremely large sarcomas, or in cases in which recurrences of tumors with critical boundaries could cause considerable morbidity (54). Regardless of the weakness of this recommendation, the stated factors can barely be said to apply to uterine LS following THE. In brief, there is currently no indication for subjecting patients whose LS have been completely resected via THE to adjuvant RT. In general, adhering to the recommendations, guidelines and approaches described for LMS (cf. Vol. 1, Chapter 2) would be adequate practice.

For R1/2 resected myxoid round cell LS, postoperative RT is said to reduce the rate of local recurrence without having any effects on survival (51). Therefore, the NCCN Guidelines for retroperitoneal and abdominal STS make the (albeit weak) 2B recommendation to take postoperative RT into consideration as a therapeutic option for those extremely rare cases in which tumors have been subjected to uterus-sparing R1 resections. Reresection is recommended for cases in which only R2 resection margins could be achieved in primary surgery (53, 54).

Analogous to retroperitoneal/abdominal STS and STS of the extremities, it is not common practice to apply adjuvant CHT. To date, it has not yet been reliably scientifically proven that undergoing adjuvant CHT has a positive impact on DFS and OS (1, 11, 24). The same applies to cases in which LS of various sites arise in patients under 22 years of age. In fact, one study has revealed that, for the latter group, adjuvant RT and/or CHT was associated with shorter survival, though attention must also be drawn to selection biases that were far from insignificant (76). In a larger retrospective study on extrauterine myxoid round cell LS, adjuvant CHT was found to have no influence on DFS and OS (51). Accordingly, the current NCCN Guidelines for uterine sarcomas and soft tissue sarcomas do not recommend it (54). Well-differentiated LS are deemed non-chemosensitive anyway (54), and dedifferentiated and pleomorphic LS show little to no responsivity to CHT (78). This perspective alone already suffices to exclude the administration of adjuvant therapy to patients with these tumor types.

In general, treating LS with hormones is not established or common in practice.

There is no indication for subjecting uterine liposarcoma patients who have had a hysterectomy leaving R0 resection margins to postoperative radiation therapy. Postoperative radiation therapy can be considered in cases in which conservative surgery has left R1 margins. Doing so has no influence on survival.

It is not established or common in practice to subject uterine liposarcomas to adjuvant chemotherapy or hormone therapy.

2.1.9 Primary radio-, chemo- and hormone therapy, approach in cases of general inoperability

No data are available on this issue for uterine LS specifically. We must thus critically refer to what is known about extrauterine LS in this context. The data that follow therefore primarily refer to LS of extrauterine sites. First and foremost, the data suggest that patients with extrauterine myxoid round cell LS (all sites) whose tumors are inoperable can be subjected to preoperative RT. There are accounts in which such a strategy has successfully effected tumor diameter shrinkage, but also in which disease progressed during therapy (51). For retroperitoneal and intraabdominal sarcomas, the current NCCN Guidelines on soft tissue sarcomas recommend neoadjuvant RT, however only in the form of a weak 2B recommendation (54). Therefore, exceptional cases in which patients are inoperable or where effecting tumor shrinkage is deemed necessary can be referred to primary RT.

Well-differentiated LS are not chemosensitive (54, 70), making them ineligible for primary CHT. Dedifferentiated, myxoid round cell, and pleomorphic LS all exhibit differing degrees of responsivity to doxorubicin and ifosfamide (36, 70). Dedifferentiated and pleomorphic LS have rather poor response rates (78). Particularities are discussed in the subsection on palliative CHT. The current NCCN recommendations on soft tissue sarcomas and on retroperitoneal and abdominal sarcomas lend support to the adequacy of neoadjuvant CHT in the form of a 2A recommendation (54), albeit for all STS and not LS in particular. In one study, subjecting patients with myxoid round cell LS to neoadjuvant therapy with doxorubicin and ifosfamide effected a PR in 41.6 % of cases. Tumors shrank by 26.5 % on average. However, more than two-thirds of patients in the cohort also underwent additional RT. Following surgery, median PFS was 50 mo and the 5-year PFS was 0.68 % (for further information cf. Vol. 1, Chapter 2) (40). An attempt at therapy with doxorubicin and/or ifosfamide with or without additional RT can thus be considered. A further study revealed that subjecting patients with myxoid round cell LS to primary or neoadjuvant CHT yields no recognizable benefits as of yet (51). Doxorubicin was administered in the majority of cases covered.

In another study, 46 % of patients with advanced myxoid round cell LS who underwent neoadjuvant trabectedin therapy showed a PR, including one case in which imaging still revealed a mass but that mass could not be found during surgery (26). These experiences combined with the low rate of side effects occurring make primary or neoadjuvant CHT with trabectedin a highly adequate option. Particularities pertaining to the administration of trabectedin are discussed in the subchapter on palliative therapy. If the good results that can be achieved by subjecting LMS patients to a combination of trabectedin and doxorubicin (63) were equally valid for LS (for details see Vol. 1, Chapter 2), then said regimen would have to be considered the option of choice for neoadjuvant CHT. In Germany and the USA, the use of trabectedin in preoperative settings currently remains “off-label”.

According to a randomized study on STS including LS (33), the efficacy of CHT can be improved by subjecting patients to local hyperthermia. The study compared a relatively toxic neoadjuvant CHT combination regimen of etoposide (125 mg/m^2 d 1 a. d 4), ifosfamide (1,500 mg/m^2 d 1–4), and doxorubicin (50 mg/m^2 d 1) to patients who were administered the same CHT regimen plus local hyperthermia (42 °C at the tumor over 60 minutes) at three week intervals on d 1 and 4 of each CHT cycle. While higher response rates could be achieved using the CHT-hyperthermia combination compared to standalone CHT (28.8 vs. 12.7 %), for both groups the rate was only 37 % for patients in whom R0 resection was subsequently achieved in surgery. After resection of the tumor, all patients underwent up to another 4 cycles of CHT with or without hyperthermia, and roughly 60 % of patients in both groups had additional RT. Overall, the additional application of hyperthermia to retroperitoneal sarcomas had a statistically significant positive impact on median PFS. The greatest benefit was a longer recurrence-free period during the first two years. However, it must also be critically noted that the hyperthermia group underwent considerably more CHT cycles, that nowadays etoposide is hardly ever used for uterine LMS, and that additional regional hyperthermia had no beneficial effects on OS. The working group in question (33) currently only uses doxorubicin plus ifosfamide. In light of the numerous imponderables, administering a combination of CHT plus hyperthermia as a neoadjuvant or primary therapeutic strategy should not yet be regarded as standard practice (for further information cf. Vol. 1, Chapter 2). However, said combination should be considered in individual exceptional cases. There are no indications for neoadjuvant HT in cases of LS.

In absolutely exceptional cases, neoadjuvant radiotherapy or neoadjuvant therapy with doxorubicin can be considered for patients with very large uterine liposarcomas. Trabectedin or trabectedin plus doxorubicin are most likely to yield positive effects. However, trabectedin is currently not yet certified and permitted for use in primary therapeutic settings.

In individual cases, primary or neoadjuvant therapy can involve a combination of hyperthermia plus chemotherapy. There are no indications for neoadjuvant HT.

2.1.10 Aftercare, recurrences, metastases

The aftercare strategy for LS should be clinically guided by symptomatology via gynecological and general examination. Check-ups should be scheduled every 3 months for the first 2 years, every 6 months for the next 3 years, and every 12 months thereafter. It has yet to be proven that undergoing complex and laborious laboratory-chemical, technical and/or imaging examinations like CT, MRI and PET-CT, has positive effects on patients.

This is primarily footed in the fact that, to date, early intervention in cases of metastases and recurrences that are only traceable via imaging diagnostics has yet to be scientifically proven as beneficial for survival. Since patients with solitary isolated metastases in the lung or the liver could possibly benefit from surgery in terms of survival, it could be sensible to perform yearly imaging examinations on these two organs. Accordingly, the current NCCN Guidelines make a category 2A recommendation to perform radiography or CT on the thorax every 6 to 12 months over 5 years, in addition to the clinical follow-up examinations (53). There are, however, currently no valid data of which we are aware that would support of such a course of action. The NCCN Guidelines go on to state that other imaging techniques should only be resorted to in cases in which symptoms give rise to a clinical indication for such practice (53). Atypical lipomatous tumors and well-differentiated LS do not metastasize. Accordingly, pulmonary CT is not indicated in the context of aftercare.

Overall, for the reasons stated above, more intensive diagnostic steps should only be taken when clinical examination and/or symptoms make such measures necessary. When there is the clinical suspicion of recurrence or of metastasis to the pelvis, the abdominal cavity or the abdominal wall, patients must undergo an abdominal CT or an abdominal MRI in order to assess spread and to derive a respective therapeutic strategy. PET-CT is not an adequate means for examining and determining metastatic spread due to the incidence of false-negative results with which said measure is associated (71). No adequate or usable tumor markers have yet been determined that could serve to monitor the course of the disease.

Well-differentiated LS virtually never develop metastases, while recurrences are common. Recurrences can also occur as dedifferentiated LS. Further details are provided in the subsection on prognosis. Brain metastases are extremely rare, regardless of whether patients have undergone prior resection with or without RT/CHT, and are usually only discovered 10 years after primary therapy. They are usually preceded by lung metastases (74), and are so rare that there is no justifiable need to purposefully look for them. Brain metastases apparently most commonly occur in patients with pleomorphic LS, and are least commonly found in cases of myxoid LS.

Symptom-guided clinical aftercare is recommended. Check-ups should be scheduled for every 3 months in the first 2 years, every 6 months the following 3 years, and every 12 months thereafter. Performing complex and laborious laboratory-chemical and imaging examinations has not been to proven to be associated with benefits for survival. Semiannual to annual follow-up imaging examinations of the lung could be beneficial, except in cases of well-differentiated liposarcoma, if any metastases uncovered by doing so will also be removed.

The most fundamental problem with liposarcomas is the frequency with which they locally recur. For predominantly round celled and pleomorphic liposarcomas in particular, distant metastases should also be reckoned with.

2.1.11 Surgical management of and postoperative additive therapy for recurrences and metastatic disease

Well-differentiated LS show virtually no response to CHT, and dedifferentiated and pleomorphic LS respond only poorly (78). This in itself already suffices to underline that resection is the method of choice for dealing with recurrences and metastases (78). As there are essentially no data specific to uterine LS in terms of their surgical management, one must resort to the data and procedures pertaining to retroperitoneal and intraabdominal LS or other STS. Overall, subjecting LS patients to therapeutic treatment for recurrences and metastases yields more positive results than for LMS patients, also in terms of OS (29). The resectability of recurrences and metastases is regarded as an important prognostic factor. Resected retroperitoneal and intraabdominal sarcomas, including LS, have a median OS of 60 mo versus 20 mo among non-resected tumors. Fifty-five percent of recurrences are still resectable. Diffuse intraperitoneal sarcomatosis or intensive vascular involvement are the most common causes for a lack of resectability. Tumor grade, multifocality, and tumor growth rate are important post-resection prognostic factors (29). Extensive tumor spread within the abdomen is the most common tumor-related cause of death in LS patients (and the only one for well-differentiated LS patients), rather than distant metastatic disease. Resecting repeat recurrences is particularly adequate in cases in which the first recurrences could be completely removed (29). For patients who have undergone primary resection of local recurrence, disease specific OS is 100 mo for patients with tumor growth rates < 1.0 cm/mo, compared to only 21 mo for patients with growth rates equal to or greater than 1 cm/mo (1 cm/mo rule) (62).

There are no data pertaining to the question of when is the most adequate point in time to actually perform surgery on recurrent tumors. Resection is deemed indicated when symptoms are present and/or continued tumor growth poses a threat to tumor resectability. For cases to which this does not apply, adopting an observant, patient approach is regarded as the most adequate approach. This also applies in cases of repeat recurrence (29). Symptomatic tumors that cannot be completely resected due to the anatomical circumstances at hand can also be subjected to palliative cytoreductive methods. Doing so has been shown to improve median OS to 9 mo versus 3 mo for cases subjected only to biopsy (46). When the growth rate is equal to or above 1 cm/mo, performing renewed surgery on local recurrences no longer has an influence on OS. Such cases are deemed inadequate for renewed cytoreduction and should be referred to systemic therapy (29, 62). Therapeutic interventions for symptomatic treatment, e.g. in order to alleviate intestinal/bowel obstructions or hemorrhaging, are exceptions of this rule if the symptoms cannot be treated via other means. Growth rates of < 1 cm/mo serve as an indication for immediate surgery if strong symptoms persist or critical organs are at risk. In all other scenarios, and especially in cases of well-differentiated LS, a more reserved, observant approach that includes imaging-based monitoring/check-ups can be adopted (62).

In brief, the following approach is recommended for treating local recurrences in cases in which there is no CT-based evidence of distant metastases (29): asymptomatic recurrent tumors that are unresectable according to the results from imaging diagnostics can be either observed or subjected to systemic CHT. Where patients are symptomatic, they should be administered CHT and/or referred to targeted RT (unifocal masses). Should patients present with acute symptoms, they can undergo cytoreductive surgery without the aim of or need for achieving complete resection, i.e. it is not necessary to know with certainty prior to surgery that R0 resection margins will be achieved in such cases. Asymptomatic masses that appear to be resectable according to the results from imaging diagnostics can be either resected or subjected to observation. Observation is most likely to be indicated in cases in which prior PFI has been short, multiple resections have been performed/when recurrence is multifocal, and when there is no risk that the tumor will become unresectable in the near future. Symptomatic resectable tumors, in contrast, should always be resected. Systemic therapy can be considered when previous PFI has been short, the tumor could lose resectability in the near future, the tumor is classified as highly malignant (high-grade), or if there have already been multiple resections or recurrence is multifocal.

No particular or special approaches to aftercare and follow-up of R0 resections have yet been established. Applying targeted palliative RT to the region in which residual tumor remains could be considered. Reliable data to this end are, however, not available.

Resection, if need be multiple resections, is the therapeutic method of choice for treating recurrences and metastases. Resection is indicated when patients are symptomatic and/or future resectability is jeopardized by increased and continued tumor growth. In all other cases, adopting an observant, more reserved stance is regarded as being adequate practice. Palliative cytoreductive surgery can be considered in acutely threatening cases. Repeat resections are no longer indicated when the growth rate exceeds 1 cm/month. For R0 resections no particular or special aftercare strategies have yet been established in practice. For R1/2 resections, targeted postoperative RT can be considered.

2.1.12 Palliative radio-, chemo- and hormone therapy, therapy with small molecules, supportive therapy

Valid data are not known to exist according to which undergoing RT can be beneficial.

Currently there are no prospective studies on the efficacy of subjecting patient with uterine LS to palliative CHT using conventional substances. The data presented below, therefore, primarily refer to retroperitoneal and intraperitoneal LS or STS of all sites.

Well-differentiated LS are not chemosensitive (54, 70), so that such cases are only exceptionally eligible for palliative CHT. For dedifferentiated and myxoid round cell LS, anthracyclines (doxorubicin, liposomal doxorubicin) appear to be the most effective agents. Notwithstanding, a study covering well-differentiated and dedifferentiated LS measured a rather disappointing RR of 12 %, 3-month and 6-month PFI of 59 % and 44 %, respectively, and median PFI and OS of 4.6 and 15.2 mo, respectively (CBR 45 %). Combining doxorubicin with another agent (usually ifosfamide) yielded the best results (34). However, the higher RR had no impact on PFI and OS. It is possible that the results were negatively influenced by the fact that chemoresistant well-differentiated LS were also included. A further study has revealed an RR of 37 % and a median OS of 14 mo among patients with pleomorphic LS who were administered doxorubicin or doxorubicin plus ifosfamide. Interestingly, further remission could be achieved in all patients in whom disease had progressed while on the first-line anthracycline-containing regimens by subsequently treating them with a gemcitabine-docetaxel combination (35).

On the basis of the data at hand, patients with mild symptoms and in whom recurrences and/or metastases are not located critically should first undergo mono-CHT, most likely using doxorubicin.

Strong symptoms and/or critically located recurrences/metastases serve as an indication for combination therapy. However, in doing so, the higher levels of toxicity must be borne in mind, not least because opting for combination therapy has no beneficial effects on either PFI or OS.

According to one study, despite the fact that well-differentiated LS of all sites are usually chemoresistant, effects could still be achieved by administering high-dose CHT using ifosfamide (14 g/m^2 continuous over 14 days i.v.) – a CBR of 60 % with a median PFI of 7 months (68).

Currently, administering trabectedin yields the best results. In contrast to conventional chemotherapeutic agents, this substance has been examined and investigated in several extensive, well-designed studies. The promising results for myxoid round cell LS are likely a consequence of the trabectedin interacting with the FUS-CHOP and FUS-DDIT3 fusion genes or their oncoproteins (14, 21, 26). Neoadjuvant administration of trabectedin to patients with myxoid round cell LS effected a CR in 13 % of cases and an RR of 24 %. The other tumors exhibited SD, while no cases of PD were observed during the administration of trabectedin (26). FUS-CHOP translocations were verified in all tumors prior to therapy. In cases in which CR was achieved, the translocation was no longer traceable in the surgical specimens. A further study on a sample of previously CHT-treated advanced STS, including 476 LS without more detailed classification, revealed a CBR of 54 % (1 % CR, 6 % PR, 47 % SD) with a median OS of 16.2 mo. Overall, the results were better for LS than for all other STS (66). In another STS study, within a sample of 27 advanced or metastasized myxoid round cell LS, 15 % showed PR and 52 % of cases exhibited SD. Median PFI was 19 mo and median OS was 18.3 mo, with a 2-year OS of 41 % (45). Furthermore, among 32 advanced and metastasized CHT-treated myxoid round cell LS, an RR of 50 % (including 2 CR) and a CBR of 90 % could be achieved, along with a PFI of 17 months. Three-month and 6-month PFI were 96 % and 90 %, respectively. Effects could still be achieved by re-administering trabectedin to patients who had aborted initial treatment and whose disease had subsequently progressed. The surgical specimens obtained in cases that have been subjected to trabectedin therapy exhibit an increase in mature lipoblasts. Remissions show up as a loss of density in CT or as enhancement decreases in T1WC (28). It is possible that the excellent results associated with administering a combination of trabectedin plus doxorubicin to LMS patients (63) could also apply to LS. More detail is provided to this end in the chapter on LMS (cf. Vol. 1, Chapter 2).

A randomized trial evaluated first-line trabectedin therapy versus doxorubicin-based CHT (doxorubicin monotherapy and doxorubicin plus ifosfamide) in patients with non-resectable/metastatic translocation-related sarcomas, including myxoid round cell LS (6). While the trabectedin group had a superior PFS to the doxorubicin group (16.1 mo vs. 8.8 mo), the difference was not statistically significant. The respective CBR of 82.4 % and 86.4 % were virtually identical. However, in the doxorubicin group, more patients had to stop treatment because they had reached the maximum cumulative dose or because LVEF was abnormally low. In contrast, the more promising side effect profile of trabectedin allowed the patients in the trabectedin group to continue their treatment for longer. Consequently, it could almost have been suspected from the onset that trabectedin would achieve a superior OS.

There are no indications for palliative HT in cases of LS.

Some data do suggest that eribulin mesylate (1–4 mg/m^2 i.v. d 1 & 8, q 3 weeks) is effective for treating LS. One phase II trial largely covering dedifferentiated, myxoid and pleomorphic LS revealed a 3-mo-PFI of 46.9 % (69).

In cases of advanced disease or diffuse metastasis in patients whose overall condition is poor, providing best supportive therapy and care could be an adequate option (34, 53, 54).

Subjecting liposarcoma patients to palliative radiotherapy is not established or routine practice. Well-differentiated liposarcomas do not respond to chemotherapy. For all other types of liposarcoma, doxorubicin is among the most effective agents. While combining doxorubicin with ifosfamide does improve remission rates, said combination is also considerably more toxic and does not serve to prolong the progression free interval. The best results can currently be achieved using trabectedin, either as a monotherapy or in combination with doxorubicin.

2.2 Extrauterine liposarcomas

2.2.1 Liposarcoma of the vulva and the vagina

General, pathogenesis, pathologico-anatomical features

Of the few cases in which LS arise in extrauterine sites of the female genital tract, the vast majority occur in the vulva. The vagina is only rarely primarily affected. Vulvar sarcomas account for 1.2 % of malignant vulvar tumors, and only 11 % of all vulvar sarcomas are LS (37). Vulvar LS do not constitute an independent genital tumor type and must be categorized as superficial STS of the trunk, while vaginal LS belong to the retroperitoneal STS. Current WHO Classification lists vulvar LS under soft tissue sarcomas as "other sarcoma (liposarcoma)", and makes no mention of vaginal LS at all (58).

The mean age of women with vulvar LS is 52 years (56). When occurring in the vulva, well-differentiated LS are termed "atypical lipomatous tumors". The vulva in fact serves as an exception of sorts, since most well-differentiated LS occur in the deep soft tissue. Myxoid round cell LS and pleomorphic LS seem to arise even more rarely in the vulva than they already do in the uterus. Fewer than 1 % of all dedifferentiated LS are subcutaneous (81). One quarter of pleomorphic LS develop in the skin or the subcutis (32). Patients are aged between 5 and 39 years (22). Therefore, in principle, the vulva can also be affected by this tumor type (37).

Little is known in terms of etiology and pathogenesis. Nowadays, there is consensus that LS do not develop from lipomas via malignant transformation (25). LS of the vagina are extremely rare. A lipoleiomyosarcoma in the vicinity of the vaginal wall has recently been described in the literature (7).

Staging occurs in accordance with the rules for STS (cf. Vol. 1, Chapter 2).

> Adipocytic tumors as STS of the trunk also occur in the vulva on rare occasions. Well-differentiated LS are referred to as atypical lipomatous tumors when they arise at this site. Dedifferentiated, myxoid round cell and pleomorphic liposarcomas have also been encountered.
>
> Staging for both vulvar and vaginal LS is in accordance with that for soft tissue sarcomas. Tumors arising in the vagina must be categorized as retroperitoneal liposarcomas.

The vulvar tumors are usually well delineated macroscopically and are normally >3 cm. They can be situated either only in the dermis, in both the dermis and the subcutis, or only in the subcutis (22). Cutaneous and subcutaneous pleomorphic LS reach sizes between 0.8 and 15 cm (34).

The microscopic appearance of atypical lipomatous tumors is characterized by adipocytes of various sizes with adipocytic nuclear atypia as well as by the presence of lipoblasts (56). Histological data pertaining to dedifferentiated, myxoid round cell, and pleomorphic LS are described at length under "uterine LS" above. All subcutaneous pleomorphic LS contain pleomorphic lipoblasts, but can also exhibit primarily pleomorphic spindle cell and epithelioid growth patterns. Intracutaneous pleomorphic LS are almost always well and clearly delineated/circumscribed, while subcutaneous tumors usually have infiltrative margins. Necroses occasionally occur, and the MI can range between 1–48 M/10 HPF with a mean MI of 5 (23).

> Adipocytic tumors of the vulva usually appear to have well delimited margins and have a soft consistency. They can grow to a considerable size. Histologically, they do not differ from uterine and retroperitoneal liposarcomas.

Clinical presentation, diagnostics, imaging, differential diagnostics

Clinically, the tumors usually appear to be relatively soft and are well delineated. They are usually mistaken for benign vulvar lesions or Bartholin's cysts. Due to the given risk that subcutaneous vulvar tumors could also be malignant or semi-malignant mesenchymal neoplasms, any tumor should be excised leaving macroscopically clear/free margins, not least for diagnostic purposes. Every tumor that is found in the vulva should at the very least be subjected to sonography so as to reduce the risk of misdiagnoses that can be fatal when they result in inadequate surgery being performed.

Common lipoma has to be taken into consideration as a possible DD for atypical lipomatous tumors, i.e. that a lipoma could be mistaken for an atypical lipomatous tumor. However, it appears to occur more frequently in practice that atypical lipomatous tumors are mistaken for lipomas (24). The reason why this occurs is that, in order for an atypical lipomatous tumor to be diagnosed as such, the presence of adipocytes of varying sizes, of lipoblasts, and of fibrous septa (that in turn also contain cells with atypical nuclei) must be verified. Since these characteristics often only occur focally, they can be easily and quickly missed. Verifying MDM2 amplification using FISH can be helpful. The presence of lipoblasts also allows a clear differentiation from angiomyofibroblastoma (57). Myxoid LS in the vulva can histologically bear resemblance to myxoid dermatofibrosarcoma protuberans. Angiomyxoma, myxoid chondrosarcoma, and myxoid malignant fibrous histiocytoma are further differential diagnostic considerations (24). Overall, DD for vulvar LS essentially mirrors DD for vulvar LMS and can be read up on there in more detail. So-called lipoblastoma have been observed in the inguinal region during childhood. They are also referred to as fetal/embryonal lipoblastoma. They consist of hypocellular lobules of adipocytes in various stages of differentiation. The lobules are separated by fibrous septa that may be cellular. Affected children are usually younger than 3 years, recurrences are known to have occurred (48).

The imaging characteristics of vaginal and vulvar LS do not differ significantly from those of uterine/retroperitoneal LS. In terms of differential diagnosis, lipogenic tumors can be easily discerned from non-lipogenic tumor types via imaging diagnostic procedures. However, securely and accurately differentiating lipoma from atypical lipomatous tumors is not possible, especially when sited in the area of the vulva (59). Vulvar and vaginal tumors should always be subjected to sonography. Hyperechoicity is strongly suggestive of an adipocytic tumor and should be further clarified via MRI. However, just because a tumor is hypoechoic need not automatically exclude LS as a possibility (80). The CT and MRI characteristics of vulvar and vaginal LS are essentially congruent with those of their uterine/retroperitoneal counterparts. Preoperative MRI or CT are generally indicated as means for establishing potential resection margins (54).

Vulvar LS are often mistaken for Bartholin's cysts. The tumor is usually solid and soft. Bartholin's cysts can usually be excluded from consideration via anamnesis, clinical examination, and sonography. Once a Bartholin's cyst has been ruled out, as a matter of principle vulvar tumors should be fully excised with a wide disease-free margin. Leiomyosarcoma and other soft tissue sarcomas are the most important differential diagnoses.

The imaging characteristics of vulvar and vaginal adipocytic tumors do not differ from those of their uterine counterparts. Imaging procedures are indicated for extrauterine lipogenic tumors as means for determining where the resection margins should be.

Course, prognosis, operative, systemic and radiogenic therapy

Analogous to their counterparts at other sites, vulvar and vaginal atypical lipomatous tumors only develop locoregional recurrences – distant metastasis practically never arises. When metastatic disease does occur, it is rather likely that a dedifferentiation has been overlooked. Recurrences of completely excised atypical lipomatous tumors have not been reported. However, the number of known cases in which such tumors have been fully resected is very small. Superficial pleomorphic LS have a better prognosis than such located at other sites. Distant metastasis is not known to occur. The median DFS is 26 mo (22). One can thus assume that all subtypes of vulvar LS have a superior prognosis compared to retroperitoneal LS. Patient age and tumor size are further prognostic factors. For patients with lipogenic tumors, a prognostic forecast can be made by using a nomogram (4, 12).

The prognosis for all vulvar adipocytic tumors appears to be more promising than that associated with their retroperitoneal counterparts. No cases of distant metastasis have yet been described in the literature.

As for all STS of the trunk, the primary therapeutic option for vulvar LS is extirpation with clear/free resection margins, i.e. excision well outside/beyond the so-called pseudo-capsule (27). For vaginal LS, achieving this aim may well require the partial resection of neighboring organs or an anterior and/or posterior exenteration (7). The pseudo-capsule consists of compressed tumor and neighboring tissue, and thus always contains tumorous microsatellites. Accordingly, cutting or damaging the "capsule" or drawing the resection margins to close to the capsule are associated with an increased rate of local recurrence (27). Resection margin positivity is generally associated with shorter DFS and OS (60). For atypical lipomatous tumors/well-differentiated LS, the resection margins can be defined a little more tightly/held narrower if the tumor borders vital or critical structures (e.g. rectum and/or bladder) (54). There is currently no indication for performing an LNE, as is already the case for uterine, retroperitoneal, and abdominal LS. There are no data that suggest that doing so would potentially offer any benefits. Likewise, there have to date been no studies on the effects of adjuvant CHT or postoperative RT on R0 resected dedifferentiated, myxoid round cell, or pleomorphic LS. Postoperative RT is deemed a sensible option in cases in which tumor residuals remain following resection (38). Such course of action is apparently associated with a longer DFS (8). Postoperative RT has no effect in cases of R0 resected atypical lipomatous tumors (8).

According to the current NCCN Guidelines for soft tissue sarcomas, whether or not postoperative RT should be applied depends on grading, tumor size, margin status, and location (superficial vs. deep) (see also staging of STS in the chapter on LMS, Vol. 1, Chapter 2) (54). Low-grade vulvar tumors (tumors of the trunk) (G1/2 $<$ and $>$ 5 cm) that have been resected with final margins of $>$ 1.0 cm and in which the (pelvic) fascial plane has remained intact need not be referred to postoperative RT. Except for atypical lipomatous tumors, reresection is required if the tumor reaches right up to the cut margin of the surgical specimen or if the fascial plane is not intact (waiving reresection is possible for 1a tumors). The guidelines strongly recommend (category 1) considering RT for patients whose tumors have infiltrated or breached the fascial plane (stage 1b/2b) (54). For high-grade tumors (G3), further therapeutic intervention can only be abstained from when they are small, superficial, in stage 1a, and have been resected with wide clear resection margins. However, the NCCN Guidelines are unspecific in terms of which size thresholds this recommendation exactly applies to. The NCCN Guidelines make the category 1 recommendation that patients with all other types of high-grade tumors should undergo postoperative RT. In principle, the same rules apply as have been stated for LMS (cf. Vol. 1, Chapter 2) and ANS (cf. Chapter 1).

Where LS are very large and in immediate proximity to critical structures, neoadjuvant RT can be performed as a means for achieving better conditions and circumstances for surgery. According to one study on myxoid round cell LS (which also included tumors of the posterior and the groin), administering neoadjuvant RT served to effect a significant reduction in tumor diameter by 59 % (64). Referring patients to neoadjuvant RT or neoadjuvant RT-CHT is also supported by the current NCCN recommendations (54).

For vaginal LS, reference can be made to the recommendations pertaining to retroperitoneal STS. The respective approach and strategy to be adhered to is elaborated in detail in the subchapters on vaginal ANS (cf. Chapter 1 and Vol. 1, Chapter 2).

Referring patients whose vulvar and vaginal LS have been subjected to surgery to adjuvant CHT or RT-CHT is only given a weak 2B recommendation. In fact, the benefits of doing so have yet to be substantiated in scientific trials and studies. For more details, please refer to the respective sections on LMS of the vagina and the vulva (Vol. 1, Chapter 2).

Aftercare, recurrences, metastases and their treatment

Aftercare and follow-up are identical to what is recommended for uterine LS further above. Regarding the therapeutic approach to be adopted in case of recurrence and/or metastasis, performing a metastasectomy is regarded as the method of choice. It has yet to be proven that further measures offer any benefits when R0 resection margins have been achieved; accordingly, further measures are not routinely recommended (54). The further course of action has been described in detail in the chapter on uterine adipocytic tumors.

Recurrences of atypical lipomatous tumors should be subjected to surgery as often as is necessary until clear, i.e. R0 resection margins have been achieved. Patients can subsequently expect to remain tumor-free for several years (56). No reliable data suggest that undergoing RT following the resection of recurrences would be beneficial. Retrospective data suggest that postoperative RT might be beneficial following resection of atypical lipomatous tumors (38). Very large lesions can be subjected to radiation so as to effect tumor shrinkage. There is currently no indication for subjecting patients whose recurrences have been resected to postoperative CHT.

Tumor extirpation with wide/clear resection margins is the therapeutic method of choice for all vulvar and vaginal adipocytic tumors. Cases of unclear margins should be subject to reresection or to postoperative radiation therapy. Superficial low-grade tumors with clear (i.e. R0) resection margins do not require postoperative irradiation. Liposarcomas that have breached the fascia and/or that are classified as high-grade tumors should be subjected to postoperative radiation therapy. For vaginal liposarcomas, the same course of action applies as does for vaginal leiomyosarcomas. No further adjuvant therapeutic measures have been proven to be effective. Larger tumors can be subjected to neoadjuvant radiation therapy or radio-chemotherapy as means for improving operability/resectability. For recurrences and metastasis, resection is the therapeutic option of choice. The particularities pertaining to palliative therapy for vulvar and vaginal liposarcomas do not deviate from those pertaining to liposarcomas of other sites.

2.2.2 Peritoneal liposarcoma

LS occasionally also occur in the abdominal cavity. When they do, they are usually well-differentiated LS (Fig. 2.2.1) and can grow to a considerable size.

Dedifferentiation occurs only exceptionally (52). The histological and imaging-related characteristics have already been described comprehensively in the context of uterine LS. Clinical appearance, sonographic findings, and DD most closely resemble those of retroperitoneal LS.

Retroperitoneal LS are in the surgeons' ballpark. Definite R0 resection is the therapeutic method of choice. Particularities pertaining to recurrence can be read up on in the respective section on uterine LS.

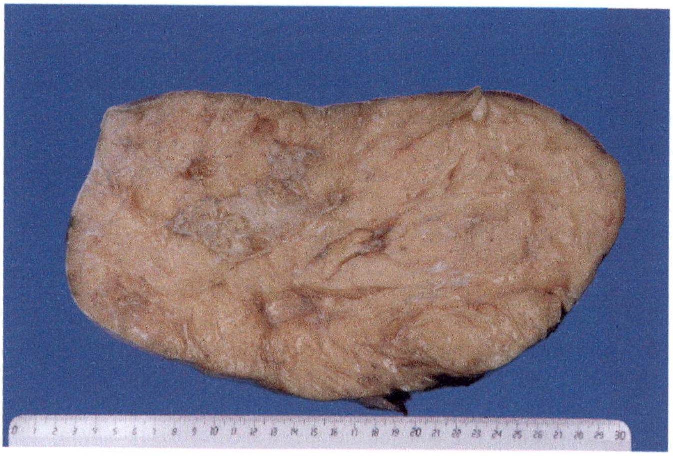

Fig. 2.2.1: Well-differentiated liposarcoma originating in the mesentery.

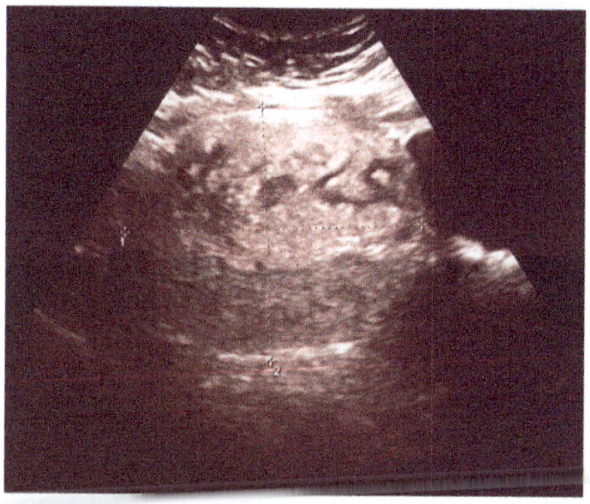

Fig. 2.2.2: Sonographic image of mesenteric lipoma with regressive alterations, the hypoechoic spaces within the hyperechoic tumor most likely correspond to histologically verified necroses.

References

(1) Al-Zaid T, Somaiah N, Lazar AJ. Targeted therapies for sarcomas: new roles for the pathologist. Histopathology 2014; 64: 119–133

(2) Amann G. Weichteiltumoren aus pathologischer Sicht – allgemein. In: Breitenseher M, Dominkus M, Amann G (eds). Bildgebende Diagnostik und Therapie der Weichteiltumoren mit pathologischer Klassifikation, Nuklearmedizin, interventioneller Therapie. Georg Thieme: Stuttgart New York, 2008, pp. 17–29

(3) Aman G. Weichteiltumoren aus pathologischer Sicht – Systematik nach WHO-Klassifikation 2002. In: Breitenseher M, Dominkus M, Amann G. (Hrsg.): Bildgebende Diagnostik und Therapie der Weichteiltumoren mit pathologischer Klassifikation, Nuklearmedizin, interventioneller Therapie. Georg Thieme: Stuttgart New York, 2008, pp. 30–71

(4) Ardoino I, Miceli R, Berselli M, Mariani L, Biganzoli E, Fiore M, Collini P, Stacchiotti S, Casali PG, Gronchi A. Histology-specific nomogram for primary retroperitoneal soft tissue sarcoma. Cancer 2010; 116: 2429–2436

(5) Beger C, Sclgelberger G. In: Schlag p, Hartmann JT, Budach V. Weichgewebetumoren. In: Schlag P, Hartmann JT, Budach V. Weichgewebetumoren. Springer: Berlin Heidelberg, 2011, pp. 37–42
(6) Blay JY, Leahy MG, Nguyen BB, Patel SR, Hohenberger P, Santoro A, Staddon AP, Penel N, Piperno-Neumann S, Hendifar A, Lardelli P, Nieto A, Alfaro V, Chawla SP. Randomised phase III trial of trabectedin versus doxorubicin-based chemotherapy as first-line therapy in translocation-related sarcomas. Eur J Cancer 2014; 50: 1137–1147
(7) Byrd L, Sikand K, Slade R. Lipoleiomyosarcoma of the vagina. J Obstet Gynaecol 2007; 27: 334–335
(8) Cassier PA, Kantor G, Bonvalot S, Lavergne E, Stoeckle E, Le Pechoux C, Meeus P, Sunyach MP, Vaz G, Coindre JM, Linassier C, Labib A, Delcambre C, Bay JO, Leyvraz S, Duberge T, Lagrange JL, Duret A, Blay JY. Adjuvant radiotherapy for extremity and trunk wall atypical lipomatous tumor/well-differentiated LPS (ALT/WD-LPS): A French Sarcoma Group (GSF-GETO) study. Ann Oncol 2014; 25: 1854–1860
(9) Choi AH, Barnholtz-Sloan JS, Kim JA. Effect of radiation therapy on survival in surgically resected retroperitoneal sarcoma: A propensity score-adjusted SEER analysis. Ann Oncol 2012; 23: 2449–2457
(10) Chu CY, Tang YK, Chan TS, Wan YH, Fung KH. Diagnostic challenge of lipomatous uterine tumors in three patients. World J Radiol 2012; 4: 58–62
(11) Cormier JN, Huang X, Xing Y, Thall PF, Wang X, Benjamin RS, Pollock RE, Antonescu CR, Maki RG, Brennan MF, Pisters PW. Cohort analysis of patients with localized, high-risk, extremity soft tissue sarcoma treated at two cancer centers: Chemotherapy-associated outcomes. J Clin Oncol 2004; 22: 4567–4574
(12) Dalal KM, Kattan MW, Antonescu CR, Brennan MF, Singer S. Subtype specific prognostic nomogram for patients with primary liposarcoma of the retroperitoneum, extremity, or trunk. Ann Surg 2006; 244: 381–391
(13) Dei Tos AP. Liposarcomas: diagnostic pitfalls and new insights. Histopathology 2014; 64: 38–52
(14) D'lncalci M, Galmarini CM. A review of trabectedin (ET-743): An unique mechanism of action. Mo l Cancer Ther 2010; 9: 2157–2163
(15) Dixit D, Akin O. Etraperitonela sarcoma. In: Hricak H, Akin O, Sala E, Ascher SM, Levine D, Reinhold C. Diagnostic Imaging Gynecology. 1st edn. AMIRSYS 2007; 1/32–1/35
(16) Fadare O. Heterologous and rare homologous sarcomas of the uterine corpus: A clinicopathologic review. Adv Anat Pathol 2011; 18: 60–74
(17) Fadare O, Khabele D. Pleomorphic liposarcoma of the uterine corpus with focal smooth muscle differentiation. Int J Gynecol Pathol 2011; 30: 282–287
(18) Fletcher CDM, Rydholm A, Singer S, Sunderam M, Coindre JM. Soft tissue tumours: epidemiology, clinical features, histopathological typing and grading. In: Fletcher CDM, Unni K, Mertens F (eds). World Health Organization Classification of Tumours of Soft Tissue and Bone. Lyon: IARC Press: 2002, pp. 12–18
(19) Fletcher CD. The evolving classification of soft tissue tumours – an update based on the new 2013 WHO classification. Histopathology 2014; 64: 2–11
(20) Folpe AL, Weiss SW. Lipoleiomyosarcoma (well-differentiated liposarcoma with leiomyosarcomatous differentiation): A clinicopathologic study of nine cases including one with dedifferentiation. Am J Surg Pathol 2002; 26: 742–749
(21) Forni C, Minuzzo M, Virdis E, Tamborini E, Simone M, Tavecchio M, Erba E, Grosso F, Gronchi A, Aman P, Casali P, D'Incalci M, Pilotti S, Mantovani R. Trabectedin (ET-743) promotes differentiation in myxoid liposarcoma tumors. Mol Cancer Ther 2009; 8: 449–457

(22) Gardner JM, Dandekar M, Thomas D, Goldblum JR, Weiss SW, Billings SD, Lucas DR, McHugh JB, Patel RM. Cutaneous and subcutaneous pleomorphic liposarcoma: A clinicopathologic study of 29 cases with evaluation of MDM2 gene amplification in 26. Am J Surg Pathol 2012; 36: 1047–1051

(23) Gebhard S, Coindre JM, Michels JJ, Terrier P, Bertrand G, Trassard M, Taylor S, Château MC, Marquès B, Picot V, Guillou L. Pleomorphic liposarcoma: clinicopathologic, immunohistochemical, and follow-up analysis of 63 cases: A study from the French Federation of Cancer Centers Sarcoma Group. Am J Surg Pathol 2002; 26: 601–616

(24) Gholami S, Jacobs CD, Kapp DS, Parast LM, Norton JA. The value of surgery for retroperitoneal sarcoma. Sarcoma 2009; 2009:605840. DOI: 10.1155/2009/605840

(25) Goldblum JR, Folpe Al, Weiss SW. Liposarcoma. In: Enzinger and Weiss's Soft Tissue Tumors. 6th edn., Mosby Elsevier Internet Ausg. 2014; Pos. 17520–18448

(26) Gronchi A, Bui BN, Bonvalot S, Pilotti S, Ferrari S, Hohenberger P, Hohl RJ, Demetri GD, Le Cesne A, Lardelli P, Pérez I, Nieto A, Tercero JC, Alfaro V, Tamborini E, Blay JY. Phase II clinical trial of neoadjuvant trabectedin in patients with advanced localized myxoid liposarcoma. Ann Oncol 2012; 23: 771–776

(27) Gronchi A, Colombo C, Raut CP. Surgical management of localized soft tissue tumors. Cancer 2014 DOI: 10.1002/cncr.28715

(28) Grosso F, Sanfilippo R, Virdis E, Piovesan C, Collini P, Dileo P, Morosi C, Tercero JC, Jimeno J, D'Incalci M, Gronchi A, Pilotti S, Casali PG. Trabectedin in myxoid liposarcomas (MLS): A long-term analysis of a single-institution series. Ann Oncol 2009; 20: 1439–1444

(29) Gyorki DE, Brennan MF. Management of recurrent retroperitoneal sarcoma. J Surg Oncol 2014; 109: 53–59

(30) Henricks WH, Chu YC, Goldblum JR, Weiss SW. Dedifferentiated liposarcoma: A clinicopathological analysis of 155 cases with a proposal for an expanded definition of dedifferentiation. Am J Surg Pathol 1997; 21: 271–281

(31) Hong R, Lim SC, Jung H. A myxoid liposarcoma arising in a leiomyoma of the uterus: A case report. Arch Gynecol Obstet 2008; 277: 445–448

(32) Hornick JL, Bosenberg MW, Mentzel T, McMenamin ME, Oliveira AM, Fletcher CD. Pleomorphic liposarcoma: clinicopathologic analysis of 57 cases. Am J Surg Pathol 2004; 28: 1257–1267

(33) Issels RD, Lindner LH, Verweij J, Wust P, Reichardt P, Schem BC, Abdel-Rahman S, Daugaard S, Salat C, Wendtner CM, Vujaskovic Z, Wessalowski R, Jauch KW, Dürr HR, Ploner F, Baur-Melnyk A, Mansmann U, Hiddemann W, Blay JY, Hohenberger P. Neo-adjuvant chemotherapy alone or with regional hyperthermia for localised high-risk soft-tissue sarcoma: A randomised phase 3 multicentre study. Lancet Oncol 2010; 11: 561–570

(34) Italiano A, Toulmonde M, Cioffi A, Penel N, Isambert N, Bompas E, Duffaud F, Patrikidou A, Lortal B, Le Cesne A, Blay JY, Maki RG, Schwartz GK, Antonescu CR, Singer S, Coindre JM, Bui B. Advanced well-differentiated/dedifferentiated liposarcomas: role of chemotherapy and survival. Ann Oncol 2012; 23: 1601–1607

(35) Italiano A, Garbay D, Cioffi A, Maki RG, Bui B. Advanced pleomorphic liposarcomas: Clinical outcome and impact of chemotherapy. Ann Oncol 2012; 23: 2205–2206

(36) Jones RL, Fisher C, Al-Muderis O, Judson IR. Differential sensitivity of liposarcoma subtypes to chemotherapy. Eur J Cancer 2005; 41: 2853–2860

(37) Jones ISC, Crandou A, Sandav K. Vulvar sarcomas: A 25 plus-year experience from Queensland. Open Journal of Obstetrics and Gynecology 2013; 3: 37–40

(38) Kang J, Botros M, Goldberg S, Giraud C, Nielsen GP, Chen YL, Raskin K, Schwab J, Yoon SS, Hornicek FJ, Delaney TF. The use of radiation therapy in the management of selected patients with atypical lipomas. Sarcoma 2013; 2013: 485483 DOI: 10.1155/2013/485483

(39) Katenkamp D, Katenkamp K. Pathologie maligner Weichgewebetumoren. In: Schlag P, Hartmann JT, Budach V. Weichgewebetumoren. Springer: Berlin Heidelberg, 2011, pp. 7–22
(40) Katz DP, Boonsirikamchai RS, Benjamin S, Patel JA, Ludwig JC, Trent L, Xiao V, Ravi H, Choi D, Araujo M. Efficacy of neoadjuvant doxorubicin and ifosfamide (AI) in myxoid/round cell liposarcoma (MRCL): The M. D. Anderson Cancer Center experience (MDACC). J Clin Oncol 2010; 28: Suppl Abstr. 10080
(41) Kilpatrick SE, Doyon J, Choong PF, Sim FH, Nascimento AG. The clinicopathologic spectrum of myxoid and round cell liposarcoma. A study of 95 cases. Cancer 1996; 77: 1450–1458
(42) Köhler G, Belau, A, Dennis K, Evert K, Evert M, Hesse J, Hegenscheid K, Köller M, Krichbaum J, Kühnast M, Lehnhoff H, Lehr A, Linke L, Marcinek A, Müller S, Riechmann C, Schalitz S, Simon J, Spring P, Schädler, J, Ständer C, Trojnarska D, Wilcke S, Witte N, Zygmunt M. Deutsches klinisches Kompetenzzentrum für genitale Sarkome und Mischtumoren an der Universitätsmedizin Greifswald (DKSM) und Kooperationspartner VAAO Deutschland und FK Frankfurt/Sachsenhausen. Datenbank und Promotions- und Forschungsgruppe genitale Sarkome, Greifswald 2016, www.medizin.uni-greifswald.de/gyn/dksm/
(43) Kumarasamy NA, Gayer G. Retroperitoneal sarcomas. Semin Ultrasound CT MR 2011; 32: 422–432
(44) Le Cesne A, Cresta S, Maki RG, Blay JY, Verweij J, Poveda A, Casali PG, Balaña C, Schöffski P, Grosso F, Lardelli P, Nieto A, Alfaro V, Demetri GD. A retrospective analysis of antitumour activity with trabectedin in translocation-related sarcomas. Eur J Cancer 2012; 48: 3036–3044
(45) Lee HP, Tseng HH, Hsieh PP, Shih TF. Uterine lipoleiomyosarcoma: report of 2 cases and review of the literature. Int J Gynecol Pathol 2012; 31: 358–363
(46) Lehnert T, Cardona S, Hinz U, Willeke F, Mechtersheimer G, Treiber M, Herfarth C, Buechler MW, Schwarzbach MH. Primary and locally recurrent retroperitoneal soft-tissue sarcoma: local control and survival. Eur J Surg Oncol 2009; 35: 986–993
(47) Levine PH, Wei XJ, Gagner JP, Flax H, Mittal K, Blank SV. Pleomorphic liposarcoma of the uterus: case report and literature review. Int J Gynecol Pathol 2003; 22: 407–411
(48) Liu Q, Xu Z, Mao S, Zeng R, Chen W, Lu Q, Guo Y, Liu J. Perineal lipoblastoma: A case report and review of literature. Int J Clin Exp Pathol 2014; 7: 3370–3374
(49) McDonald AG, Dal Cin P, Ganguly A, Campbell S, Imai Y, Rosenberg AE, Oliva E. Liposarcoma arising in uterine lipoleiomyoma: A report of 3 cases and review of the literature. Am J Surg Pathol 2011; 35: 221–227
(50) Miettinen M. Immunohistochemistry of soft tissue tumours – review with emphasis on 10 markers. Histopathology 2014; 64: 101–118
(51) Moreau LC, Turcotte R, Ferguson P, Wunder J, Clarkson P, Masri B, Isler M, Dion N, Werier J, Ghert M, Deheshi B. Canadian Orthopaedic Oncology Society (CANOOS). Myxoid/round cell liposarcoma (MRCLS) revisited: An analysis of 418 primarily managed cases. Ann Surg Oncol 2012; 19: 1081–1088
(52) Nascimento AF, Nucci MR. Disorders of the peritoneum. In: Crum CP, Nucci MR, Lee KL (eds.). Diagnostic Gynecologic and Obstetric Pathology. Elsevier Saunders, 2011, pp. 717–757
(53) National Comprehensive Cancer Network: NCCN Clinical Practice Guidelines in Oncology – Uterine neoplasms. Version 2.2016 www.nccn.org
(54) National Comprehensive Cancer Network: NCCN Clinical Practice Guidelines in Oncology – Soft tissue sarcomas. Version 2.2016 www.nccn.org
(55) Noël P, Reinhold C. Lipomatous uterine tumors. In: Hricak H, Akin O, Sala E, Ascher SM, Levine D, Reinhold C. Diagnostic Imaging Gynecology. 1st edn. AMIRSYS 2007, 2/124–2/127
(56) Nucci MR, Fletcher CD. Liposarcoma (atypical lipomatous tumors) of the vulva: A clinicopathologic study of six cases. Int J Gynecol Pathol 1998; 17: 17–23

(57) Nucci MR. Soft tissue lesions of the vulva and vagina. In: Crum CP, Nucci MR, Lee KL (eds.). Diagnostic Gynecologic and Obstetric Pathology. Elsevier Saunders, 2011, pp. 165–184
(58) Nucci MR, Ganesan R, McCluggage WG, Nielsen GP. Soft tissue tumors. In: Kurman RJ, Carcangiu ML, Herrington, CS, Young RH (eds.). WHO Classification of tumors of female reproductive organs. International Agency for Research on Cancer, Lyon 2014, pp. 243–249
(59) O'Donnell PW, Griffin AM, Eward WC, Sternheim A, White LM, Wunder JS, Ferguson PC. Can experienced observers differentiate between lipoma and well-differentiated liposarcoma using only MRI? Sarcoma 2013; 2013: 982784. DOI: 10.1155/2013/982784
(60) O'Donnell PW, Griffin AM, Eward WC, Sternheim A, Catton CN, Chung PW, O'Sullivan B, Ferguson PC, Wunder JS. The effect of the setting of a positive surgical margin in soft tissue sarcoma. Cancer 2014; DOI: 10.1002/cncr.28793
(61) Oliva E, Carcangiu ML, Carinelli SG, Ip P, Loening T, Longacre TA, Nucci MR, Prat J, Zaloudek CJ. Mesenchymal tumors. In: Kurman RJ, Carcangiu ML, Herrington, CS, Young RH (eds.) WHO Classification of tumors of female reproductive organs. International Agency for Research on Cancer: Lyon 2014, pp. 135–147
(62) Park JO, Qin LX, Prete FP, Antonescu C, Brennan MF, Singer S. Predicting outcome by growth rate of locally recurrent retroperitoneal liposarcoma: the one centimeter per month rule. Ann Surg 2009; 250: 977–982
(63) Pautier P, Floquet A, Chevreau C, Penel N, Guillemet C, Delcambre C, Cupissol D, Selle F, Isambert N, Piperno-Neumann S, Thyss A, Bertucci F, Bompas E, Alexandre J, Collard O, Lavau-Denes S, Soulié P, Toulmonde M, Le Cesne A, Lacas B, Duffaud F; French Sarcoma Group. Trabectedin in combination with doxorubicin for first-line treatment of advanced uterine or soft-tissue leiomyosarcoma (LMS-02): A non-randomised, multicentre, phase 2 trial. Lancet Oncol 2015 Mar 17. pii: S1470-2045(15)70070-7. DOI: 10.1016/S1470-2045(15)70070-7
(64) Pitson G, Robinson P, Wilke D, Kandel RA, White L, Griffin AM, Bell RS, Catton CN, Wunder JS, O'Sullivan B. Radiation response: An additional unique signature of myxoid liposarcoma. Int J Radiat Oncol Biol Phys 2004; 60: 522–526
(65) Sampath S, Hitchcock YJ, Shrieve DC, Randall RL, Schultheiss TE, Wong JY. Radiotherapy and extent of surgical resection in retroperitoneal soft-tissue sarcoma: multi-institutional analysis of 261 patients. J Surg Oncol 2010; 101: 345–350
(66) Samuels DL, Chawla S, Patel S, von Mehren M, Hamm J, Kaiser PE, Schuetze S, Li J, Aymes A, Demetri GD. Clinical outcomes and safety with trabectedin therapy in patients with advanced soft tissue sarcomas following failure of prior chemotherapy: results of a worldwide expanded access program study. Ann Oncol 2013; 24: 1703–1709
(67) Sandberg AA. Updates on the cytogenetics and molecular genetics of bone and soft tissue tumors: liposarcoma. Cancer Genet Cytogenet 2004; 155: 1–24
(68) Sanfilippo R, Constantinidou A, Bertulli R, Coco P, Fumagalli E, Scurr M, Morosi C, Pilotti S, Judson IR, Casali PG. Sensitivity of well-differentiated/dedifferentiated liposarcoma (WD/DD) and myxoid round cell/liposarcoma (MRCL) to high-dose ifosfamide: Combined analysis from two European referral institutions. J Clin Oncol 2011; 29: Suppl Abstr. 10023
(69) Schöffski P, Ray-Coquard IL, Cioffi A, Bui NB, Bauer S, Hartmann JT, Krarup-Hansen A, Grünwald V, Sciot R, Dumez H, Blay JY, Le Cesne A, Wanders J, Hayward C, Marreaud S, Ouali M, Hohenberger P. European Organisation for Research and Treatment of Cancer (EORTC) Soft Tissue and Bone Sarcoma Group (STBSG). Activity of eribulin mesylate in patients with soft-tissue sarcoma: A phase 2 study in four independent histological subtypes. Lancet Oncol 2011; 12: 1045–1052
(70) Scurr M. Histology-driven chemotherapy in soft tissue sarcomas. Curr Treat Options Oncol 2011; 12: 32–45

(71) Sheah K, Ouellette HA, Torriani M, Nielsen GP, Kattapuram S, Bredella MA. Metastatic myxoid liposarcomas: imaging and histopathologic findings. Skeletal Radiol 2008; 37: 251–258
(72) Shin YR, Rha SE. Miscellaneous tumors of the uterus. In: Kim SH (ed). Radiology Illustrated Gynecologic Imaging. 2nd edn. Springer, 2012, pp. 249–297
(73) Shiraev T, Pasricha SS, Choong P, Schlicht S, van Rijswijk CS, Dimmick S, Stuckey S, Anderson SE. Retroperitoneal sarcomas: A review of disease spectrum, radiological features, characterisation and management. J Med Imaging Radiat Oncol 2013; 57: 687–700
(74) Shweikeh F, Bukavina L, Saeed K, Sarkis R, Suneja A, Sweiss F, Drazin D. Brain metastasis in bone and soft tissue cancers: A review of incidence, interventions, and outcomes. Sarcoma 2014; 2014: 475175. DOI: 10.1155/2014/475175
(75) Song T, Shen J, Liang BL, Mai WW, Li Y, Guo HC. Retroperitoneal liposarcoma: MR characteristics and pathological correlative analysis. Abdom Imaging 2007; 32: 668–674
(76) Stanelle EJ, Christison-Lagay ER, Sidebotham EL, Singer S, Antonescu CR, Meyers PA, La Quaglia MP. Prognostic factors and survival in pediatric and adolescent liposarcoma. Sarcoma 2012; Article ID 87091076.
(77) Toro JR, Travis LB, Wu HJ, Zhu K, Fletcher CD, Devesa SS. Incidence patterns of soft tissue sarcomas, regardless of primary site, in the surveillance, epidemiology and end results program, 1978–2001: An analysis of 26,758 cases. Int J Cancer 2006; 119: 2922–2930
(78) Tseng WH, Martinez SR, Do L, Tamurian RM, Borys D, Canter RJ. Lack of survival benefit following adjuvant radiation in patients with retroperitoneal sarcoma: A SEER analysis. J Surg Res 2011; 168: e173–180
(79) Tseng WW, Somaiah N, Lazar AJ, Lev DC, Pollock RE. Novel systemic therapies in advanced liposarcoma: A review of recent clinical trial results. Cancers (Basel) 2013; 5: 529–549
(80) Yang DM, Kim HC, Lim JW, Jin W, Ryu CW, Kim GY, Cho H. Sonographic findings of groin masses. J Ultrasound Med 2007; 26: 605–614
(81) Yoshikawa H, Ueda T, Mori S, Araki N, Myoui A, Uchida A, Fukuda H. Dedifferentiated liposarcoma of the subcutis. Am J Surg Pathol 1996; 20: 1525–1530

Image references

Dieckmann, Frauenärztliche Praxis, Torgelow. Fig. 2.2.2
Evert M, Evert K. Universitätsmedizin Greifswald, Institut für Pathologie, Greifswald. Figs. 2.1.1 (B), (C); 2.1.3
Evert M, Evert K. Pathologisches Institut Universität Regensburg, Regensburg. Figs. 2.1.1 (D); 2.1.2 (A), (B); 2.2.1
Forner M. Evangelisches Krankenhaus Köln Kalk, Gynäkologie und Geburtshilfe, Köln. Fig. 2.1.3 (A)
Roth HJ. MVZ RNR Remscheid am Sana-Klinikum, Radiologie und Nuklearmedizin, Remscheid. Fig. 2.1.3 (B)–(F)
Schmidt A. Evangelisches Krankenhaus Mülheim a. d. Ruhr, Frauenklinik, Mühlheim. Fig. 2.1.1 (A)

Günter Köhler, Katja Evert, Marek Zygmunt and Matthias Evert

3 Rhabdomyosarcoma

The overall incidence of all subtypes of rhabdomyosarcoma (RMS) of all sites of the body is 0.17 per 100,000 for white and 0.2 per 100,000 for black women. The rarity of RMS becomes clear when compared to the incidence of uterine LMS, which is at 0.55/100,000 women (119). About one quarter of all RMS originate in the urogenital system, and they can affect the vulva, the vagina, the cervix, the uterus, the fallopian tube and the ovary in adult women (30). In general, one differentiates between embryonal RMS (ERMS), alveolar RMS (ARMS), pleomorphic RMS (PRMS) and, since more recently, spindle cell RMS. Botryoid RMS (sarcoma botryoides) constitutes a special variant of ERMS (132). While 20 % of RMS in children occur in the genital region, RMS only rarely occur there in adult women. In contrast, RMS occur rather frequently as the sarcomatous component in uterine CS and AS.

The presentation that follows refers to genital RMS in adult women. Most of the findings, insights, clinical experiences, and therapeutic recommendations for RMS in adults are primarily rooted in data gathered in the context of pediatric oncology, in particular the so-called CWS studies (Cooperative Soft Tissue Sarcoma Study Group), the studies conducted by the Intergroup Rhabdomyosarcoma Study Group (IRSG) and those of the European Paediatric Soft Tissue Sarcoma Study Group. Regarding therapy and therapeutic management, the boundaries between RMS in children, adolescents, and adults are blurred and rather indefinite. RMS in children and adolescents should be placed in the hands of pediatric oncologists or pediatric surgeons. The approach to treating virtually all RMS of the female genital tract needs to be an interdisciplinary one. Due to the need for multimodal therapeutic approaches, responsibility for devising and guiding treatment strategies should primarily lie in the hands of hematologist-oncologists in close cooperation with pediatric oncologists, radiologists, and gynecologists. Potentially dangerous CHT is in the hemato-oncologists' and pediatric oncologists' ballpark. Accordingly, determining the need for and necessary regimen of CHT, administering it, and monitoring it should be their responsibility. The complex CHT charts are thus only addressed parenthetically here. RMS patients should be included in scientific studies as a matter of course. Uterine PRMS in adult women constitutes a more or less independent tumor variant and belongs primarily in the hands of gynecologists. Perineal and perianal RMS as well as RMS of the bladder are not discussed. However, it is inevitable that the presentation that follows at least in part refers to RMS of all sites and in patients of all age groups.

Genital rhabdomyosarcomas are extremely rare in adult women. Diagnostic and therapeutic strategies are based in particular on the experiences gathered in the context of rhabdomyosarcomas in children. They must be subjected to an interdisciplinary treatment strategy without exception.

3.1 Uterine rhabdomyosarcoma

3.1.1 General, epidemiology, etiology, pathogenesis, staging

Among all RMS of all sites in children and adolescents (age ≤ 19 years), ERMS, ARMS, PRMS, and RMS-NOS account for 57.3 %, 25.7 %, 1.1 %, and 13.2 % of all cases, respectively. For adult women, the numbers (ERMS: 20.4 %, ARMS: 14.5 %, PRMS: 19.1 %, RMS-NOS: 43.4 %) show a significant and clear shift towards PRMS and RMS-NOS. Overall, the urogenital system (excl. bladder and prostate) is affected slightly more frequently in adults than in non-adults (116).

Of the uterine RMS arising in patients aged ≤ 20, 65.3 % are initially diagnosed before the patients' 10th birthday (2). Uterine RMS are generally heterologous malignant mesenchymal tumors showing evidence of skeletal muscle differentiation (97). It is unlikely that they originate from striated/skeletal muscle cells (49).

A number of genetic syndromes have come to be associated with RMS in children, including Li–Fraumeni syndrome (49, 101). There have also been accounts of ERMS arising in siblings (2 and 22 years old, 14 and 17 years old), however without any underlying genetic cause being discernible (89, 120). Cervical ERMS are not seldom observed to be associated with Sertoli–Leydig cell tumors (27, 29, 69).

ERMS are often characterized by a loss of heterozygosity at the 11p15 locus and recurrent chromosome 8 gains (80, 113). Somatic mutations become more frequent as age progresses (113).

ARMS are known to have t(2;13)(q35;q14) and t(1;13)(p36;q14) translocations that in turn effect an expression of various fusion genes, for instance PAX3-FKHR or PAX7-FKHR (114). As is also the case for numerous other types of uterine sarcoma, there are accounts that suggest an association between the development of PRMS and tamoxifen use (96).

Fifty-three percent of genital RMS in adult women are primarily localized in the uterine cervix, 20 % in the uterine corpus, 13 % in the vulva, 7 % in the fallopian tube, and 7 % in the ovaries (41). Only 6 % of all sarcomas that arise in the vagina of adult women are RMS. At the same time, the vagina is also the rarest site of genital RMS in adult women (124). In contrast, during puberty, 50 % of all genital RMS arise in the vagina (48). According to current SEER data, 38.8 % of all RMS of the female reproductive tract (age ≤ 19 years) are localized in the cervix or the uterus (64), of which 65.5 % occur in patients aged 10 and above.

In one study, ERMS, ARMS, and PRMS accounted for 73.3 %, 13.3 %, and 13.3 % of all RMS of the adult female genital tract (41).

Up until 2013, there were 130 accounts of RMS of the corpus and the cervix in patients aged 5 mo to 90 years (72). RMS is the most common type of sarcoma to arise in the cervix of adult women (36, 37). More recent data (6) suggest that cervical RMS is the third most common sarcoma variant, behind LMS and AS. Women with cervical

RMS are aged between 7 and 87 years (median 27), and 90 % of affected women are white (6). Other sources have measured a median age of 18.4 years (2.9–51.9 years) (69).

Botryoid ERMS is the most common form of cervical RMS (73 % of all RMS at that site), while PRMS are only occasionally encountered in the cervix (69). In total, only four cases of cervical ARMS have been described in the literature (11, 13, 33, 93).

Among botryoid ERMS, the ratio of cervical ERMS to ERMS of the uterine corpus is roughly 4:1 (72). According to a meta-analysis (85), ERMS and PRMS each account for around 50 % of all RMS of the corpus uteri. ARMS most frequently arise in the vulvar region, and only exceptionally occur in the area of the cervix or the corpus uteri (41, 132). Women are aged between 16 and 80 years (85). Among 8 uterine RMS covered in the DKSM materials database, 7 were ERMS and only 1 was ARMS (65). Patient age, including one case of cervical RMS, was between 13 and 57 years (mean 41.7, median 44.5) (65). ERMS of the corpus uteri are known to have arisen in patients aged 76 years (117). Uterine RMS in patients aged less than 20 years are ERMS or botryoid tumors in 80.7 % of cases, while the remainder are accounted for by alveolar and undifferentiated tumors (2).

PRMS arise in women aged between 35–87 years (mean 66.3). The majority of affected women are postmenopausal (38). Uterine PRMS have an incidence rate of 0.05 cases/100,000 women (85) which is thus ten times lower than for LMS. In children, PRMS account for less than 1 % of all RMS. PRMS differ substantially from ERMS and ARMS, both clinically and in terms of the therapeutic approach they require, and should thus rather be classified as STS. Classifying and staging RMS is relatively complicated, and what is known primarily refers to RMS in children. That being said, classification and staging for pediatric RMS are also applied to adult cases, not least because the transitions are fluid between pediatric and adult tumors in terms of their behavior and characteristics as well as their classification and staging, rather than abrupt or sudden.

Together with RMS of the efferent urinary tracts, RMS of the female genital tract (excluding the urinary bladder) are deemed favorable sites (91). This includes vaginal, vulvar, and uterine RMS. It is not entirely clear how the rare RMS of the tube and the ovaries should be classified. What can be said, though, is that perineal and perianal RMS do not fall within the category of genital tumors. Differentiating between vulvar, perineal and perianal RMS can be challenging, but is very important from a therapeutic and prognostic perspective. The term "vulvar RMS" only encompasses tumors of the minor and major labia and of the vulvar vestibule, but excludes RMS arising between the vaginal introitus and the anus.

The staging criteria for RMS are defined according to local spread/confinement (confined to site of origin or infiltration of surrounding tissue), tumor diameter, regional LN status, and the presence of distant metastasis (Tab. 3.1.1). What needs to be noted in this regard is that LN status primarily refers to results from clinical and imaging diagnostics, and not to histological findings. Classification as N1 thus implies that LN are positive both clinically and in imaging. On the basis of the criteria listed in

Tab. 3.1.1, RMS are staged using the "Pretreatment Staging System" (Tab. 3.1.2) of the Soft Tissue Sarcoma Committee of the Children's Oncology Group. This system in turn considers primary tumor site, presence or absence of infiltration of surrounding tissue, tumor diameter, clinical/imaging-derived LN status, and the presence or absence of distant metastasis.

Postoperative risk assessment and treatment are guided by the "Intergroup Rhabdomyosarcoma Study Group (IRSG) clinical group classification system" (78) and the Surgical-pathologic Group System of the Soft Tissue Sarcoma Committee of the Chil-

Tab. 3.1.1: Criteria for the pretreatment staging of rhabdomyosarcomas.

f. s.*	Orbit, head and neck, biliary tracts, urogenital system without bladder, prostate & kidney
u. s.*	All other sites
T1	Tumor confined to site of origin (no infiltration of/extension to surrounding tissue)
T2	Tumor extends to/infiltrates surrounding tissue
a	Tumor size ≤ 5 cm in largest dimension
b	Tumor size > 5 cm in largest dimension
N0	Regional lymph nodes not clinically involved
N1	Regional lymph nodes clinically involved
NX	Clinical regional lymph node status unknown (not examined; no information)
M0	No distant metastasis
M1	Distant metastasis present

f./u. s.: favorable/unfavorable site

Tab. 3.1.2: Pretreatment Staging System of the Soft Tissue Sarcoma Committee of the Children's Oncology Group. Genital RMS belong to the group of tumors with a favorable localization (91).

Stage	Site	T-stage	Tumor size	Regional lymph nodes	Distant metastasis
1	Favorable	T1 or T2	Any size	N0 or N1 or NX	M0
2	Unfavorable	T1 or T2	a ≤ 5 cm	N0 or NX	M0
3	Unfavorable	T1 or T2	a ≤ 5 cm	N1	M0
			b > 5 cm	N0 or N1 or NX	
4	Any site	T1 or T2	Any size	N0 or N1 or NX	M1

It is virtually impossible for genital RMS to occur in stages 2 and 3. This does not apply, however, to retroperitoneal sarcomas.

Tab. 3.1.3: Intergroup Rhabdomyosarcoma Study Group (IRSG) clinical group classification system for rhabdomyosarcomas (20).

Group	Definition
I	A: localized disease, completely resected, confined to site of origin; no regional lymph node involvement
	B: Localized disease, completely resected, with infiltration outside site of origin; no regional lymph node involvement
II	A: localized grossly resected tumor with microscopic residual disease at the resection margins; no signs of lymph node involvement
	B: regional disease with clinically involved LN completely resected with no microscopic residual disease, most distant distal lymph nodes not involved
	C: regional disease grossly resected, involved regional lymph nodes grossly resected with microscopic residual disease or histologic involvement of the most distant distal lymph nodes
III	A: incompletely resected tumor, state/condition after biopsy
	B: gross tumor resection (debulking of > 50 % of tumor)
IV	A: any tumor size, with distant metastasis verified via imaging regardless of the surgical therapy to which the primary tumor is subjected, positive distal lymph nodes
	B: any tumor size, positive tumor cells in the liquor, in the pleural or peritoneal fluids, or pleural or peritoneal implants

dren's Oncology Group. It essentially constitutes a surgical-pathological classification or grouping system that refers to the extent of disease, the type of resection, microscopic assessment of tumor margins and LN, and the presence or absence of distant metastasis (s. Tab. 3.1.3).

Group I covers localized tumors that have been subjected to complete microscopic resection, while group II encompasses cases with evidence of regional spread that have been subjected to complete gross resection with microscopic residual disease as well as negative LN or completely resected positive LN. Group III represents tumors subjected to incomplete microscopic resection with positive yet not resected LN, or with gross residual disease independent of the tumor's localization, including malignant effusions. Group III also covers tumors that have been subjected only to biopsy, i.e. the state in which the tumor remains after biopsy has been performed. Group IV comprises cases in which there is distant metastasis and/or nodal involvement beyond the regional LN. Regional LN are defined differently than those of carcinomas of the same site: for the cervix, the corpus, and the vagina, LN of the vasa iliaca externa, interna and communes are classified as regional LN. Para-aortic lymph node involvement is already regarded as distant metastasis. For the vulva, only the inguinal lymph nodes are classed as regional LN (35).

Besides the surgical-pathological group classification system, the TNM system can also be used in the postoperative context (Tab. 3.1.4). The two classification systems can actually be correlated with each other very well (Tab. 3.1.5). The surgical-pathological group classification system in turn constitutes the foundation for RMS risk group classification (Tab. 3.1.6). For RMS-NOS, risk group is determined according to disease site (favorable, unfavorable), patient's age, tumor size, and LN involvement. RMS-NOS do not fall within the group of low risk tumors.

Tab. 3.1.4: Postoperative staging (TNM classification).

pT0	No histological evidence of primary tumor in the respective specimen/sample
pT1	Tumor confined to site/organ of origin, Completely resected with no signs of microscopic residual disease
pT2	Tumor with infiltration/extension beyond site/organ of origin, Completely resected with no signs of microscopic residual disease
pT3	Tumor with or without infiltration/extension beyond site/organ of origin, incomplete resection
pT3a	Microscopic residual disease
pT3b	Gross residual disease
pT3c	Additional malignant effusion
pTX	Tumor status cannot be assessed histologically
pN0	No histological evidence for positive regional lymph node involvement
pNl	Positive regional lymph nodes
pNla	Involved nodes considered to be completely resected
pNlb	Involved nodes considered not to be completely resected
pNX	Regional lymph nodes cannot be assessed due to lack of pathological examination or inadequate information
pM0	No microscopic evidence of distant metastasis outside/beyond the regional lymph nodes
pMl	Distant metastasis histologically confirmed
pMX	Distant metastasis cannot be assessed due to a lack of pathological examination

The aforementioned classifications are tailored to ERMS, ARMS, and RMS-NOS as they arise in children. They can, however, be adopted for the corresponding adult RMS as well, as these are usually treated in the same way as RMS in children are.

Adult, non-pediatric PRMS are classified in accordance with the TNM classification system for malignant tumors or STS. Accordingly, adult uterine PRMS should be classified using this system, not least because they are subject to different treatment strategies than their pediatric counterparts (34, 91). The attending pathologist should always inform the clinician of which classification system is being adhered to.

Tab. 3.1.5: Correlation of IRS groups and postoperative TNM stage.

IRS Group	Definition	pTNM
I	Tumor completely resected both grossly and microscopically	
IA	Tumor confined to the organ/site of origin	pTl
IB	Tumor with infiltration of/extension beyond the site/organ of origin	pT2
II	Microscopic residual disease in tumors subjected to complete gross resection	pT3a
IIA	No lymph node involvement	
IIB	Lymph nodes involved but resected	
III	Microscopic residual disease in tumors subjected to complete gross resection, lymph nodes involved but not resected	pT3a
	Gross residual disease following resection or only biopsy	pT3b
	Malignant effusion (e.g. ascites, pleural effusion)	pT3c
IV	Distant metastasis or involvement of non-regional lymph nodes	pT4

Tab. 3.1.6: Soft Tissue Sarcoma Committee of the Children's Oncology Group: rhabdomyosarcoma risk group classification.

Risk group	Histologic subtype	Clinical stage	IRS group
Low risk	Embryonal	1	I, II, III
	Embryonal	2, 3	I, II
Intermediate risk	Embryonal	2, 3	III
	Alveolar	1, 2, 3	I, II, III
High risk	Embryonal or alveolar	4	IV

An ARMS must consist of > 50 % alveolar components. If the alveolar component is ≤ 50 %, then the tumor is classified as ERMS. Pretreatment stages 2 and 3 do not apply to RMS of the female genital tract. Only ERMS fall within the intermediate risk group. RMS-NOS should be classified as intermediate risk. PRMS are not included in this risk group classification. Instead, the risk and treatment strategies for undifferentiated STS apply to PRMS.

Uterine rhabdomyosarcomas are heterologous malignant mesenchymal tumors showing evidence of skeletal muscle differentiation. Seventy-three percent of rhabdomyosarcomas of the adult female genital tract are embryonal, 13 % are alveolar, 13 % are pleomorphic, and 20 % are rhabdomyosarcomas NOS. Fifty-three percent are primarily localized in the cervix, 20 % in the uterine corpus, 13 % in the vulva, 7 % in the fallopian tube, and 7 % in the ovaries. Cervical and corporal tumors occur at a ratio of 4:1. Uterine rhabdomyosarcomas are usually embryonal or pleomorphic tumors. Different systems for pretreatment, posttreatment and risk classification exist for rhabdomyosarcomas, all of which are derived from experiences with childhood tumors. The "Intergroup Rhabdomyosarcoma Study Group (IRSG) clinical group classification system" is the most prominent.

3.1.2 Macroscopic and microscopic features

The mean diameter of all RMS of the adult female genital tract is 3.4 cm (0.8–6 cm) (41). Among 9 cases of ERMS and ARMS in the DKSM material database, said mean diameter was 5.2 cm (2.5–9 cm) (65).

ERMS usually present as polypoid tumors originating in the cervix or the cavity of the uterus. However, like PRMS, they can develop as polypoid submucosal, completely intracavitary or intramural tumors and can prolapse from/via the cervix and protrude into the vagina (127). The botryoid subtype, which is the most common form of cervical ERMS, is submucosal, completely covered by the local epithelium, and has a polypoid gross appearance with typical grape-like structures (Fig. 3.1.1 (A)). In many cases, such tumors have a smooth, glistening, hyaline macroscopic appearance, sometimes with grossly visible focal hemorrhages (27, 57, 110).

In the DKSM materials, 50 % of ERMS and ARMS were described as soft or decomposing, 25 % were necrotic, and 37 % exhibited hemorrhages (65).

PRMS can also develop well-circumscribed tumors with a pseudo-capsule. The cut surface appears fleshy and soft, commonly with visible macroscopic hemorrhages and necroses. PRMS are of a white to gray color in most cases (38, 98, 99). Uterine PRMS have a mean diameter of 8.8 cm (39).

ERMS tumor cells are predominantly small, undifferentiated round cells with minimal cytoplasm and hyperchromatic nuclei. Strap cells with eosinophilic cytoplasm and cross-striations are also common (Fig. 3.1.1 (B)).

The botryoid variant, as a special growth form, is located directly beneath the mucous membranes or epithelium, and typically exhibits varying hypercellular and hypocellular sections. The characteristic hypercellular sections develop from cellular condensation of primitive small blue cells beneath epithelial surfaces (cambium layer) or around trapped endometrial glands. They can also form islands or enclaves within hypocellular areas (72). These hypocellular areas develop on the basis of an edematous or myxoid matrix. These characteristics can be found in almost all botryoid ERMS of the cervix and the corpus (72). Aggregations of immature chondrocytes are often present and are usually located in close proximity to the hypercellular sections of the tumor (72, 86, 98, 131). Histologically differentiating the common, non-polypoid ERMS with varying degrees of cellularity in combination with an edematous and myxoid matrix from the botryoid variant is particularly challenging.

The spindle cell variant of ERMS only exceptionally occurs in the uterus. Besides focal botryoid RMS components and a myxoid matrix, this variant exhibits an ample predominance of immature bundled spindle cells, some of which have light eosinophilic cytoplasm and cross-striations (79).

In ARMS, primitive, usually round (but sometimes polygonal) mononuclear or multinuclear cells predominate. In most cases, they are arranged in a pseudoalveolar pattern or in the form of “nests” that are separated from one another by delicate strands/cords of connective tissue. The loosely connected cells contain differing levels

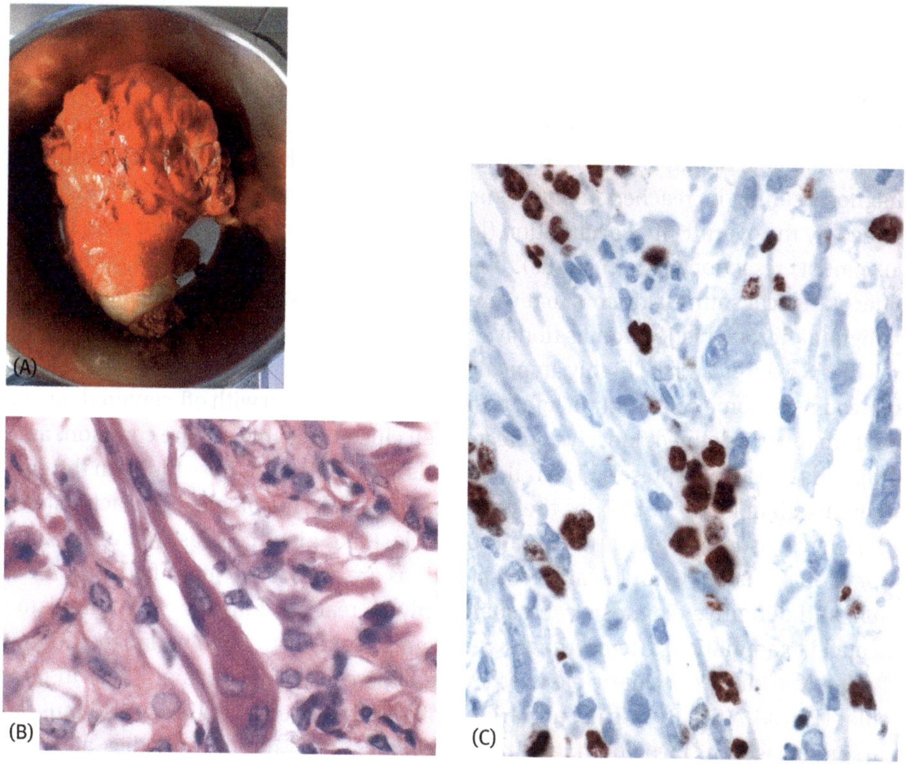

Fig. 3.1.1: (A) uterine botryoid embryonal rhabdomyosarcoma in a 42-year-old woman. The polypoid, visibly grape-like tumor has prolapsed/protrudes from the cervix; extensive intramural growth is already clearly outwardly visible; (B), (C) identical case; (B) Microscopically, besides giant cells, HE staining also clearly reveals the cross-striations in the rhabdomyogenic cells; (C) Ki-67 staining serves to visualize the ample proliferations.

of eosinophilic cytoplasm and hyperchromatic nuclei. The densely packed small tumor cells generate the appearance that is usually typically exhibited by "small round blue cell tumors". Solid sections without alveolar structures can be present that usually exhibit ample mitotic activity (45). In contrast to ERMS, the cells are generally larger and have round nuclei. Furthermore, multinuclear cells are common and cross-striations are visible in the majority of cases. The presence of light eosinophilic cytoplasm in the round cells is regarded as an important diagnostic pointer (132). Epithelial markers can occasionally be positive in ARMS (97). However, overall, differentiating between the prognostically more favorable ERMS and the more aggressive ARMS is not a simple task. Molecular-pathological verification of underlying genetic PAX/FKHR gene fusions is regarded as the gold standard for reaching an accurate diagnosis.

RMS-NOS are difficult to classify, both clinically and prognostically. They essentially reflect a group of neoplasms for which pathologists have only limited experience in terms of classification. It needs to be noted that RMS-NOS do not constitute an independent or separate entity of neoplasm. While such lesions can be diagnosed as RMS, pinpointing a specific subtype is not possible. Classification as RMS-NOS is usually the result of insufficient tissue being yielded from biopsy in combination with crushing phenomena. Biopsy should be repeated in such cases where possible. If a definitive diagnosis cannot be reached, then prognosis, risk group, and treatment should all be guided by the overall clinical situation (localization, patient's age, tumor size, LN involvement, resection/margin status). It cannot be entirely ruled out that, at least in older statistical sources, tumors that were diagnosed as RMS-NOS were in fact LMS or malignant fibrous histiocytomas (today: pleomorphic sarcomas NOS) (116).

PRMS exhibit a mix of highly atypical spindle-shaped, round, and polygonal rhabdomyoblasts. Some cells contain light eosinophilic cytoplasm with off-centered nuclei and form poorly defined, loosely connected cell clusters. Giant cells are common, and strap cells can also be present. Overall, the cells are larger than those found in the embryonal variant (38, 99). Besides the typical microscopic/histological characteristics, PRMS have also been found to contain osteoclast-like giant cells as well as myxoid stroma on occasion. Cytoplasmic cross-striations are only rarely identified (38). A reliable and definitive diagnosis can usually only be reached following immunohistochemical examinations. Hemorrhages are common and occur in all variants of RMS.

The Ki-67 index is clearly elevated in the hypercellular sections of ERMS in particular (Fig. 3.1.1 (C)). Practically all variants of RMS positively express skeletal muscle markers myogenin, myoglobin, and myoD1 (38, 45, 79). MyoD1 antibodies are very early markers for rhabdomyogenic differentiation and can be identified in practically all forms of RMS. The nuclei express the proteins myogenin and myoD1, both of which are usually not traceable in either normal cross-striated muscle cells or in other STS (15, 23). Myogenin, the most important marker in the context of pathologico-anatomical diagnostics, is a transcription factor for rhabdomyogenic differentiation. Accordingly, it can occasionally also be expressed in regenerating skeletal muscle. Similar to myoD1, myogenin is particularly relevant for tissue differentiation in the embryonic phase. Myogenin expression is thus elevated in immature RMS and RMS with low differentiation in particular, for example ARMS. In contrast, myosin and myoglobin only come to be expressed in the later stages of myogenic differentiation. Up to 96 % of RMS also test positive for desmin and muscle-specific actin (15, 23, 72). In contrast to the other aforementioned markers, both desmin and muscle-specific actin are not monospecific to RMS.

Immunohistochemical testing also facilitates the differentiation between ERMS and ARMS. While ARMS exhibit diffuse and ample myogenin and myoD1 staining, ERMS and RMS-NOS show a significantly weaker, usually focal reaction (88, 107). Notwithstanding, identifying translocations in ARMS is deemed important, in particular in cases in which precise subgroup typification is gene-fusion dependent. For more detail pertaining to further differentiation and differing fusion gene expressions, reference should be had to the specialist pathologico-anatomical literature (132).

The majority of PRMS also express calponin and CD56. Undifferentiated tumors of different histogenesis (e.g. sarcomatoid carcinomas) can usually be easily immunohistochemically discerned, since PRMS generally do not express cytokeratins and other similar markers (38). Accurately differentiating PRMS from high-grade LMS is both highly important and not always straightforward. Besides the common absence of SMA in PRMS (72), another method that can be helpful in this regard is assessing the presence of myogenin or myoD1 and the absence of caldesmon, the best leimyogenic marker of tumor cells. Extensive dedifferentiation in RMS can lead to a loss of myogenin and myoD1 expression. By definition, these markers are never expressed in undifferentiated sarcomas (88).

ERMS only focally express ER and PGR, and this only in 25 % and 12.5 % of cases, respectively (72).

Rhabdomyosarcomas can be histologically differentiated into embryonal, alveolar, pleomorphic rhabdomyosarcomas, as well as rhabdomyosarcomas NOS. Embryonal rhabdomyosarcomas include the botryoid and spindle cell subtypes. All of these tumor types exhibit rhabdomyogenic differentiation and express the skeletal muscle markers myogenin, myosin, myoglobin, and myoD1. Myogenin and myoD1 can be found neither in normal cross-striated muscle cells, nor in other soft tissue sarcomas.

3.1.3 Clinical presentation, diagnostics, screening

Postmenopausal bleeding, or AUB in form of prolonged and heavy and intermenstrual bleedings in premenopausal women, are the most important symptoms. Potentially malodorous vaginal discharge can also occur. In the majority of cases, ERMS of the cervix and the corpus present as cervical, occasionally endometrial polyps (46, 72, 127). These polypoid tumors can grow and extend all the way to the introitus vaginae. They range in size from 2 to 9.5 cm, and some tumors are pedunculated (27, 57). Due to their size, they can occasionally lead to or be associated with uterine inversion (13). What is rather striking about these tumors is their predominantly smooth surface (84). Botryoid ERMS polyps usually have a grape-like appearance, but can also bear resemblance to common mucosal polyps.

If technically feasible, primary extirpation with wide clear margins is the generally recommended diagnostic method of choice (cf. RMS of the vulva and the vagina). Histological diagnosis of cervical RMS is reached via tumor extirpation with wide clear margins or, if this course of action is not feasible or possible, via standalone biopsy. RMS of the corpus are usually incidental findings made during or following curettage performed in response to AUB. PRMS, in particular, are not rarely intramurally located and can thus often not be diagnosed as such via curettage. Sometimes the tissue specimens gathered via curettage only reveal necroses (127). In the DKSM material database, curettage was performed on 7 of 8 uterine RMS because of AUB, and in five of those cases an RMS was actually diagnosed. Thirty-eight percent of RMS were incidentally diagnosed as such postoperatively (65). When clinical examination and sonography reveal suspicious intramural findings, the same approach should be adopted as applies to LMS (Vol. 1, Chapter 2). A diagnostic flowchart is discussed in detail in the chapter on prevention of inadequate sarcoma operations (Vol. 1, Chapter 6). For cases that are highly suspicious, both clinically and in terms of their imaging characteristics, THE without injuring the uterus is the method of choice for women who are postmenopausal or who have no desire for (further) reproduction. In unclear cases, in cases in which patients wish to preserve their reproductive capacity, as well as in cases in which patients reject THE for other reasons, performing ultrasound-guided transcervical punch biopsy with an 18 or 16 (1.2–1.6 mm) gauge needle is indicated, if the results yielded from curettage are deemed unsuspicious (cf. Vol. 1, Chapter 6). The PDQ Guidelines and study protocols are in favor of the aforementioned measures (35, 91).

CA-125 can be elevated in ARMS and PRMS (56, 98). Analogous to LMS, accounts of elevated LDH levels have also been described in adult uterine PRMS (129) and pediatric ARMS (87). In both instances, the LDH values correlated with extent of disease.

When an RMS is either suspected or has been diagnosed as such, the next necessary step is to perform imaging diagnostic procedures for pretreatment staging, as well as for assessing LN status in ERMS and ARMS in particular (91). The imaging methods applied should at the very least include thoracic CT. PET-CT is recommended in cases in which difficulties are encountered in assessing LN status via other imaging diagnostic procedures (40, 118, 121). PET-CT is also said to improve prognostic accuracy. The identification of positive LN involvement and of distant metastasis as well as a high SUV ($SUV_{max}/SUV_{liver} > 4.5$) in PET-CT are relevant prognostic factors (7). Where possible, LN that appear abnormal, either clinically or in imaging diagnostic procedures, should be biopsied (cf. primary surgery) (32).

There are no particular screening methods for rare RMS. Since cervical ERMS develop beneath the mucous membranes, cytological swabs will only very rarely yield positive results. There is one account in which cells were found in the swab taken from a patient with polypoid intracaval uterine ERMS that could at the very least be interpreted as constituting sarcoma cells (127).

Additional or postmenopausal bleeding are the most important symptoms of uterine rhabdomyosarcomas. Embryonal RMS of the cervix and the corpus clinically present as "polyps" in the majority of cases. Diagnosis is reached on the basis of biopsy, curettage or – for cervical RMS – via resection with wide clear margins, where deemed technically feasible. Where the diagnosis is clear, imaging diagnostics using CT or MRI are necessary for pretreatment staging and for assessing lymph node status.

3.1.4 Imaging

There is only very little literature on the imaging characteristics of genital RMS. Results from sonography, CT, and MRI are all highly unspecific and do not allow safe or accurate distinctions to be made from other types of pure genital sarcoma.

In sonography, RMS exhibit heterogeneous echoicity with hyperechoic and hypoechoic regions as well as anechoic sections that most likely correspond to necroses (52). The boundaries between the different echogenicities are either washy or sharp/clear with bizarre structures overall (Fig. 3.1.2 (A), (B)). The aforementioned characteristics, while not specific to RMS, give rise to suspect the presence of a malignant mesenchymal tumor and are not shown by regular LM in sonography.

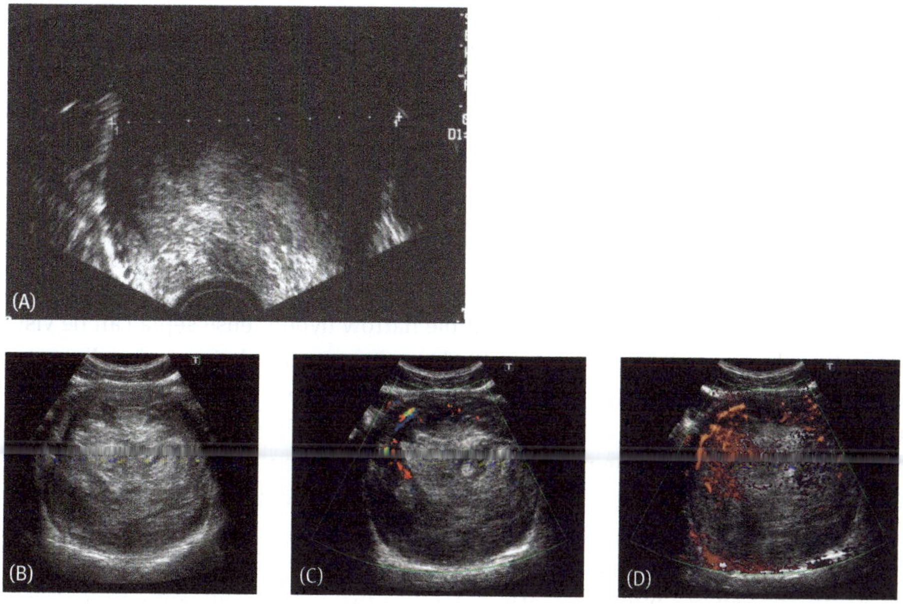

Fig. 3.1.2: (A) vaginal sonography of the rhabdomyosarcomas depicted in Fig. 3.1.1. The tumor has heterogeneous echogenicity with sometimes diffuse, sometimes irregular bizarre margins between the regions of different echogenicity; (B) embryonal uterine rhabdomyosarcoma with a diameter of 13 × 10 cm and positive lymph node involvement in a 19-year-old woman. The heterogeneous and inhomogeneous echogenicity with diffuse boundaries/margins between the areas of different echogenicity is striking; (C), (D) color Doppler sonography shows that the anechoic voids in (C) in part correspond to vessels and serve to evidence the tumor's massive degree of central vascularity.

CT reveals a heterogeneous tumor that is isodense to soft tissue, and that shows a strong heterogeneous enhancement in CECT (52, 57). While these characteristics are common in soft tissue sarcomas, they do not allow a specific diagnosis as RMS to be reached (Fig. 3.1.3 (A), (B)).

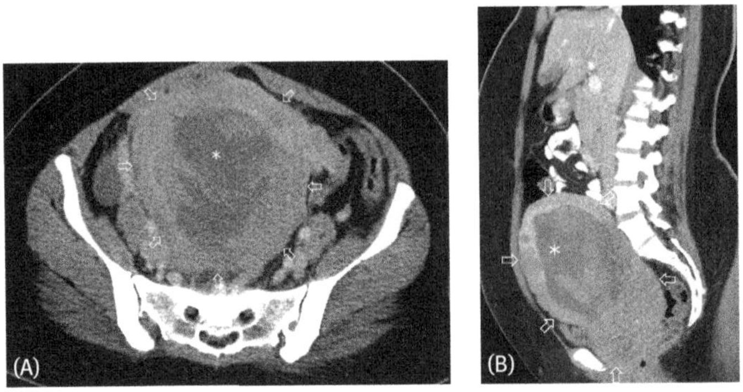

Fig. 3.1.3: Botryoid embryonal rhabdomyosarcoma from Fig. 3.1.1. (A), (B) axial (A) and sagittal (B) abdominal CECT in the portal venous phase show a clearly enlarged uterus (13 × 14 × 20 cm) (bold arrows) with polypoid, solid and necrotic tumor components. The hyperdense border area resembles viable tumor components. The central hypodense area corresponds to necrotic sections (stars) resulting from rapid growth. The tumor appears to be clearly delineated from its surroundings (bold arrows).

The air bubbles that seem to occur quite frequently (Fig. 3.1.4 (A)) apparently constitute small air entrapments that are predominantly located at the margins of the tumor between the macroscopically polypoid or grape-like (botryoid) structures.

T2W MRI shows high or intermediate SI. In intermediate SI, numerous pockets of hyperintensity are visible. In ERMS, multiple narrow hypointense septa can be visible within the tumor that confer a marbled appearance and that occasionally serve to visualize the tumor's botryoid structures. The ample hemorrhages are also visible in MRI. RMS have low SI in T1W. Strong heterogeneous enhancement is recognizable in T1WC images, though the necroses that are often present show no enhancement (52, 109, 127). These characteristics combined with a polypoid clinical appearance are at the very least suggestive of RMS. Advanced cervical carcinomas can be rather easily differentiated from advanced cervical RMS in MRI in particular – while cervical carcinoma usually exhibits infiltration of/extension to the vaginal wall, RMS, in contrast, only cause the vaginal wall to distend (Fig. 3.1.4 (A), (B)).

In light of the fact that these tumors exhibit early spread/growth, MRI or CT of the pelvis/abdomen and a CT scan of the lung are indicated as means for primary staging, assessing LN status, and determining optimal treatment (30). For RMS in adults, PET-CT can be considered to securely and reliably assess LN status and to detect unusually localized metastases. For uterine RMS at least, the reasonability of PET-CT is indeed questionable, not least because such tumors should be subjected to THE in combination with selective LNE of intraoperatively suspicious (!) LN (cf. primary surgery). For PRMS, both clinically and therapeutically, performing an LNE has yet to be proven beneficial, so that the respective diagnostic procedures become redundant for this tumor variant. Notwithstanding, there have been considerations as to whether

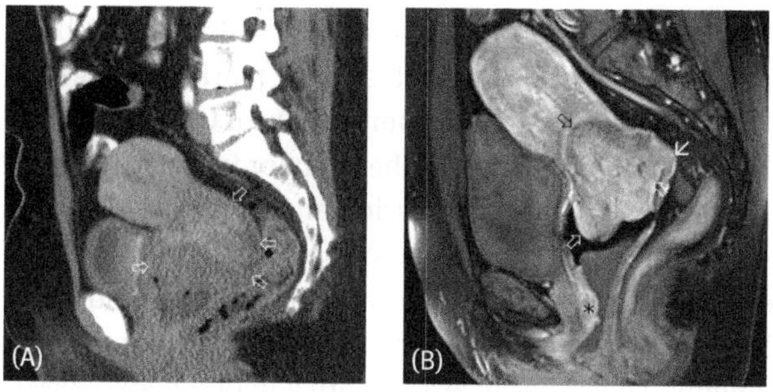

Fig. 3.1.4: Comparison between a cervical botryoid rhabdomyosarcoma (A) in a 54-year-old patient, and a cervical carcinoma (B) in a 50-year-old patient; (A) abdominal sagittal CECT shows the significant degree to which the rhabdomyosarcoma has distended the vagina (bold arrows), further some air bubbles are visible within the tumor; (B) In contrast, sagittal T1 weighted MRI with i.v. administration of contrast agent plus fat suppression reveals no vaginal distension by the tumor (open arrows). Due to superior local resolution and soft tissue contrast compared to CT, MRI allows for more precise local staging. Here, infiltration of the posterior fornix and a drop metastasis on the anterior vaginal wall in the lower third of the vagina (star) are visible.

diagnostic selective LNE could be replaced by a PET-CT examination (43). However, PET-CT should be performed in cases in which there is the suspicion of bone or bone marrow involvement (32, 40).

The imaging characteristics of rhabdomyosarcomas are nonspecific and correspond to those of other soft tissue sarcomas. Sonography reveals a heterogeneous echogenicity with hyper- and hypoechoic areas, as well as anechoic sections. CT shows a tumor that is isodense to soft tissue that usually contains clearly discernible necroses. Rhabdomyosarcomas have high or intermediate signal intensity in T2W MRI. Signal intensity is low in T1W. PET-CT is recommended where imaging diagnostic procedures fail to provide a reliable assessment of lymph node status.

3.1.5 Differential diagnostics

On occasion, polypoid vaginal and cervical RMS can be difficult to macroscopically discern from common mucous membrane polyps. There are even known cases of microscopic misdiagnoses (84). An RMS must always be considered a plausible possibility in child and adolescent patients.

CS and AS, which occur much more frequently than RMS, are the most important histological DD for uterine RMS. In AS with stromal overgrowth, the epithelial component may only be focally present, which in turn increases the likelihood that it is missed/overlooked and subsequently not diagnosed in biopsy and curettage specimens. On the other hand, an ERMS with trapped endometrial glands may be difficult to discern from an AS with an RMS component. ERMS also often exhibit similar growth patterns (botryoid, phylloid) to AS and often also show cellular condensation (cambium layer in ERMS, "cuffing" in AS) at the margins to epithelial structures (cf. Chapter 6). DD is further compounded by the fact that the RMS-specific markers myogenin and myoD1 are also expressed in the rhabdomyogenic components of CS, AS, and occasionally LG-ESS. Myogenin and myoD1 expression in these tumor types is a typical differential diagnostic pitfall. Strong ER and PGR expression are rather suggestive of AS and serve to reduce the likelihood of an RMS (72). Therefore, every uterine RMS, and especially PRMS, must be rigorously subjected to extensive tissue and immunohistochemical examinations (cytokeratin markers) with a view to assessing the presence or absence of epithelial components. This is because a CS with a heterologous PRMS component will always be more likely than a pure PRMS until there is proof to the contrary, especially in postmenopausal women. This notwithstanding, there are cases in which a reliable differentiation between an AS with SO by an RMS (cf. AS) and an ERMS is not possible (72). Spindle celled RMS can easily be mistaken for LMS. However, to date only two cases of spindle cell RMS arising in adult women (28 and 76 years old) have been described in the literature (63). Without immunohistochemical analyses, an ERMS could also be misdiagnosed as myxoid LMS or myxoid components of an LG-ESS (41). Misdiagnoses in the opposite direction are also possible.

PRMS can bear close resemblance to pleomorphic LMS. However, in contrast to RMS, LMS are almost always primarily localized within the uterine wall. Both of these tumor types express desmin. Myogenin, by contrast, is only expressed in PRMS, and caldesmon is almost only expressed in LMS. Another difference is that LMS cells do not exhibit any cross-striation. While UUS can also bear resemblance to RMS, the former can be reliably excluded from consideration on the basis of its lack of expression of myogenic markers. Undifferentiated carcinomas can also be microscopically similar to PRMS, but compared to the latter, they express cytokeratins but no myogenic markers.

Cervical or corporal polyps are the most important clinical differential diagnostic options for uterine rhabdomyosarcomas. Histological differentiation from carcinosarcomas and adenosarcomas with sarcomatous overgrowth can be extremely challenging. Pleomorphic rhabdomyosarcomas bear close microscopic resemblance to pleomorphic leiomyosarcomas and undifferentiated uterine sarcomas. Exclusion of these options occurs on the basis of specific skeletal and smooth muscle markers.

3.1.6 Course, prognosis

The data pertaining to the prognosis of RMS largely come from studies focusing on pediatric RMS. However, they have often also included adolescent and adult women. The majority of these studies have focused on ERMS and ARMS. Childhood and adult PRMS and RMS-NOS have only been the subject of relatively few studies.

A recent SEER analysis (128) of RMS (ERMS, ARMS, PRMS, RMS-NOS) in patients aged up to 19 years revealed 5-year and 10-year OS of 64.5 % and 61.8 %, respectively, for the entire cohort. Five-year OS continuously worsened as tumor diameter increased – tumors with a diameter of 0–4 cm had a 5-year OS of 79.5 % that dropped to 61.6 % for tumor diameters of 5–9 cm, and to only 45.9 % for tumor diameters ≥ 10 cm. Likewise, prognosis worsened as patient age increased. Children aged 0–4 had a 5-year OS of 71.3 %, while for adolescents aged 15–19 the figure was only 47.9 %. ERMS have a more favorable 5-year OS compared to ARMS (73.5 vs. 46.3 %). Localized tumors, regionally spread RMS, and patients with distant metastatic disease had 5-year OS of 84.0 %, 72.4 %, and 35.7 %, respectively. RMS in favorable locations had a significantly better prognosis than such at unfavorable sites (cf. Tab. 3.1.1). The same also applies to the comparison of whether resection was or was not performed. Patients who underwent RT had better 5-year OS than patients who did not (65.6 % vs. 62.7 %), though the difference was only of weak statistical significance. A useful nomogram for assessing 5-year and 10-year OS has been published (128) that was developed on the basis of these SEER data as well as on the findings from the IRSG (102). It must be noted that said nomogram only refers to RMS in women aged ≤ 19. RMS in older women are said to have a clearly less favorable prognosis. In one study, RMS in patients aged > 50 years (all variants and types, 33 % in urogenital sites) were associated with a significantly poorer DFS and OS than in younger patients (31). These findings notwithstanding, the aforementioned nomogram and the SEER data on which it is largely based nonetheless provide good leads for prognostically assessing adult patients. A further SEER analysis (116) compared adult RMS (> 19 years, n = 1,071) to childhood and adolescent RMS (≤ 19 years, n = 1,529) for both genders. With a 5-year OS of 27 %, adult RMS were statistically associated with significantly poorer survival compared to non-adult RMS (61 %). More specifically, pediatric tumors of all stages and all RMS variants and subvariants had a better prognosis. Regionally advanced tumors and the presence of distant metastasis were much more frequent in the adult cohort. A comparison was not possible for PRMS as these occurred too rarely in the children/adolescent group.

In a current study on adult RMS of all variants and sites, upon multivariate analysis, only risk group (low vs. high) and primary localization (favorable vs. unfavorable) remained as significant factors pertaining to OS (47). Even in IRS group IV, favorable primary localizations have a far better prognosis than those in unfavorable primary sites (20). According to further sources (24, 58, 81), the following constitute favorable prognostic factors for all RMS: absence of distant metastasis, urogenital localization (without bladder and prostate), localized tumor subjected to complete surgical resection at primary diagnosis, ERMS or botryoid histology, tumor size < 5 cm, and patient age > 1 and < 10 years.

Eighty-six percent of all genital RMS in adult women present as IRSG group I–III at the time of initial diagnosis (41). Roughly 82 % of patients with cervical RMS had disease classified as IRSG group I (69). Ten percent of adult women with uterine and vaginal RMS had developed distant metastasis at the time of primary diagnosis (28). All childhood urogenital RMS in IRSG groups I/II had a better 3-year DFS than those in IRSG group III (83 % and 86 % versus 73 %). ERMS, ARMS, undifferentiated RMS, and RMS-NOS had respective 3-year DFS of 83 %, 66 %, 55 % and 66 % (22). Applying postoperative CHT to children with RMS of all types yielded an overall 3-year DFS of 77 % and a 3-year OS of 86 % (22).

Genital ERMS without distant metastasis all fall within the low-risk group, while respective ARMS are classified as "intermediate risk" (Tab. 3.1.6). All ERMS and ARMS that are accompanied by primary distant metastatic disease belong in the high-risk group. PRMS are not included in the table.

Disease-free OS for childhood ERMS and ARMS depends on the respective risk-group to which they are allocated. Patients at low risk have an estimated 3-year PFS rate of 88 %, while those at intermediate risk have rates between 55–76 %. For high-risk patients, the estimated 3-year PFS rate is at < 30 %. It must be generally assumed that adults have less favorable rates by comparison (32).

The LN are involved in 22 % of all patients with histological RMS variants of all types at favorable sites/localizations. Among ARMS and ERMS of all localizations, the LN were positive in 45 % and 43 % of cases, respectively. In the same study, the LN were only involved in 10 % of PRMS cases (108). These data serve to underline the clinical data that suggest that PRMS are more closely related to STS than to ERMS and ARMS. ARMS with LN positivity have a significantly poorer prognosis than such with N0 status (5-year disease-free OS of 43 % vs. 73 %). Their prognosis resembles that of cases in which there is just one isolated distant metastatic tumor.

For ERMS, whether the LN are positive or negative is of no prognostic influence, which stands in stark contrast to ARMS. However, the presence of just one solitary distant metastatic tumor already significantly impacts negatively on prognosis (108).

Positive LN are detected in 18 % of all patients with all variants of cervical RMS, which is significantly higher than the rates for both LMS (0 %) and AS (2.9 %) (6). In contrast, no positive LN were found – neither clinically, nor intraoperatively or via imaging diagnostics – in any of the patients with cervical ERMS and PRMS covered in two further studies (2, 69).

Interestingly, in a study covering all variants of vaginal and uterine RMS, the LN were both pathologico-anatomically and clinically free of disease (108). Yet another study revealed that the LN were affected in 27 % of uterine RMS in children and adolescents (≤ 20 years). Of the 6 uterine ERMS in the DKSM material database, 2 had positive LN (33.3 %), while the one ARMS in the database showed no LN involvement (65). No definitive conclusions can be drawn from the LN status of uterine RMS, neither from a prognostic nor from a therapeutic perspective, because the data that are currently available, when taken together, are inconsistent, conflicting, and stem from too small a number of studies (69).

At least for under 21-year-olds, it can be said that genital RMS have a better prognosis than such at other sites (22, 78). RMS of all variants, types, and sites in adult women have a median DFS of 9 mo (1–24 mo), a 2-year DFS of 15 %, and a 5-year disease-specific OS of only 29 % (41). This outstandingly poor prognosis for RMS in adults stands in sharp contrast to the 5-year OS rate among children with gynecologic RMS

(2, 75). Young women over 20 already have a noticeably poorer prognosis than younger women (53). Regarding these age-specific prognostic differences, it is assumed that childhood RMS and RMS in adults are biologically different tumors, an assumption that is somewhat reflected in the different histological variants (PRMS common in adult women!). For instance, adult RMS behave similarly to other STS in that they show a poor response to CHT (53), which apparently is connected with an elevated level of chemoresistancy in adult tumors (66). It is indeed so that expression of the "multidrug resistance proteins" in adult ERMS and PRMS becomes stronger as patient age increases. By contrast, ARMS showed no increased levels of expression of these proteins despite exhibiting poor chemoreactivity (66). However, it has been assumed that RMS in adults have not been treated with modern CHT regimens with the same frequency and consistency as childhood RMS (42). A small study covering only cervical RMS revealed no influence of patient age on prognosis (69).

Five-year OS for all stage I cervical sarcomas lies between 80 % and 67 %, while the rates for stages II and III are 42 % and 20 %, respectively, and 33 % resp. 11 % for stages IVA and IVB (6). Cervical RMS do not have a significantly less favorable DFS and OS compared to all other cervical (!) sarcoma types. However, higher stages of disease are indeed associated with poorer prognostic data (6).

ERMS of all sites in female patients aged ≤ 19 years have a 5-year OS of 69 % (116). For genital ERMS in girls and women aged up to 21 years, 5-year DFS and OS are 52 % and 92 %, respectively (105). Cervical RMS, which are in fact ERMS in the vast majority of cases, are considered to have a relatively promising prognosis (72), with a DFS that is considerably and an OS that is by trend longer than for RMS localized at other genital (!) sites (41). Deceased patients died within 1–96 mo (median 8 mo) (72). At a median follow-up of 23 mo, only 27 % of patients with cervical ERMS had local recurrence without distant metastasis (69). According to another source, the prognosis for cervical RMS is considerably poorer than for patients with vaginal RMS (55). The latter, however, do not occur in adult women, so that a comparison or transfer of these data to patients beyond childhood is essentially not possible. Overall, ERMS is deemed a favorable histological finding.

In one study, ARMS of all sites in girls and young women aged ≤ 19 years had a 5-year OS of 47 % (116). Cervical ARMS are only rarely encountered (93) and are deemed to have a poorer prognosis than ERMS do (2). According to one source, ARMS that express the PAX3-FKHR fusion gene apparently have a less favorable prognosis than tumors in which the PAX7-FKHR fusion gene is found (114). In further studies, the observation has been made that non-metastatic, PAX3/FOX01 positive ARMS have a significantly poorer course compared to ARMS patients whose tumors test positive for PAX7/FOX01 expression. As already stated above, it is thus recommended that fusion gene status be taken into account in risk assessments for ARMS patients. The prognostic behavior of ARMS is said to resemble that of ERMS, according to some sources (83, 125), a finding that was not mirrored in the results from another study (115). Overall, ARMS is regarded as an unfavorable histological finding (20).

Independent from whether they are classified as favorable or unfavorable histologies but depending on age, both ERMS and ARMS are said to exhibit good chemoreactivity.

PRMS have the worst prognosis. PRMS of all sites have a 5-year OS of 47 % in patients aged ≤ 19 years, while the rate for adults accounts for 53.4 % (42). Prognosis for adult PRMS is in fact even worse than for adult ARMS (116). Eighty-six percent of all adult PRMS already exceed 5 cm in their widest dimension at the time of primary presentation (Fig. 3.1.5) (42).

Fifty-nine percent of 27 women already had extrauterine dissemination at the time of initial presentation. Only 19.2 % of women remained recurrence-free during follow-up. Seventy-three percent had deceased, of whom 53 % had died within 6.5 mo. Disease stage, and whether disease was confined to the uterus or had spread beyond the uterus, had no impact on overall survival in the observed sample (39). ARMS and

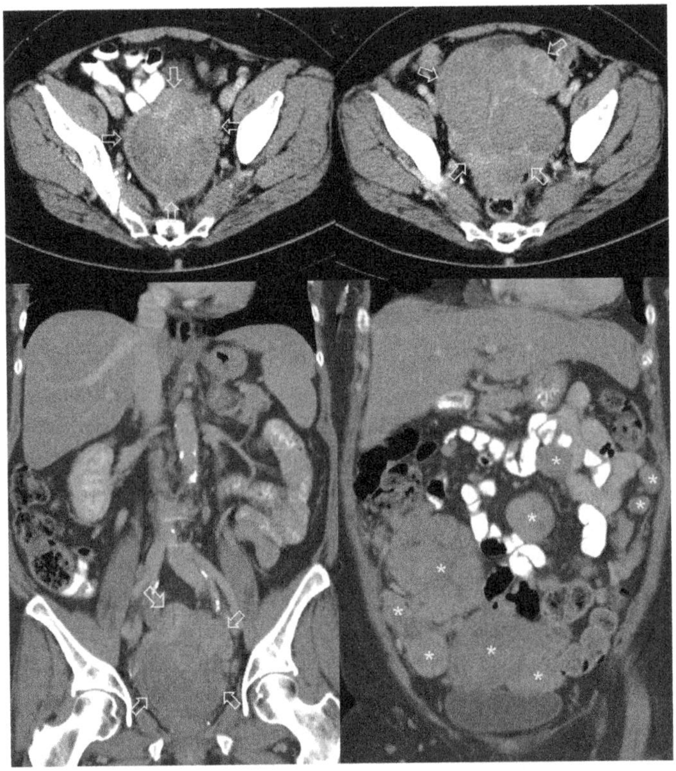

Fig. 3.1.5: 64-year-old patient with pleomorphic rhabdomyosarcoma of the uterus. Axial and coronal abdominal CT in the portal venous phase (top and bottom left) reveal a knotty, nodulated tumor, with inhomogeneous contrast agent enhancement (arrows), that originates from the uterus and that extends far into the vagina (8 × 9 × 11 cm); two months later (top and bottom right), the primary tumor had grown substantially (14 × 11 × 13 cm) and peritoneal metastases could be observed (stars).

PRMS generally have a poorer prognosis than ERMS and its different variants (2). Overall, both clinically and biologically, PRMS apparently more closely resemble high-grade STS than they do pediatric RMS (42).

All genital rhabdomyosarcomas belong to the group of rhabdomyosarcomas in favorable localizations. Generally, localized embryonal rhabdomyosarcomas of the female genital tract have a promising prognosis, regardless of lymph node and resection status. All patients with alveolar rhabdomyosarcomas are classified as being at intermediate risk. Pleomorphic rhabdomyosarcomas are always deemed high-risk tumors. The presence of distant metastasis is always an unfavorable prognostic factor. Lymph node positivity and/or positive resection margins are further adverse prognostic factors for non-embryonal rhabdomyosarcomas. For all variants of rhabdomyosarcoma, a patient age of > 20 years, a tumor diameter ≥ 5 cm, and non-subjection to chemotherapy are further negative prognostic variables. Radiation therapy only has an insignificant influence on overall survival. The prognostic factors pertaining to pleomorphic genital rhabdomyosarcomas are largely congruent to those of the other types of high-grade genital sarcoma.

3.1.7 Primary surgery

Recommendations differ between the USA and Europe in terms of whether primary resection or primary CHT with/without RT should be preferred. One substantial reason for this lies in the differing assessments of the surgical risks that an R0 resection involves. The primary approach in cases of childhood RMS must be individually tailored and planned in close cooperation with pediatric oncologists. It is strongly advised that such children be brought into respective studies. Children and adolescents with vaginal RMS (see below) are usually first started on CHT so as to avoid/prevent mutilating surgical interventions (2). Such cases belong exclusively in the hands of pediatric oncologists. Accordingly, more details are not provided here to this end.

In general, ERMS, ARMS, and RMS-NOS should only be subjected to surgical resection prior to CHT if such surgery will not result in genital mutilation or severe reductions in organ functionality, and if complete resection with sufficient surrounding tissue (i.e. a sufficiently wide margin of resection) can be achieved. Affected LN should be subjected to sampling where possible (91). Since adult uterine RMS are generally surgically accessible, surgery is deemed the first treatment method to be considered. As is also the case for the other forms and variants of uterine sarcoma, for uterine RMS, too, the overarching surgical goal is achieving complete resection. Besides tumor size, regional and distant metastasis, and patient age, resection margin status is regarded as one of the key predictors for the further course of disease in adult RMS patients (54). The general minimum requirement is a 0.5 cm wide healthy tissue margin. This recommendation must be adhered to in cases of uterus-sparing surgery. Reresection is indicated if the primary resection margins were not located sufficiently far into non-diseased neighboring tissue (91). If R0 margins are achieved via reresection or if no residual disease can be traced, an RMS can be classified under group I under the condition that primary surgery caused no contamination or tumor cell dissemination (e.g. morcellation). For RMS of the uterine corpus that are subjected to THE, the resection/tissue margins play only a subordinated role, since the entire compartment “uterus” is removed anyway in such cases. Morcellation is contraindicated in all cases. ERMS and ARMS of the uterine corpus should be treated with primary CHT when patients wish to preserve fertility. However, adhering to the necessary disease-free tissue margin of 0.5 cm would barely be possible in such cases anyway. Performing these surgical methods anyway could make postoperative RT necessary that otherwise might not have been necessary beforehand.

Among the 8 adult uterine ERMS/ARMS in the DKSM material database, 4 were surgically treated via TAH, 2 via RAH, 1 via LAVH, and 1 via TVH (65). In a further study (72), 20 ERMS of the cervix and 5 ERMS of the corpus in adult women were surgically removed via THE, tumor resection, conization or “polypectomies”. There is no visible evidence to suggest that adopting conservative surgical approaches had adverse effects on patient prognosis. In an additional survey covering 52 cases of cervical and uterine adult ERMS, for all 10 cases in which the women died, there was no evidence to suggest that their deaths were connected to the surgical method (tumor resection, TAH, RAH, LNE) to which they had been subjected. There were 2 deaths among 12 cases that had been subjected to local resection, and 1 of those 2 patients who died had not received postoperative CHT.

Overall, from the available data, one can conclude that total THE or organ-sparing R0 tumor resection can be regarded as adequate methods of surgical treatment in adult women with ERMS. Accordingly, when there is an urgent desire to preserve fertility and in cases of girls and female adolescents, organ-sparing cervical operations are indeed possible so long as secure R0 resection margins (0.5 cm disease-free tissue margin) can be and are achieved. If these conditions cannot be met in cases of RMS in the cervical region, then primary CHT and radical trachelectomy are further options. Adopting a conservative surgical approach to treating cervical ERMS is also supported and reinforced by numerous casuistics (9, 29, 50, 59, 61, 68). In fact, no residual tumor was traceable in 6 out of 7 patients who underwent “polypectomies” or curettage (72). In addition, for ERMS of the corpus, an SAH leaving R0 resection margins is another possible option. There is currently no indication for performing RAH or RVH on patients with ERMS that are confined to the cervix. Individual case histories have served to provide no evidence that such procedures are beneficial (110).

Only 4 cases of cervical ARMS have been reported to date. In two cases, the patients died of disease within a very short period of time despite having undergone radical HE and subsequent postoperative ERT or CHT (11, 33). The other two patients (21 and 39 years old) both underwent TAH with BSO. One was subsequently put on an adjuvant CHT regimen consisting of VAC (vincristine, actinomycin, cyclophosphamide) and remained disease-free for 20 mo from initial diagnosis (13). In the other case, the patient underwent both VAC CHT and additional ERT (93), and remained free of recurrence or relapse for 3 years after initial presentation (end of follow-up period).

There are no data to suggest that performing a simultaneous BSO offers any benefits for patients with any variant of genital non-ovarian RMS. Doing so could be difficult to justify given the fact that HR expression is essentially always negative in these types of neoplasm. However, in Germany, both adnexa are removed in 75 % of patients with uterine RMS (65). If postoperative RT is planned (see adjuvant therapy) for women who have undergone organ-preserving cervical surgery and who desire to preserve fertility, then the ovaries should be surgically relocated away from the area that is to be irradiated (91).

To date, there is no evidence that subjecting patients with genital RMS to therapeutic systematic (!) pelvic and para-aortic LNE offers any favorable effects in terms of DFS and OS. Among 6 cases of cervical and uterine ERMS (all IRSG group I) that were subjected to pelvic and para-aortic LNE, 3 died within one year, while the others remained recurrence-free for up to 125 mo (41). Another study analyzed 11 cases of cervical RMS (10 ERMS, 1 PRMS), 5 of which were found in adult women (86). Conization was performed in 7 cases, 1 patient underwent a polypectomy, and four were subjected to TAH with or without BSO. None of the patients underwent an LNE. Only one patient died of disease during the follow-up period. The extent of surgery to which patients were subjected appeared to have no influence on survival. According to a further meta-analysis (72), among 26 women with uterine and cervical ERMS who underwent LNE, there were a total of 6 deaths. In contrast, only 2 of the 12 women who merely underwent tumor resection died. In a further study, among women aged > 40 years with cervical RMS (all group I), the same number of deaths were registered for women who underwent LNE as among those who did not (4).

Genital RMS generally have a relatively promising prognosis, even when there is LN involvement (67). Since the available data suggest that performing an LNE per se has no apparent effect on DFS and OS, there is no indication for subjecting ERMS and ARMS patients to therapeutic systematic (!) pelvic and para-aortic LNE. Besides, the para-aortic LN are not regional LN for these tumor variants. According to the German Guidelines for STS, the practice of performing systematic LNE under the indication of therapeutically treating LN metastases is deemed obsolete (112).

These data notwithstanding, the extent and mode of adjuvant therapy in cases of ERMS and ARMS are dependent on LN status (cf. Tab. 3.1.6). Primary classification as N0 or N1 is made first and foremost on the basis of the results from clinical and imaging diagnostic examinations (cf. Tab. 3.1.1). It is, therefore, necessary that imaging diagnostic examinations via pelvic CT, MRI, or PET-CT (where applicable) are performed prior to subjecting ERMS and ARMS to definitive therapeutic intervention. The current PDQ recommendation and study protocols (35, 91) explicitly recommend that LN status be confirmed through LN biopsy or sampling of LN that appear suspicious either clinically or in imaging. SLN biopsies should be performed whenever doing so appears to be possible (35). There is no indication for a systematic LNE. Such intervention can, however, be considered if subsequent RT is contraindicated (35). Positive LN above/beyond the communis vessels are already classified as distant metastasis.

Cases in which ERMS or ARMS are incidentally discovered postoperatively should be referred to imaging diagnostic examinations in order to assess LN status. PET-CT should be included in unclear cases. Otherwise, performing selective LNE is a sensible option to opt for. Attention must be drawn to the fact that postoperative RT should also be performed in such cases in which removed LN are histologically found to be without disease, despite having been classified as "positive" via prior clinical and imaging diagnostic examination (91).

No data or information are available pertaining to endoscopic procedures like TLH or LAVH without injury to the uterus. The downside of these procedures is that they do not allow for clinically suspicious LN to be palpated. Therefore, such surgical procedures must be viewed critically in cases in which no imaging procedures have been conducted or in which the results from such procedures are unclear.

The approach to be applied in cases of ERMS and ARMS in children, young women, and women who wish to preserve fertility is described in the subchapter on primary CHT.

The data situation pertaining to the surgical approach to be adopted for PRMS is very bleak. In one metastudy (39) that included 27 PRMS, an LNE was performed in 10 cases. Of these women, 3 had no recurrence, 2 survived despite recurrence, and 5 died during the follow-up period. Individual case reports indicate that RAH apparently has no influence on survival in PRMS patients (96). The same analysis also revealed no benefits from performing a BSO (39). There is one account of a child with PRMS undergoing a successful "polypectomy" and subsequent CHT (12). However, the results stemming from this case cannot be transferred or translated to PRMS in adult women.

Current NCCN Guidelines for soft tissue sarcomas envisage that PRMS be treated like the other forms of uterine sarcoma and STS (92, 112), which categorically excludes organ-sparing surgical strategies from being opted for PRMS patients. Consequently, THE without injuring or damaging the uterus is the therapeutic method of choice. Analogous to the other pure uterine sarcomas and STS, there is no justification for a systematic LNE. The same also applies to selective LNE, not least because no generally accepted conclusions pertaining to adjuvant therapy can be drawn from the results of said procedure. Details are provided in the respective chapters on the other forms and variants of uterine sarcoma.

In advanced ERMS and ARMS, primary tumor debulking should not be opted for if it is or becomes clear prior to or during surgery that there will be residual disease (group III) (91). This recommendation is founded in the fact that there is no evidence to suggest that such intervention offers more favorable OS compared to biopsy with subsequent CHT (14). Therefore, for localized cervical ERMS and ARMS in children and young women, it is sensible to first opt for CHT (62), a strategy that is in line with the generally preferred approach to treating the genitalia of children.

Subjecting advanced RMS to primary resection is only recommended under the condition that the tumor appears to be R0 resectable and that injury to vital neighboring organs and tissue can be ruled out (14, 71). This recommendation only refers to the surgical approach for children and cannot generally be carried over to adult patients. Attention is and should be drawn to the fact that primary debulking, even when postoperative residual disease would be the consequence (R1/2 situation, group III), is indicated in cases in which retroperitoneal or otherwise localized tumors could cause or already have caused dysfunctions (e.g. intestinal obstruction, ureteral compression) (14, 91). This can apply to adult women with pelvic retroperitoneal or abdominal RMS. Accordingly, indications for extensive surgical procedures (e.g. bowel resections) must be addressed differently than in pediatric cases in which CHT would first be attempted. The PDQ recommendations do not even exclude exenterations for adult genital RMS, if such a procedure appears to be successfully performable in the given case. However, if there is already distant metastatic disease, tumor debulking is not deemed a sensible approach (except in acutely threatening situations) (91).

Surgical management of advanced uterine PRMS should be approached analogous to other high-grade uterine sarcomas like LMS and UUS (cf. Vol. 1, Chapters 2 and 5).

Total hysterectomy is the therapeutic method of choice for uterine embryonal and alveolar rhabdomyosarcomas in adult women. For young women and women who desire to preserve fertility, organ-sparing operations leaving a 0.5 cm wide disease-free tissue margin are possible. For cervical tumors, local resections, conizations or even trachelectomies are eligible surgical procedures in this regard. Tumors in the uterine corpus can be excised via supracervical hysterectomy. Morcellation is contraindicated in any case. Reresection is indicated in cases in which primary resection fails to achieve the required resection margin status. Performing an ovarectomy is not necessary. It is generally recommended that lymph nodes that appear suspicious in clinical and imaging diagnostic examinations be subjected to selective lymphonodectomy. Said procedure is also important for the context of planning adequate adjuvant therapy. There is no indication for performing a (therapeutic) systematic pelvic and para-aortic lymphonodectomy. The aforementioned procedure can be indicated if postoperative radiation therapy is contraindicated and lymph nodes are positive.

Advanced tumors can be subjected to primary cytoreduction if fulfilling the conditions of an R0 resection appears to be possible either intraoperatively or according to the results from imaging diagnostics. Cytoreductive operations with residual tumor should only be carried out in cases of jeopardized organ functionality.

Surgical management of uterine pleomorphic rhabdomyosarcomas should be approached analogous to other uterine sarcomas. Hysterectomy without injuring or damaging the uterus is the therapeutic method of choice.

3.1.8 Adjuvant and additive radio-, chemo- and hormone therapy

Which forms of adjuvant therapy are necessary is guided by the RMS risk groups (cf. Tabs. 3.1.6 and 3.1.7). In contrast to the other types of genital sarcoma, RT is regarded as an important component of the multimodal treatment of childhood ERMS, ARMS, and RMS-NOS. The current recommendations in this regard almost exclusively refer to pediatric patients. There are currently no standards for adult ERMS and

ARMS, and there is a lack of adequate studies to this end. Due to the lack of data that specifically pertain to adult ERMS and ARMS, one can largely draw on studies that are devoted to childhood sarcomas, not least because women up to the age of 40 who have ERMS or ARMS should be treated in accordance with the criteria that are in place for children and adolescents (112).

Postoperative RT is not necessary in cases in which group I ERMS have been fully resected (78). In contrast, such treatment is indicated for all group I ARMS and RMS-NOS as well as for all ERMS patients who are LN positive and/or in whom only R1/2 resection margins have been achieved (all group IIA, IIB, IIC, III) (cf. Tab. 3.1.7) (104, 106, 126).

The field of irradiation is generally determined by the extent of disease prior to surgery or CHT, and includes the regions in which affected LN are located. Maintaining a safety margin of 2 cm is generally recommended (91, 126). Potentially necessary CHT should be performed prior to RT. The common dose of irradiation is 1.8 Gy/d 5 d per week over 5–6 weeks (91), while the cumulative dose should be between 36 and 50 Gy. The total cumulative dose to be administered in an individual case depends on the extent of residual disease and on LN status (105). During ERT, the administration of actinomycin D should be suspended when patients are on VAC-CHT (123). In the IRSG studies, RT was initiated after 6 weeks in group II, and after 12 weeks in group III (2).

RT for patients with cervical and uterine tumors can also take the form of VBT. Standalone VBT is deemed sufficient for cases of tumors at applicators wall with a size of < 4 cm, while tumors that exceed these dimensions should be subjected to a combination of VBT and ERT. This approach serves to keep the rate to which side effects arise low. Standalone ERT will be performed if VBT is not feasible (73).

To date, there are no adequate studies that specifically refer to the use of adjuvant CHT in adult uterine RMS. In one meta-analysis covering 52 operated adult cervical ERMS, 3 out of 5 (60 %) patients who received no postoperative treatment whatsoever died. Two of 4 (50 %) women who only underwent postoperative RT died, as did 2 of 8 (25 %) patients who were postoperatively treated with RT-CHT. These data allow the conclusion to be drawn, albeit with caution, that subjecting women with cervical ERMS to clinical observation or postoperative RT alone constitutes inadequate practice. Of 25 evaluable cases in which the patient received adjuvant CHT, only 2 (8 %) were deceased during the follow-up period.

One study on a sample of 10 cervical RMS was unable to prove beyond doubt that adjuvant CHT has a beneficial effect on patient prognosis (69). In another study, 12 of 14 child and adult patients with cervical ERMS remained disease-free following local resection and VAC-CHT (29). Only very few cases of cervical ARMS have been adequately described in the literature. In one account, a patient who underwent TAH plus adjuvant RT and CHT remained disease-free for three years (end of follow-up), while in another case, a patient who had been subjected to RAH with adjuvant pelvic ERT plus VAI-CHT relapsed and subsequently succumbed to her disease within 3 mo. However, in the latter case, the parametria and the uterine serosa had already been primarily involved. Genital RMS that are already advanced at the time of primary diagnosis/presentation appear to have a poor prognosis even when subjected to surgery and adjuvant CHT (48).

Overall 3-year DFS and 3-year OS for childhood (aged ≤ 19 years) RMS of all types and variants subjected to postoperative CHT are 77 % and 86 %, respectively. CHT effects a more favorable prognosis for patients with tumors in the groups I and II in particular.

In one study, adult RMS of all sites (!) that were treated with pediatric CHT regimens had a 5-year OS that was superior to that measured for patients who did not undergo CHT or who received inadequate CHT regimens (60 % vs. 40 %) (42). Among 16 girls with genital ERMS who received CHT, the 5-year DFS was 52 % and 5-year OS was 92 %. Putting patients with RMS of all variants and all genital (!) localizations on adjuvant CHT regimens thus tends to have beneficial effects on both PFS and OS. However, the differences are not statistically significant (41). A different study came to the conclusion that adjuvant CHT does not serve to significantly improve OS in adult women (53). The disappointing results, despite adequate surgical treatment, were most likely a result of adjuvant CHT being applied too rarely, the administration of inadequate CHT regimens, and a relatively large proportion of PRMS in the samples. However, virtually identical response rates and survival data are achieved when adult RMS are stratified according to the prognostic factors for pediatric RMS (42).

It is, therefore, insistently recommended that pediatric CHT protocols also be applied to adult ERMS and ARMS patients (42). Accordingly, all ERMS, ARMS, and RMS-NOS patients should receive adjuvant CHT. The approach suggested in Tab. 3.1.7 also corresponds to what is recommended for RMS of the female genital tract (2). The time period between surgery and adjuvant CHT should not exceed 8 weeks.

For low-risk cases (ERMS group I, IIA), the two-drug VA-regimen is deemed sufficient (Tab. 3.1.7) (105), a regimen that is relatively uncomplicated and that will effect a reaction in most uterine RMS (cf. therapy proposal). The total time period of CHT

Tab. 3.1.7: Adjuvant/additive chemo- or radiochemotherapy for genital embryonal and alveolar rhabdomyosarcomas and RMS-NOS (2, 22, 82, 91, 105, 106, 126).

Chemotherapy VA	Chemotherapy VAC	Plus radiotherapy
ERMS	All ARMS/RMS-NOS*	All ARMS/RMS-NOS*
Group I, IIA	All N1	All N1
		All group IIA - III#

VA Vincristine plus actinomycin (abbreviated protocol with reduced cyclophosphamide dose is possible), **VAC** Vincristine plus actinomycin plus ifosfamide, * due to their unclear typification, RMS-NOS should be allocated to ARMS in order to prevent undertreatment (35), # does not apply to ERMS N0 that have been R0 resected either primarily or following chemotherapy; radiotherapy can also be omitted in cases of R0 resected N0 ARMS.

administration is 22 weeks. Collaboration with hemato-oncologists and/or pediatric oncologists should be categorically sought.

For all other cases (except PRMS), three-drug VAC-CHT in accordance with "Intergroup Rhabdomyosarcoma Study Protocol IV" is the standard CHT regimen to be administered (3, 22, 91). Cyclophosphamide can be replaced with ifosfamide (VAI-CHT). A combination of vincristine, ifosfamide, and etoposide is deemed equally effective (22). Alternating VAC with vincristine, topotecan, and cyclophosphamide yielded no difference in effect (3). The relatively high levels of toxicity, especially in the "three-drug regimens", must be borne in mind, and the maximum permissible doses must be strictly adhered to. CHT was administered over a period of 42 to 45 weeks depending on protocol, but usually over a 25-week period. More recent data suggest that stage I group IIB/C ERMS can also be treated under a reduced treatment protocol in which the cumulative cyclophosphamide dose is reduced from 26.4 to 4.8 g/m^2. The study in question covered patients aged up to 50 years with tumors of all sites (123).

The discussed CHT and CHT-RT regimens are highly toxic and can bear lethal consequences for the patients subjected to them. Accordingly, they should only be administered by experienced medicinal oncologists. In contrast to the other types of uterine sarcoma, additive CHT or CHT-RT is also indicated for cases in which there is postoperative residual disease (group III) (22).

The few known case studies of PRMS do not allow any definitive conclusions to be drawn as to the effects that adjuvant CHT and RT have on DFS and OS in patients with these tumors (96). No impact on survival could be identified in a group of 27 women with PRMS (38, 39). Among 12 women who received adjuvant CHT, 10 died during the 12 mo follow-up period, 1 relapsed, and only 1 remained disease-free. One patient with uterine PRMS (IRSG group III) who underwent TAH with BSO and postoperative RT relapsed after 3 mo and died of disease within 5 mo. In a different, smaller study, 2 of 12 (16 %) patients who received adjuvant CHT and 7 of 23 (30 %) who did not developed distant metastasis (42). However, the share of genital PRMS in said study could not be discerned. Overall, it has yet to be evidenced in valid, reliable scientific studies that adjuvant CHT has a beneficial effect on DFS and OS in PRMS patients. Furthermore, it is known that the chemosensitivity of ARMS and PRMS in patients aged > 20 years is significantly lower than in younger patients and roughly corresponds to that of adult STS (53). The study comes to the overall conclusion that it remains scientifically unproven that CHT has positive prognostic effects on adult ARMS and PRMS, though it must be borne in mind that the sample of said study did not include any urogenital RMS.

In light of the fact that PRMS almost exclusively arise in adult women, the poor prognosis with which PRMS are associated, the lack of specific standards, and the fact that PRMS are predominantly not included in scientific studies, the NCCN Guidelines for soft tissue sarcomas (92) recommend that treatment strategies be designed in accordance to the criteria for STS. Against this backdrop, analogous to the other forms of uterine sarcoma and in contrast to ERMS and ARMS, administering adjuvant CHT cannot be regarded as standard practice, not least because adequate studies have yet to provide evidence that doing so offers any benefits in terms of DFS and OS. Therefore, the recommendations and guidelines pertaining to uterine LMS or UUS (cf. Vol. 1, Chapters 2 and 5) can be adhered to in such cases.

Therapy proposal VA-CHT regimen for low-risk embryonal rhabdomyosarcomas

Vincristine 1.5 mg/m² i.v. (max. single dose 2 mg) d 1, 8, 15, 22, 3 wk interv., tot. 4 cycles +
Actinomycin-D 1.5 mg/m² (max. single dose 2 mg) d 1 and 22, 3 wk interv., tot. 4 cycles

The highly toxic to life threatening three-drug regimens, especially when combined with RT, belong in the hands of hemato-oncologists. They are, however, set out in the (albeit confidential) "CWS-Guidance for risk adapted treatment of soft tissue sarcoma and soft tissue tumours in children, adolescents, and young adults" of the Cooperative Weichteilsarkom Studiengruppe (CWS) of the Gesellschaft für Pädiatrische Onkologie und Hämatologie (GPOH) (Version 1.6. from 12/12/2012; Stuttgart, Germany 2012). If required, they can be requested from the Studienzentrum: Olgahospital, Klinikum Stuttgart, Bismarckstraße 8, D-70176 Stuttgart or the responsible hemato-oncologist or pediatric oncologist and be discussed in lieu of the specific case at hand.

There is no indication for adjuvant or additive HT.

With the exception of definitively R0 resected embryonal rhabdomyosarcomas without lymph node involvement, postoperative radiotherapy is indicated for all uterine embryonal and alveolar rhabdomyosarcomas. All rhabdomyosarcomas except pleomorphic rhabdomyosarcomas should be subjected to adjuvant chemotherapy. For R0 resected embryonal rhabdomyosarcomas without lymph node involvement, a combination of vincristine and actinomycin is deemed sufficient. A combination of vincristine, actinomycin D, and cyclophosphamide is indicated for all other cases. Radiotherapy should be incorporated into chemotherapy. Adjuvant chemotherapy with/without radiotherapy is also indicated when cytoreductive surgery has been performed.

Pleomorphic rhabdomyosarcomas are generally not subjected to postoperative radiotherapy and/or adjuvant chemotherapy in practice. In general, an approach should be adopted that is analogous to the approach envisaged for soft tissue sarcomas or the other types of uterine sarcoma.

3.1.9 Primary radiation, hormone and chemotherapy, approach in cases of general inoperability

For children and adolescents, THE is classified as a mutilating surgical intervention. Accordingly, pediatric uterine RMS are primarily treated via CHT. In these cases, securing of the histological diagnosis is followed by neoadjuvant or primary CHT/RT-CHT. There are known accounts in which CR or PR with only small residual disease were observed after or during CHT (18, 92, 106). Among 11 cases of uterine RMS, CHT served to spare the uterus in 8, though additional ERT or BT were administered in some of these cases (75). High levels of toxicity through CHT and RT and also deaths must be reckoned with (18). THE must follow if CHT or CHT-RT do not effect a CR. Respective cases are matters for pediatric oncologists and are not elaborated further here. R0 resectable cervical ERMS and ARMS can also be subjected to primary surgery.

One study (14) showed that performing biopsy and subsequently administering neoadjuvant CHT to patients with locally advanced ERMS and ARMS did not result in a significantly poorer PFI or OS compared to patients who underwent biopsy with consecutive cytoreductive surgery that left gross residual disease (group III). Notwithstanding, both PFI and OS were marginally better in the group subjected to primary debulking. This is likely to be because CHT administered after cytoreduction achieves better response rates than primary CHT (14). Primary cytoreductive surgery leaving residual disease is nonetheless not recommended except for exceptional cases (91). If locally advanced tumors do not pose an acute threat to organ functionality and an R0 resection thereof appears to be unachievable, it is indicated that securing the diagnosis via biopsy should be followed by neoadjuvant CHT, usually in combination with RT (71). There is currently no evidence that interval surgery following primary CHT or CHT-RT has favorable effects on OS. PFI is apparently only improved when no viable tumor tissue can be found following CHT (103). Administering RT after residual viable tumor tissue has been R0 resected can serve to increase PFI, but not OS (103).

Analogous to the recommendations pertaining to pediatric tumors, primary CHT is a viable possibility for cases of ERMS and ARMS in young women and/or women with an urgent desire to preserve fertility. Both MRI and preoperative PET-CT are urgently recommended for such cases so as to be able to safely exclude possible LN involvement and the presence of distant metastasis. If the tumor cannot be detected via imaging diagnostics after administration of CHT, then resection is no longer necessary, analogous to the pediatric treatment protocols. Cases have been reported in which complete remissions were achieved in children and adolescents (18). In one study, administering primary CHT served to reduce the frequency of HE by 48 % in group I/II and by 22 % in group III/IV (2). Regarding women who desired to preserve their fertility, it must be borne in mind that RT was also undergone in many cases and that the data refer to persons up to the age of 17.

Primary CHT, possibly in combination with RT, is indicated for cases of generally inoperable disease. Standalone RT can be opted for in cases of genital RMS in which CHT is contraindicated. However, there are no studies that are devoted specifically to this question.

The VAC-CHT protocol is generally the method of choice to be applied in the context of primary or neoadjuvant CHT (91). One report describes an account of an ERMS in which primary VAC-CHT and subsequent combination therapy with cisplatin and etoposide yielded no response (57). In contrast, one study reports a case of uterine ARMS in which application of the VAC-regimen effected a clear preoperative remission that allowed subsequent resection to be performed. Following additional postoperative VAC-CHT, the patient remained disease-free for 20 mo (end of follow-up) (13). Required surgery is usually performed after the 12th week of CHT in the majority of cases. In the neoadjuvant context, patients are generally not given RT prior to undergoing planned resection (2). RT is no longer indicated if R0 resection is successful and there is no LN involvement (2). When there is residual disease or when patients are N1, RT should be applied 12 weeks after surgery (2).

Overall, the benefits of interval surgery (delayed primary operation, second-look intervention) are disputed. The primary advantage of such an approach is that it allows for remaining viable tumor tissue to be detected. However, when viable tumor tissue is detected, only the PFI is shortened, but not OS (103). Interval surgery is thus only deemed sensible if an R0 resection appears to be achievable. If this succeeds, RT can possibly be omitted or the RT dose can be reduced (91). This is of relevance for cases in which the patient wishes to retain the functionality of the ovaries. Primary CHT should be administered by medicinal oncologists due to the potentially lethal risks with which the measure is associated.

There is no recommended course of action for cases in which there is primary distant metastatic disease. Uterine or cervical tumors that are operable should be subjected to surgery. If the metastases are open to R0 resection according to imaging diagnostic criteria, then they, too, can be resected, usually in a second surgical session. When patients have already developed lung metastases at the time of primary diagnosis, the primary tumor should be subjected to multimodal treatment. Applying CHT in this context usually also effects metastatic remission. Additionally, resecting the lung metastases is not said to improve prognosis (25). For the majority of cases, the most sensible course of action would therefore be to follow up the uterine operation with CHT, and to then reassess the operability of the metastases. Primary CHT could also be an adequate option. Such cases should be elaborately discussed in multidisciplinary tumor conferences involving gynecologists, the specialists responsible for metastasis surgery, radiologists, and hemato-oncologists.

One publication reports that an RR of > 50 % was yielded in a sample of 7 adult patients with PRMS by administering vincristine, doxorubicin, and ifosfamide in the additive and neoadjuvant contexts (95). This regimen thus also appears to be suitable for primary or neoadjuvant CHT in PRMS patients. Further chemotherapeutic options are discussed under palliative CHT. If no response can be achieved, CHT regimens should be resorted to in line with the NCCN Guidelines for soft tissue sarcomas (92) that are also effective for treating STS.

A combination of doxorubicin and ifosfamide should most likely be considered in such cases.

There is no indication for primary hormone therapy for all kinds of rhabdomyosarcoma.

In cases of uterine embryonal and alveolar rhabdomyosarcomas, when surgery is contraindicated or if patients wish to preserve their fertility, primary chemotherapy using a combination of vincristine, actinomycin D, and cyclophosphamide can be administered. Complete remission makes resection unnecessary. In cases of advanced localized disease in which organ functionality is not acutely jeopardized and for which successful R0 resection does not appear to be achievable, securing the diagnosis via biopsy and subsequent neoadjuvant CHT is generally indicated. R0 resection should be aspired to via interval surgery in cases of residual disease. Radiotherapy is indicated if R0 resection is not possible or if residual disease remains. Pleomorphic rhabdomyosarcomas can be treated with the same aforementioned chemotherapeutic regimen, both primarily and in the neoadjuvant context. Overall, however, the rules and guidelines described for the other types of uterine sarcoma apply. There is no indication for primary hormone therapy for all kinds of rhabdomyosarcoma.

3.1.10 Aftercare, recurrences, metastases

There are no evidence-based data concerning aftercare. Aftercare should, therefore, be arranged analogous to the other types of uterine sarcoma, which includes clinical examination, an x-ray of the thorax, and sonographic examination of the genital region every 3 mo plus an MRI of the tumor bed every 6 mo in years 1 to 3. Conventional x-ray diagnostics of the lung should be complemented with a CT when there is suspicion of disease recurrence. In isolated cases (ARMS in particular), a bone scintigraphy or an F-18-fluoride-PET(/CT) can be performed. Depending on the individual case, PET(/CT) can also be applied as a means for monitoring treatment response or in cases in which there is concrete suspicion of relapse. In years 4 and 5, the intervals between the aforementioned measures should be 6 mo, though MRI can optionally be conducted every 12 mo. From year 6 onwards, intervals of 12 mo are deemed sufficient, and can be extended to 24 mo as of year 11. However, more intensive diagnostics should be undertaken if patients present with symptoms (71, 92, 112).

Among pediatric RMS (excluding PRMS) that have been subjected to primary treatment, recurrences and/or distant metastasis occur as local or locoregional recurrences (including LN recurrences) in 76 %, as only distant metastatic disease in 15 %, and as both locoregional recurrences and distant metastases in 9 % of cases (17). However, these figures refer to all primary disease localizations and can only be said to apply to genital RMS to a limited degree.

According to one larger study, poor prognosis for metastatic ERMS, RMS-NOS, and ARMS is strongly linked to the following factors: prior RT, initial tumor size > 5 cm, time of relapse < 18 mo from primary diagnosis, unfavorable primary disease site, nodal involvement at the time of primary diagnosis, ARMS and previous 3- or 6-drug CHT (17). The chance of cure can be estimated on the basis of these factors using a respective nomogram (17). However, the estimations are based on pediatric and adolescent RMS and exclude PRMS.

Aftercare for uterine rhabdomyosarcomas largely corresponds to aftercare for other uterine sarcoma types. Recurrences and metastases arise as local or locoregional recurrences in 76 %, as distant metastases in 15 %, and as both locoregional recurrences and distant metastases in 9 % of cases.

3.1.11 Surgical management and postoperative additive therapy for recurrences and metastatic disease

The following data almost exclusively refer to pediatric ERMS and ARMS of all sites. As is also the case with primary therapy, the conclusions drawn from the data can also be applied to adult RMS. Among all uterine RMS with local recurrence or regional LN involvement, ERMS that were small, in stage 1 and in group I at initial presentation had the most promising prognosis (24, 77). Distant metastasis, prior RT, a primary tumor size of > 5 cm, and a PFI of < 18 mo are deemed unfavorable prognostic factors for OS following relapse (17, 26).

There are currently no standards concerning the approach to be adopted in cases of recurrent disease or metastasis. For adult RMS of all sites that are accompanied by distant metastasis, applying a multimodal treatment strategy consisting of resection, CHT, and RT is associated with significant benefits for both PFI and OS (31). Treatment in these situations should thus be approached as it is in the context of primary treatment, in that it adheres to a respective concept, for which several options are available. These include: CHT with/without local therapeutic intervention (resection with/without RT); primary resection with subsequent CHT; or RT with subsequent surgical intervention. Case-specific decisions on which alternative to opt for should be made on the basis of operability/resectability in cooperation with pediatric or medicinal oncologists. Patients who have an estimated chance of cure below 10 % according to the prognostic nomogram for recurrences (17) should be offered experimental therapy (17).

Multimodal therapeutic strategies for locally recurrent or metastatic tumors that include resection have a noticeably better prognosis than those that do not (28, 54). The time period until death is significantly longer for patients (all localizations, ≤ 18 years) who receive both surgery and CHT than for those whose treatment plan does not include surgery (54). Thirty-seven percent of patients who underwent surgery were disease-free after a mean follow-up period of 4.9 years, while 42 % had died within the same time frame. Ninety-two percent of patients who did not undergo resection died (54).

Local recurrences should generally be resected. More radical surgical methods, even exenterations, are indicated in cases in which there is no distant metastasis (extensive bone metastases in particular) (28, 54). Resecting isolated lung metastases also appears to be a sensible option (54), though an R0 resection needs to be achievable in such cases in order to opt for said approach. Where radical surgery is being considered, the possibility and tenability of the surgical complications that can potentially arise must be balanced against overall prognosis. Whether primary resection or primary CHT should be preferred is thus also dependent on the localization and resectability/operability of disease (34). Notwithstanding, CHT should constitute part of any treatment strategy for recurrent disease. RT should first be applied to the region that is to be operated on, unless said region has previously already been irradiated. In those rare cases in which the region in question has already been subjected to irradiation and where surgical resection is not possible in said region, repeat RT can be considered (91).

The combinations CHT plus successful R0 resection without RT, and R1/2 resection with RT are regarded as adequate approaches to the local treatment of ARMS. According to one study, 50 % of ARMS patients who have a circumscribed recurrence survive if treated with adequate local relapse therapy including CHT (26). Disseminated recurrences and/or metastases that are not accessible to adequate local treatment generally have a poorer prognosis.

CHT regimens in this context should use effective agents that have not yet been tried in the given case, and can be administered either as a monotherapy or combination therapy. Adequate CHT regimens are discussed in the following section.

Local recurrences and distant metastases of PRMS should be treated in accordance with the principles and guidelines for the other types of soft tissue or uterine sarcomas (e.g. LMS and UUS, Vol. 1, Chapters 2 and 5) (92).

Treatment of recurrences and metastases of embryonal and alveolar rhabdomyosarcomas should be multimodal. Chemotherapy with/without secondary resection and/or radiation therapy, primary resection with subsequent chemotherapy, or radiation therapy with subsequent surgery are the respective options in this regard. Deciding which of these strategies to opt for must be guided by the operability of the findings. Local recurrences should rather be subjected to surgical therapy. More extensive surgical procedures can be adequate in individual cases. Local recurrences and metastases of pleomorphic rhabdomyosarcomas should be treated in accordance with the principles in place for the other types of soft tissue sarcoma and uterine sarcoma.

3.1.12 Palliative radiotherapy, chemotherapy and hormone therapy, therapy with small molecules

RT is indicated in cases of general inoperability or when there is a solitary recurrence and/or metastasis. Regions that have previously already been irradiated can be re-subjected to irradiation upon consultation of the radiologist (91). Such RT should be administered in combination with CHT as a general rule. Patients with inoperable or diffuse recurrences and metastases should be referred to systemic therapy. In the majority of cases, patients with ERMS and ARMS will have previously already undergone VAC or VAI-CHT, either adjuvantly or in the context of treating recurrence. If they have not, then the aforementioned regimens constitute the treatment method of choice. If they have, a combination of cyclophosphamide plus topotecan can be applied, which has been shown to have an RR of 66 % in recurrent or otherwise CHT refractory ARMS and ERMS (as well as 20 % SD) (111). Irinotecan plus vincristine is another possible combination. One study measured a 1-year PFI and 1-year OS of 38 % and 60 % for this regimen, respectively (76). PR and SD were observed in 36 % resp. 30 % of cases. In a phase II trial, subjecting patients with metastatic RMS to topotecan monotherapy yielded an RR of 46 % (4 % CR, 42 % PR). ARMS showed better responses than ERMS. Nothing could be said in terms of survival, as topotecan constituted but one element of a larger CHT package (100). A CR was achieved in one isolated case of recurrent uterine ERMS with a combination of ifosfamide and mitomycin D (5).

In one trial, administering a regimen of vincristine, doxorubicin, and ifosfamide to patients with extragenital PRMS yielded an RR of 86 % (95). However, only 55 % of patients were still alive after a follow-up period of 2 years.

According to the results from one piece of research, patients with locally recurrent or distantly metastatic RMS (all histological types, all sites) who showed a CR to CHT had a 5-year OS of 57 %, compared to only 7 % among those patients who responded poorly or not at all (34). Treatment for patients with ERMS and ARMS should be planned and given in cooperation with hemato-oncologists and pediatric oncologists.

For PRMS, those CHT regimens should be applied to which the other STS are also responsive (92), most prominently a combined doxorubicin and ifosfamide regimen. Further options are described in the chapter on LMS (Vol. 1, Chapter 2).

There is a report of one account in which a PR was achieved in an ARMS patient by administering the TKI pazopanib following unsuccessful treatment with VAC-CHT (51).

Therapy proposal (embryonal and alveolar rhabdomyosarcomas) upon exhaustion of the standard therapeutic options

Irinotecan 50 mg/m^2 i.v. d 1–5, wks 1; 4; 13; 25; 34; 49 + Vincristine 1.5 mg/m^2 d 1, wks 1; 2; 4; 5; 13; 14; 25; 26; 34; 35; 46; 47; 49; 50

Cyclophosphamide 250 mg/m^2 i.v. + Topotecan 0.75 mg/m^2 i.v. d 1–5, q 3 wks

Therapy proposal (pleomorphic rhabdomyosarcoma)

Doxorubicin 25 mg/m^2 i.v. d 1–3 + Ifosfamid 2.5 g/m^2 i.v. d 1–4 q 3 wks

There is no indication for palliative hormone therapy.

Radiotherapy is indicated in cases of general inoperability or when local recurrences and metastases are inoperable. Radiotherapy in such cases should, as a general rule, be accompanied by chemotherapy. Persistently inoperable or diffuse recurrences and metastases must be referred to modes of systemic therapy that are effective in achieving responses in rhabdomyosarcomas. Pleomorphic rhabdomyosarcomas are largely treated analogous to the other types and variants of soft tissue sarcoma.

3.2 Extrauterine rhabdomyosarcoma

3.2.1 Rhabdomyosarcoma of the ovary and the fallopian tube

General, pathogenesis, pathologico-anatomical features

Primary ovarian RMS are the absolute exception. Ovarian and vulvar RMS account for 19.4 % of RMS of the female genital tract in patients aged up to 19 years (64). Ovarian RMS occur both in children and in adults. One overview reported 13 known cases up to 1998. Patients were aged between 2 and 86 years (mean 35 years) (94). A further 10 pediatric cases were reported up until 2008 (19). RMS of the fallopian tube are extremely rare (10, 44).

There have only been isolated cases of rhabdomyosarcomas arising in the ovary and the fallopian tube in adult women.

The size of ovarian RMS observed to date has ranged between 5–30 cm (mean 16 cm). The tumors are described as being solid or gelatinous and generally exhibit hemorrhages. The cut surface can be grayish-white, yellowish or pink (90, 94). Ovarian RMS are largely ERMS, while ARMS arise in this site more rarely (19, 95). ERMS can exhibit focal pleomorphic components in up to one third of cases (95). Purely ovarian PRMS are the exception (90). In one case, the precise subtype of an RMS located in the tube could not be accurately determined, while another was identified as PRMS (41).

Analogous to uterine RMS, in cases of ovarian RMS, it should first be assumed that the tumor is in fact a CS with a rhabdomyogenic sarcomatous component, not least because CS arise in the ovaries relatively frequently by contrast. The epithelial component can be barely traceable. It is, therefore, imperative that the whole specimen is meticulously examined using cytokeratin markers. This equally applies to ovarian AS with rhabdosarcomatous overgrowth. A large proportion of RMS are in fact merely a component of rare malignant teratomas (62), other malignant mixed germ cell tumors (8), and Sertoli–Leydig cell tumors.

Ovarian rhabdomyosarcomas can only barely be macroscopically discerned from carcinoma. Embryonal, alveolar, and pleomorphic rhabdomyosarcomas can all arise in the ovaries. Carcinosarcomas and germ cell tumors are the most important histologic differential diagnoses.

Clinical presentation, diagnostics, imaging, differential diagnostics

Abdominally palpable, often grossly visible lesions, sometimes accompanied by acute pains, are the fundamental characteristics and symptoms of ovarian RMS (94). Depending on their size, such tumors can cause considerable displacement of neighboring organs and even constrictions of the large veins (19). There have been accounts of ovarian RMS rupturing and causing subsequent bleeding (19, 94). It must generally be borne in mind that an RMS in the ovary could in fact be an ovarian metastasis stemming from an RMS located at a different site (130, 131). In one study on pediatric RMS, the primary tumor was only discovered after the ovarian RMS had been diagnosed as such (131). In children, RMS is said to be the histological tumor type that most frequently metastasizes to the ovaries. Metastasis can occur either bilaterally or unilaterally (131). Pediatric ovarian RMS are almost exclusively embryonal or alveolar. In some cases, the ovarian metastases were only discovered during surgery (131). Metastasis of only the sarcomatous component of a uterine CS is another differential diagnostic option.

A tumor should only be diagnosed as primary ovarian RMS if all DD options – including metastatic tumors emanating from primary tumors at other sites – have been ruled out with a high degree of certainty.

Sonography reveals septate cystic or primarily solid tumors that cannot be safely differentiated from OC (90). Similarly, in CT, lesions are unspecific and heterogeneous, and their ovarian primary origin can sometimes be discerned (19). MRI characteristics are also rather unspecific (cf. uterine RMS).

Ovarian rhabdomyosarcomas are practically indiscernible from carcinomas, neither clinically nor in terms of their imaging characteristics. They often constitute metastatic disease of rhabdomyosarcomas at other primary sites. Carcinosarcoma with a rhabdomyogenic sarcomatous component must be considered as a differential diagnostic option. Respective appropriate diagnostic measures are always required in this regard.

Course, prognosis, operative, systemic and radiogenic therapy

The majority of RMS are confined to one ovary (94). Roughly 50 % of patients present with stage II or stage IV disease at the time of initial presentation (94). Isolated metastases can occur in the greater omentum (90). It is not rarely the case that ovarian RMS already exhibit extensive spread and are inoperable at first. There are accounts of RMS spontaneously rupturing (19, 94). It is not clear whether or not ovarian RMS can be classified as tumors with a favorable primary localization. So long as this question has not been resolved, in the context of determining adequate subsequent treatment, it appears to be pertinent and safer to place ovarian RMS in the "unfavorable" category. Accordingly, all patients with ovarian RMS must be deemed at intermediate risk. The fact that ovarian RMS generally have a poor overall prognosis serves to support such an approach. As only very few cases of ovarian RMS are known, median and mean PFI and OS as well as 5-year OS cannot be calculated or estimated with any degree of accuracy. In one study, patients who did not survive died within 10 days to 26 mo (94). In one case of RMS of the fallopian tube, the LN were already involved at the time of primary diagnosis.

There are no data pertaining to adequate surgical therapy. This is exacerbated by the fact that the diagnosis "ovarian RMS" is usually only reached intraoperatively. Based on the general standards, guidelines and recommendations for the treatment of RMS, primary ovarectomy must be regarded as the therapeutic method of choice for ovarian RMS that are confined to the ovary. Analogous to ERMS and ARMS of other genital sites, it is indicated that patients with ovarian RMS undergo selective LNE or that clinically suspicious LN be sampled so as to determine an adequate adjuvant therapeutic strategy. There is currently no evidence to suggest that performing an ovarectomy on the uninvolved ovary or systematic LNE offer any benefits for patient outcomes. In a similar vein, the utility of selective or systematic LNE in PRMS cases lacks any scientific substantiation.

In one case, a patient with PRMS of the tube (IRS group I) who underwent a TAH with BSO did not relapse during the 7 mo follow-up period (41).

Ovarian rhabdomyosarcomas generally have a poor prognosis. It is not clear whether or not they can be assigned to the group of tumors with a favorable primary localization. Treatment consists of performing an ovarectomy on the involved ovary. It is indicated that patients undergo selective lymphonodectomy as a means for assessing the need for and determining the particularities of potential chemotherapy and/or radiotherapy. There is no evidence that a lymphonodectomy achieves more favorable outcomes in patients with pleomorphic rhabdomyosarcomas.

The case studies at hand give no rise to assume that undergoing adjuvant CHT yields more promising outcomes. It must be critically noted in this regard, though, that some of the individual cases occurred several decades ago, that different chemotherapeutic agents were administered, and that modern concepts of systemic treatment were applied either only rarely or not at all (94). Adjuvant CHT involved use of the Mayo protocol (vincristine, cyclophosphamide, doxorubicin, and ifosfamide) in the majority of cases. In the case of one patient with RMS of the fallopian tube, adjuvant therapy using the VAC protocol yielded no response (44).

Larger analyses have shown that adult ERMS, ARMS, and RMS-NOS should be treated in the same fashion as pediatric tumors, and this also applies to the applicable CHT protocols and regimens (42). In this regard, adjuvant CHT using the VAC protocol is indicated for all ovarian ERMS, ARMS, and RMS-NOS patients who are classified as being at intermediate risk. RT should also be administered when the pelvic LN are involved and when there is residual disease (cf. Tab. 3.1.7).

PRMS should be approached analogous to the STS or the other types and variants of ovarian sarcoma (e.g. LMS).

There is no indication for adjuvant HT.

Analogous to embryonal and alveolar rhabdomyosarcomas of other sites, there is an indication to administer adjuvant chemotherapy using the respective protocols and regimens. Radiotherapy should also be performed when the lymph nodes are involved. Pleomorphic rhabdomyosarcomas should be treated in the same way as the other ovarian sarcomas.

Primarily advanced tumors can be treated analogous to uterine RMS. Patients with primarily inoperable tumors can be given CHT with vincristine, doxorubicin, and cyclophosphamide, a combination that has served to successfully achieve operability in the past (19). It is highly questionable whether additive RT serves to yield more favorable outcomes in cases in which disease has spread to the abdominal cavity. Such RT would have to take the form of whole abdomen irradiation. Due to the high level of toxicity that such a procedure implies, especially in combination with a necessary CHT and in light of the overall infaust prognosis, it should only be considered in exceptional cases.

RMS also occasionally occur in the ligamentum teres. There are known isolated accounts of ERMS, ARMS, and PRMS arising in the broad ligament (16). Treatment of such tumors is guided by the histological variant at hand as well as the IRSG and risk groups as which they are classified, analogous to uterine or ovarian RMS of the female genital tract.

Primary radiotherapy and/or chemotherapy for primarily advanced ovarian rhabdomyosarcomas should be approached in the same fashion as described for uterine rhabdomyosarcomas.

Aftercare, recurrences, metastases and their treatment

Regarding aftercare, reference can be made to what has been stated for uterine RMS. This equally applies to the treatment of recurrence and metastasis. Virtually no literature is available on this issue.

Aftercare and the treatment of recurrence and metastasis should be approached and designed in accordance with the approach described for uterine rhabdomyosarcomas.

3.2.2 Rhabdomyosarcomas of the vulva and the vagina

General, pathogenesis, pathologico-anatomical features

Vulvar and vaginal RMS account for a clearly larger share of all vulvar and vaginal sarcomas in white women than they do for black women (124). In girls and women aged up to 19 years, 41.7 % of all genital RMS originate in the vagina, while a combined 19.4 % occur in the vulva and the ovaries (64). A further study revealed that 54 % of genital sarcomas in patients aged ≤ 20 affected the vagina, 17 % arose in the uterus, 15 % were cervical, and 13 % were vulvar (2). Vulvar and vaginal RMS account for 6 % resp. 26.3 % of all vulvar and vaginal sarcomas in women aged > 18 years (124). Vaginal RMS are extraordinarily rare in adult women (41).

Vulvar RMS affect the major and minor labia, the clitoris, and the vestibulum. The transitions to perineal and perianal RMS are more fluid than abrupt, which makes a precise classification or categorization difficult in many cases. Perineal/perianal RMS no longer belong to the group of tumors classified as urogenital tumors, and thus do not belong to the group of RMS with favorable localizations. Accordingly, they are not deemed relevant to the genital tract and are not discussed any further here.

The staging, classifications, and risk groups discussed in the context of the uterine variants of RMS also apply to RMS of the vulva and the vagina. For vulvar RMS, the inguinal LN are classified as regional LN, while for RMS of the vagina, the regional LN comprise the LN of the vasa iliaca externa, interna and communes.

> Vulvar and vaginal rhabdomyosarcomas account for 6 % resp. 26.3 % of all vulvar and vaginal sarcomas in women aged > 18 years. Only tumors of the minor and major labia as well as the vestibulum are classified as vulvar rhabdomyosarcomas. Rhabdomyosarcomas of the vagina are extraordinarily rare in adult women.

The macroscopic appearance largely corresponds to that of cervical RMS. In adult women, vulvar RMS are practically always ARMS (2, 41). Ninety percent of vaginal RMS occur in children < 5 years of age and in pubescent females. They are ERMS in the majority of cases (48, 72).

Particularities pertaining to microscopic appearance are presented in the subchapter on uterine RMS.

Clinical presentation, diagnostics, imaging, prognosis

Vaginal ERMS can develop as tumors with a solid appearance that exhibit exophytic growth into the vagina (Fig. 3.2.1 (A)–(C)).

In the vulvar region, diagnosis is generally reached via complete resection leaving sufficiently wide disease-free margins. Since the requirement of leaving a disease-free resection margin of 0.5 cm cannot be fulfilled in most cases of vaginal RMS, either open biopsy or punch biopsy constitute the diagnostic methods of choice.

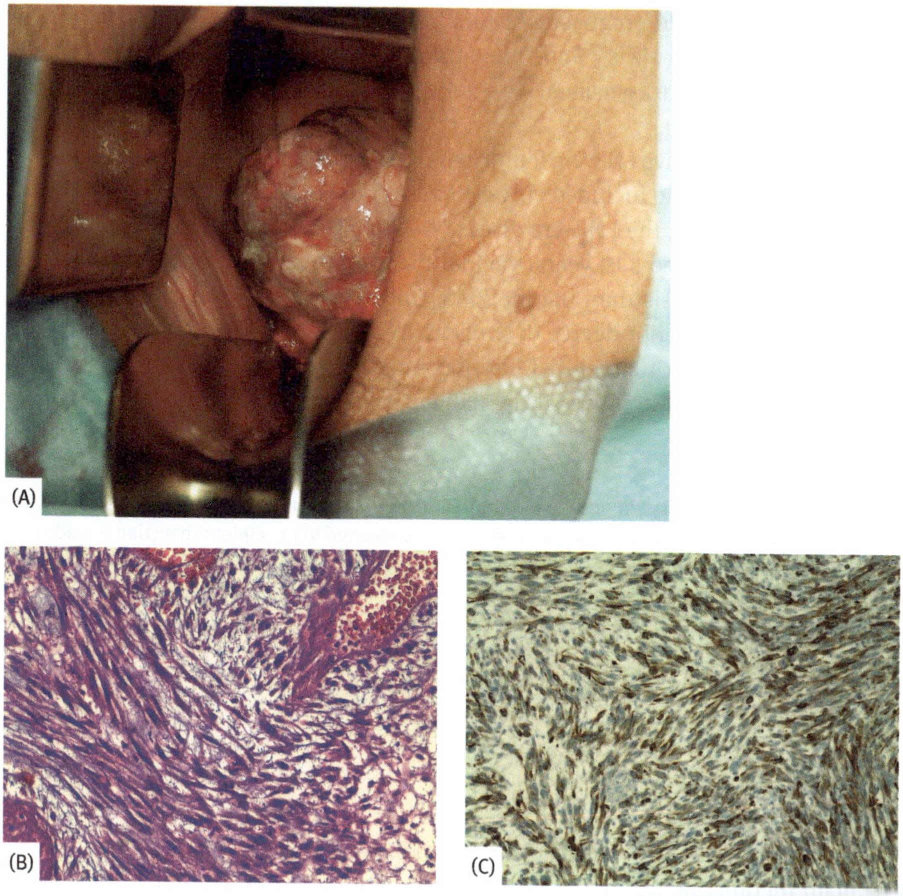

Fig. 3.2.1: Spindle celled rhabdomyosarcoma of the vagina in a 48-year-old woman, N0, R0. (A) macroscopic appearance; (B), (C) microscopically, spindle celled rhabdomyosarcoma bears resemblance to conventional leiomyosarcoma, and both of these tumor types express desmin (C), which at least allows non-myogenic spindle cell sarcomas to be ruled out. Verifying the presence of rhabdomyogenic transcription factors (such as myogenin) in the tumor cells of rhabdomyosarcomas, not depicted in this figure (though see "inset" Fig. 7.1.5 (A)), helps to differentiate rhabdomyosarcoma from leiomyosarcoma.

Analogous to uterine RMS, it is essential that imaging diagnostic examinations are conducted in order to assess whether or not there is LN involvement. Sonographic examination is deemed sufficient for assessing LN status for uterine tumors. For vulvar RMS, additional selective LNE of LN that have been found to be affected via clinical or imaging diagnostics must also be performed.

Vaginal RMS in particular are known to swiftly infiltrate neighboring structures such as the uterus and the vulva (75). According to one multivariate analysis, advanced patient age, a higher stage (regional disease vs. distant metastasis) and subjection to RT were unfavorable prognostic factors for vulvovaginal RMS. Univariate analysis revealed that tumor sizes < 5 cm, non-application of RT, and surgical resection vs. radical/no resection are associated with more favorable outcomes. Mean disease-free survival is 338 mo (124).

In one study, positive LN were found in up to 50 % of perineal RMS (108). Whether the covered sample also included vulvar RMS cannot be discerned from the publication. In another study, the LN were disease free in all covered cases of vaginal RMS (108). For patients aged < 19 years, vaginal RMS tend to yield a (albeit not significantly) poorer prognosis than uterine RMS. One assumption is that this difference is connected to a superior degree of surgical accessibility among RMS of the cervix or the corpus (64). For tumors that have been initially resected leaving gross residual disease, prognosis improves if the patient is R0 reresected prior to undergoing CHT (55).

Vulvar rhabdomyosarcomas in adult women are virtually always alveolar, while only embryonal rhabdomyosarcomas occur in the vagina. Diagnosis is reached via complete resection if said resection can be performed without injuring neighboring organs. If this cannot be achieved, open biopsy or punch biopsy are the methods of choice. Imaging diagnostics are urgently indicated for LN assessment. For vulvar RMS, LN that have been found to be affected via clinical or imaging diagnostic examination must be subjected to selective LNE. Advanced patient age, a higher stage (regional disease vs. distant metastasis) and subjection to RT are unfavorable prognostic factors for vulvovaginal RMS.

Operative, systemic and radiogenic therapy

All of the data that follow refer to vulvar and vaginal ERMS, ARMS, and RMS-NOS. The main therapeutic features mirror those pertaining to the multimodal approach described for uterine RMS. For vulvar RMS, primary resection with subsequent CHT with/without RT, neoadjuvant CHT after biopsy with consecutive interval surgery with/without subsequent RT, or primary CHT with/without RT are the available multimodal options. Analogous to uterine RMS, which of these routes should be taken depends on patient age, local and general operability, and the IRSG group. The transitions between the treatment approaches to be adopted for pediatric, adolescent, and adult patients are fluid, i.e. there are no abrupt or sudden differences at specific age thresholds. The CHT to be applied does not differ from that for uterine RMS, and generally implies the application of the protocols and regimens that are recommended for pediatric patients. In general, ERMS and ARMS in adults and children should be treated alike up to a patient age of 40. Pediatric and adolescent vulvar and vaginal RMS belong in the hands of pediatric surgeons and pediatric oncologists. Therapy for adult patients should generally be multidisciplinarily guided and the highly toxic CHT should be a matter for medicinal oncologists.

Vulvar and vaginal RMS should only receive primary surgery if it appears that R0 resection margins will be achieved and neighboring organs will not suffer injury or be impeded in their functionality (70). If these conditions cannot be fulfilled, administering CHT after performing a diagnostic biopsy is the therapeutic strategy of choice. For RMS of the vagina, it must be assumed that leaving a disease-free resection margin of 0.5 cm will inevitably cause injury to neighboring organs and severe disruption of their functionality. Against this backdrop, more extensive surgical interventions, for example a colpectomy with THE, are not indicated, especially for children, female adolescents, and young adult women. In these cases, patients should undergo primary CHT once diagnosis has been confirmed via biopsy (91). According to the European Paediatric Soft Tissue Sarcoma Study Group, local therapy in the form of secondary surgery and/or RT is no longer necessary if a CR has been achieved either during or after CHT. The tumor should be resected if CHT yields only a partial response or no response at all.

The presence of rhabdomyoblasts in surgical specimens yielded from secondary surgery that was necessary due to a previous incomplete remission is regarded as an indication for a positive reaction to CHT. CHT should be continued in such cases until further notice (1).

Consecutive RT is indicated for patients with residual disease or in whom surgical treatment is not possible or would be severely mutilating (1, 91). Such RT can also be performed as VBT with the help of a vaginal cast or mold (35, 74, 91). The advantage of the aforementioned approach is that a high dose can be applied to the tumor itself, while the surrounding tissue and organs are widely spared. Depending on the precise location, VBT can even serve to replace resection when there is only little residual tumor that does not exceed 4 cm (73). Larger tumors require resection or additional ERT (73).

There is also the recommendation that conservative therapeutic strategies for treating pediatric vaginal RMS should always include RT, since failing to do so is associated with a higher rate of recurrence in group II and III RMS (82, 122). It should be borne in mind, however, that irradiating the vagina during childhood can result in a lifelong loss of functionality of the vagina and the urethra. These consequences also arise in up to 20 % of pediatric patients subjected to VBT (75). However, RT should not be omitted for adult women with group II and III RMS. Analogous to the approach recommended for children, said RT can take the form of VBT, depending on disease localization.

Some authors regard wide primary local resection with subsequent VAC-CHT as a viable therapeutic option for vaginal RMS in pubescent patients. Three patients who underwent this treatment strategy did not relapse (48). Optimal resection with subsequent CHT is regarded as providing the best conditions for reducing the dose of or refraining entirely from RT and thus sparing patients the ample side effects with which such treatment is associated (74). In children, young women, or women of all ages who desire to preserve their fertility, the ovaries should be surgically relocated away from the region to be irradiated prior to RT.

Analogous to RMS in other sites, R0 resection is also deemed the therapeutic method of choice for vulvar RMS in adult women. If R0 resection margins cannot be achieved, or if such resection would likely result in genital mutilation, the further course of action following biopsy should be analogous to that described for vaginal RMS. BT is also a viable option for patients with vulvar RMS due to the lower dose and rate of side effects that this form of therapy entails (73).

In principle, CHT can also be administered with neoadjuvant intent in order to effect shrinkage of large tumors and to improve their operability (2).

If clinical or imaging diagnostics reveal LN involvement, biopsy or selective LNE should be performed as means for determining the type and extent of CHT and RT required (1). Study protocols state that a sentinel LN biopsy would also be an adequate option (35, 60). There is no indication for performing systematic LNE. Thought has been devoted to the question of whether or not LNE with diagnostic intent could be replaced by PET-CT (43), a course of action that would be beneficial in cases of vaginal RMS in particular.

One study recommends that patients with N1 ARMS undergo RT of both the tumor bed and the regional LN. In the opinion of the authors of this study, omitting RT in such cases would constitute patient undertreatment (108). They go on to recommend RT for LN positive ERMS as well, notwithstanding the fact that whether the LN are positive or negative has no proven prognostic implications to date. Independent of the described treatment options, the administration of RT and the choice of CHT protocol/regimen should be guided by the criteria presented in Tab. 3.1.7.

Systematic LNE should be performed in cases with LN involvement in which RT is contraindicated.

Vulvar and vaginal PRMS in adult women should be treated like other STS or the other variants and types of genital sarcoma.

Treatment of vulvar and vaginal embryonal and alveolar rhabdomyosarcomas as well as vulvar and vaginal rhabdomyosarcomas NOS should be approached analogous to the multimodal approach described for the respective uterine variants. For vulvar rhabdomyosarcomas, primary resection with subsequent chemotherapy with/without radiotherapy, neoadjuvant chemotherapy after biopsy with consecutive interval surgery with/without subsequent radiotherapy, or primary chemotherapy with/without radiotherapy, are the available multimodal options. Primary surgery is only adequate if it appears that R0 resection margins can be achieved without injuring neighboring organs (urinary bladder, rectum) or without significantly impeding their functionality. If these conditions cannot be met, securing the diagnosis via biopsy followed by primary chemotherapy is indicated. In cases in which clinical or imaging diagnostics reveal lymph node involvement, selective LNE should be performed in order to determine the type and extent of chemotherapy or radiotherapy required. There is no indication for systematic LNE.

Aftercare, recurrences, metastases and their treatment

Aftercare, diagnostics, and treatment for recurrences and metastases do not differ from what has been elaborately described for uterine RMS.

> Aftercare for and the treatment of patients with recurrent and metastatic vulvar and vaginal rhabdomyosarcomas should be approached in the same fashion as has been described for their uterine counterparts.

References

(1) Andrassy RJ, Wiener ES, Raney RB, Hays DM, Arndt CA, Lobe TE, Lawrence W, Anderson JR, Qualman SJ, Crist WM. Progress in the surgical management of vaginal rhabdomyosarcoma: A 25-year review from the Intergroup Rhabdomyosarcoma Study Group. J Pediatr Surg 1999; 34:731–734

(2) Arndt CA, Donaldson SS, Anderson JR, Andrassy RJ, Laurie F, Link MP, Raney RB, Maurer HM, Crist WM. What constitutes optimal therapy for patients with rhabdomyosarcoma of the female genital tract? Cancer 2001; 91: 2454–2468

(3) Arndt CA, Stoner JA, Hawkins DS, Rodeberg DA, Hayes-Jordan AA, Paidas CN, Parham DM, Teot LA, Wharam MD, Breneman JC, Donaldson SS, Anderson JR, Meyer WH. Vincristine, actinomycin, and cyclophosphamide compared with vincristine, actinomycin, and cyclophosphamide alternating with vincristine, topotecan, and cyclophosphamide for intermediate-risk rhabdomyosarcoma: Children's Oncology Group Study D9803. J Clin Oncol 2009; 27: 5182–5188

(4) Baiocchi G, Faloppa CC, Osório CA, Kumagai LY, Fukazawa EM, Cunha IW. Embryonal rhabdomyosarcoma of the uterine cervix in a 47-year-old woman. J Obstet Gynaecol Res 2011; 37: 940–946

(5) Ballard KS, Tedjarati SS, Robinson WR, Homesley HD, Thurston EL. Embryonal rhabdomyosarcoma: adjuvant and ex vivo assay-directed chemotherapy. Int J Gynecol Cancer 2010; 20: 561–563

(6) Bansal S, Lewin SN, Burke WM, Deutsch I, Sun X, Herzog TJ, Wright JD. Sarcoma of the cervix: natural history and outcomes. Gynecol Oncol 2010; 118: 134–138

(7) Baum SH, Frühwald M, Rahbar K, Wessling J, Schober O, Weckesser M. Contribution of PET/CT to prediction of outcome in children and young adults with rhabdomyosarcoma. J Nucl Med 2011; 52: 1535–1540

(8) Bel Haj Salah M, Brahim EB, Zidi YS, Tangour M, Kilani H, Chatti-Dey S. [Mixed germ cell tumor of the ovary with rhabdomyosarcomatous component. A case report]. Ann Pathol. 2010; 30: 394–397

(9) Bernal KL, Fahmy L, Remmenga S, Bridge J, Baker J. Embryonal rhabdomyosarcoma (sarcoma botryoides) of the cervix presenting as a cervical polyp treated with fertility-sparing surgery and adjuvant chemotherapy. Gynecol Oncol 2004; 95: 243–246

(10) Buchwalter CL, Jenison EL, Fromm M, Mehta VT, Hart WR. Pure embryonal rhabdomyosarcoma of the fallopian tube. Gynecol Oncol 1997; 67: 95–101

(11) Cakar B, Muslu U, Karaca B, Junushova B, Uslu R, Goker E. Alveolar rhabdomyosarcoma originating from the uterine cervix. Eur J Gynaecol Oncol 2011; 32: 196–198

(12) Caruso RA, Napoli P, Villari D, Starrantino M. Anaplastic (pleomorphic) subtype embryonal rhabdomyosarcoma of the cervix. Arch Gynecol Obstet 2004; 270: 278–280

(13) Case AS, Kirby TO, Conner MG, Huh WK. A case report of rhabdomyosarcoma of the uterus associated with uterine inversion. Gynecol Oncol 2005; 96: 850–853
(14) Cecchetto G, Bisogno G, De Corti F, Dall'Igna P, Inserra A, Ferrari A, Garaventa A, Scagnellato A, Carli M; Italian Cooperative Group. Biopsy or debulking surgery as initial surgery for locally advanced rhabdomyosarcomas in children? The experience of the Italian Cooperative Group studies. Cancer 2007; 110: 2561–2567
(15) Cessna MH, Zhou H, Perkins SL, Tripp SR, Layfield L, Daines C, Coffin CM. Are myogenin and myoD1 expression specific for rhabdomyosarcoma? A study of 150 cases, with emphasis on spindle cell mimics. Am J Surg Pathol 2001; 25: 1150–1157
(16) Chandarana MN, Raghu S, Bhagat M, Qureshi S. Embryonal rhabdomyosarcoma of the broad ligament. Indian J Med Paediatr Oncol. 2014; 35: 103–105
(17) Chisholm JC, Marandet J, Rey A, Scopinaro M, de Toledo JS, Merks JH, O'Meara A, Stevens MC, Oberlin O. Prognostic factors after relapse in nonmetastatic rhabdomyosarcoma: A nomogram to better define patients who can be salvaged with further therapy. J Clin Oncol 2011; 29: 1319–1325
(18) Corpron CA, Andrassy RJ, Hays DM, Raney RB, Wiener ES, Lawrence W, Lobe TE, Maurer HM. Conservative management of uterine pediatric rhabdomyosarcoma: A report from the Intergroup Rhabdomyosarcoma Study III and IV pilot. J Pediatr Surg 1995; 30: 942–944
(19) Cribbs RK, Shehata BM, Ricketts RR. Primary ovarian rhabdomyosarcoma in children. Pediatr Surg Int 2008; 24: 593–595
(20) Crist WM, Garnsey L, Beltangady MS, Gehan E, Ruymann F, Webber B, Hays DM, Wharam M, Maurer HM. Prognosis in children with rhabdomyosarcoma: A report of the intergroup rhabdomyosarcoma studies I and II. Intergroup Rhabdomyosarcoma Committee. J Clin Oncol 1990; 8: 443–452
(21) Crist WM, Gehan EA, Ragab AH, Dickman PS, Donaldson SS, Fryer C, Hammond D, Hays DM, Herrmann J, Heyn R. The Third Intergroup Rhabdomyosarcoma Study. J Clin Oncol 1995; 13: 610–630
(22) Crist WM, Anderson JR, Meza JL, Fryer C, Raney RB, Ruymann FB, Breneman J, Qualman SJ, Wiener E, Wharam M, Lobe T, Webber B, Maurer HM, Donaldson SS. Intergroup Rhabdomyosarcoma Study-IV: results for patients with nonmetastatic disease. J Clin Oncol 2001; 19: 3091–3102
(23) Cui S, Hano H, Harada T, Takai S, Masui F, Ushigome S. Evaluation of new monoclonal anti-MyoD1 and anti-myogenin antibodies for the diagnosis of rhabdomyosarcoma. Pathol Int 1999; 49: 62–68
(24) Dantonello TM, Int-Veen C, Winkler P, Leuschner I, Schuck A, Schmidt BF, Lochbuehler H, Kirsch S, Hallmen E, Veit-Friedrich I, Bielack SS, Niggli F, Kazanowska B, Ladenstein R, Wiebe T, Klingebiel T, Treuner J, Koscielniak E. Initial patient characteristics can predict pattern and risk of relapse in localized rhabdomyosarcoma. J Clin Oncol 2008; 26: 406–413
(25) Dantonello TM, Winkler P, Boelling T, Friedel G, Schmid I, Mattke AC, Ljungman G, Bielack SS, Klingebiel T, Koscielniak E; CWS Study Group. Embryonal rhabdomyosarcoma with metastases confined to the lungs: report from the CWS Study Group. Pediatr Blood Cancer 2011; 56):725–732
(26) Dantonello TM, Int-Veen C, Schuck A, Seitz G, Leuschner I, Nathrath M, Schlegel PG, Kontny U, Behnisch W, Veit-Friedrich I, Kube S, Hallmen E, Kazanowska B, Ladenstein R, Paulussen M, Ljungman G, Bielack SS, Klingebiel T, Koscielniak E; Cooperative Weichteilsarkom Studiengruppe. Survival following disease recurrence of primary localized alveolar rhabdomyosarcoma. Pediatr Blood Cancer 2013; 60: 1267–1273
(27) Daya DA, Scully RE. Sarcoma botryoides of the uterine cervix in young women: A clinicopathological study of 13 cases. Gynecol Oncol 1988; 29: 290–304.

(28) De Corti F, Bisogno G, Dall'Igna P, Ferrari A, Buffa P, De Paoli A, Cecchetto G. Does surgery have a role in the treatment of local relapses of non-metastatic rhabdomyosarcoma? Pediatr Blood Cancer 2011; 57: 1261–1265

(29) Dehner LP, Jarzembowski JA, Hill DA. Embryonal rhabdomyosarcoma of the uterine cervix: A report of 14 cases and a discussion of its unusual clinicopathological associations. Mod Pathol 2012; 25: 602–614

(30) Dome, JS, Rodriguez-Galindo C, Spunt SL, Santana VM. Pediatric solid tumors. In: Abelof MD, Armitage JO, Niederhuber JE, Kastan MB, McKenna WG (eds.). Abeloff's Clinical Oncology. 4th edn., Churchill-Livingstone Elsevier, Philadelphia 2008, pp. 2075–2129

(31) Dumont SN, Araujo DM, Munsell MF, Salganick JA, Dumont AG, Raymond KA, Linassier C, Patel S, Benjamin RS, Trent JC. Management and outcome of 239 adolescent and adult rhabdomyosarcoma patients. Cancer Med 2013; 2: 553–563

(32) Egas-Bejar D, Huh WW. Rhabdomyosarcoma in adolescent and young adult patients: current perspectives. Adolesc Health Med Ther 2014; 5: 115–125

(33) Emerich J, Senkus E, Konefka T. Alveolar rhabdomyosarcoma of the uterine cervix. Gynecol Oncol 1996; 63: 398–403

(34) Esnaola NF, Rubin BP, Baldini EH, Vasudevan N, Demetri GD, Fletcher CD, Singer S. Response to chemotherapy and predictors of survival in adult rhabdomyosarcoma. Ann Surg 2001; 234: 215–223

(35) European Paediatric Soft Tissue Sarcoma Study Group, RMS 2005 Protocol, study of the treatment on non-metastatic rhabdomyosarcoma in childhood and adolescence. Protocol EpSSg RMS 2005, Version 1.2 international – July 2008

(36) Fadare O, Ghofrani M, Stainalakos MD. Mesenchymal lesions of the uterine cervix. Pathol Case Rev. 2006; 11: 140–152.

(37) Fadare O. Uncommon sarcomas of the uterine cervix: A review of selected entities. Diagn Pathol 2006; 1: 30

(38) Fadare O, Bonvicino A, Martel M, Renshaw IL, Azodi M, Parkash V. Pleomorphic rhabdomyosarcoma of the uterine corpus: A clinicopathologic study of 4 cases and a review of the literature. Int J Gynecol Pathol 2010; 29: 122–134

(39) Fadare O. Heterologous and rare homologous sarcomas of the uterine corpus: A clinicopathologic review. Adv Anat Pathol 2011; 18: 60–74

(40) Federico SM, Spunt SL, Krasin MJ, Billup CA, Wu J, Shulkin B, Mandell G, McCarville MB. Comparison of PET-CT and conventional imaging in staging pediatric rhabdomyosarcoma. PediatrBlood Cancer 2013; 60: 1128–1134

(41) Ferguson SE, Gerald W, Barakat RR, Chi DS, Soslow RA. Clinicopathologic features of rhabdomyosarcoma of gynecologic origin in adults. Am J Surg Pathol 2007; 31: 382–389

(42) Ferrari A, Dileo P, Casanova M, Bertulli R, Meazza C, Gandola L, Navarria P, Collini P, Gronchi A, Olmi P, Fossati-Bellani F, Casali PG. Rhabdomyosarcoma in adults. A retrospective analysis of 171 patients treated at a single institution. Cancer 2003; 98: 571–580

(43) Fuchs J, Dantonello TM, Blumenstock G, Kosztyla D, Klingebiel T, Leuschner I, Schuck A, Niggli FK, Koscielniak E, Seitz G. Treatment and outcome of patients suffering from perineal/perianal rhabdomyosarcoma: results from the CWS trials—retrospective clinical study. Ann Surg 2014; 59: 1166–1172

(44) Fujiwaki R, Miura H, Endo A, Yoshino N, Iwanari O, Sawada K. Primary rhabdomyosarcoma with an epithelioid appearance of the fallopian tube: An adult case. Eur J Obstet Gynecol Reprod Biol 2008; 140: 289–890

(45) Fukunaga M. Pure alveolar rhabdomyosarcoma of the uterine corpus. Pathol Int 2011; 61: 377–381

(46) Garrett LA, Harmon DC, Schorge JO. Embryonal rhabdomyosarcoma of the uterine corpus. J Clin Oncol. 2013; 31: e48-50. DOI: 10.1200/JCO.2012.43.1841

(47) Gerber NK, Wexler LH, Singer S, Alektiar KM, Keohan ML, Shi W, Zhang Z, Wolden S. Adult rhabdomyosarcoma survival improved with treatment on multimodality protocols. Int J Radiat Oncol Biol Phys 2013; 86: 58–63

(48) Ghaemmaghami F, Karimi Zarchi M, Ghasemi M. Lower genital tract rhabdomyosarcoma: case series and literature review. Arch Gynecol Obstet 2008; 278: 65–69

(49) Goldblum JR, Folpe AL, Weiss SW. Enzinger and Weiss's Soft Tissue Tumors. 6th edn. Elsevier Saunders 2014

(50) Gruessner SE, Omwandho CO, Dreyer T, Blütters-Sawatzki R, Reiter A, Tinneberg HR, Bohle RM. Management of stage I cervical sarcoma botryoides in childhood and adolescence. Eur J Pediatr 2004; 163: 452–456

(51) Hashimoto A, Takada K, Takimoto R, Horiguchi H, Sato T, Iyama S, Murase K, Ono K, Tatekoshi A, Hayashi T, Miyanishi K, Sato Y, Kobune M, Hirayama Y, Kitamura H, Nakanishi K, Masumori N, Hasegawa T, Kato J. [Effective treatment of metastatic rhabdomyosarcoma with pazopanib]. Gan To Kagaku Ryoho 2014; 41: 1041–1044 (Abstr)

(52) Hatsiopoulou O, Sala E. In: Hricak H, Akin O, Sala E, Ascher SM, Levine D, Reinhold C. Diagnostic Imaging Gynecology. 1st edn. AMIRSYS 2007; 4/50–51

(53) Hawkins WG, Hoos A, Antonescu CR, Marshall JU, Leung DHY, Gold JS, Woodruff JM, Lewis JJ, Brennanet MF. Clinicopathologic analysis of patients with adult rhabdomyosarcoma. Cancer 2001; 91: 794–803

(54) Hayes-Jordan A, Doherty DK, West SD, Raney RB, Blakely ML, Cox CS Jr, Andrassy RJ, Lally KP. Outcome after surgical resection of recurrent rhabdomyosarcoma. Pediatr Surg 2006; 41: 633–638

(55) Hays DM, Shimada H, Raney RB Jr, Tefft M, Newton W, Crist WM, Lawrence W Jr, Ragab A, Maurer HM. Sarcomas of the vagina and uterus: the Intergroup Rhabdomyosarcoma Study. J Pediatr Surg 1985; 20: 718–724

(56) Holcomb K, Francis M, Ruiz J, Abulafia O, Matthews RP, Lee YC. Pleomorphic rhabdomyosarcoma of the uterus in a postmenopausal woman with elevated serum CA125. Gynecol Oncol 1999; 74: 499–501

(57) Jayi S, Bouguern H, Fdili FZ, Chaara H, Chbani L, Hafidi I, Kamaoui I, Arifi S, Mellas N, Bouhafa I, Hassouni K, Tizniti S, Laamartl A, Melhouf MA. Embryonal rhabdomyosarcoma of the cervix presenting as a cervical polyp in a 16-year-old adolescent: A case report. J Med Case Rep 2014; 8: 241

(58) Joshi D, Anderson JR, Paidas C, Brcncman J, Parham DM, Crist W. Soft Tissue Sarcoma Committee of the Children's Oncology Group. Age is an independent prognostic factor in rhabdomyosarcoma: A report from the Soft Tissue Sarcoma Committee of the Children's Oncology Group. Pediatr Blood Cancer 2004; 42:64–73

(59) Karaman E, Akbayir O, Kocatürk Y, Cekic S, Filiz FB, Gulkilik A. Successful treatment of a very rare case: locally treated cervical rhabdomyosarcoma. Arch Gynecol Obstet 2011; 284: 1019–1022

(60) Kayton ML1, Delgado R, Busam K, Cody HS 3rd, Athanasian EA, Coit D, La Quaglia MP. Experience with 31 sentinel lymph node biopsies for sarcomas and carcinomas in pediatric patients. Cancer 2008; 112: 2052–2059

(61) Kayton ML, Wexler LH, Lewin SN, Park KJ, La Quaglia MP, Abu-Rustum NR. Pediatric radical abdominal trachelectomy for anaplastic embryonal rhabdomyosarcoma of the uterine cervix: An alternative to radical hysterectomy. J Pediatr Surg 2009; 44: 862–867

(62) Kefeli M, Kandemir B, Akpolat I, Yildirim A, Kokcu A. Rhabdomyosarcoma arising in a mature cystic teratoma with contralateral serous carcinoma: case report and review of the literature. Int J Gynecol Pathol 2009; 28: 372–365

(63) Kim DW, Shin JH, Lee HJ, Hong YO, Joo JE, Kim EK. Spindle cell rhabdomyosacoma of uterus: A case study. Korean J Pathol 2013; 47: 388–391

(64) Kirsch CH, Goodman M, Esiashvili N. Outcome of female pediatric patients diagnosed with genital tract rhabdomyosarcoma based on analysis of cases registered in SEER database between 1973 and 2006. Am J Clin Oncol 2014; 37: 47–50

(65) Köhler G, Belau, A, Dennis K, Evert K, Evert M, Hesse J, Hegenscheid K, Köller M, Krichbaum J, Kühnast M, Lehnhoff H, Lehr A, Linke L, Marcinek A, Müller S, Riechmann C, Schalitz S, Simon J, Spring P, Schädler, J, Ständer C, Trojnarska D, Wilcke S, Witte N, Zygmunt M; Deutsches klinisches Kompetenzzentrum für genitale Sarkome und Mischtumoren an der Universitätsmedizin Greifswald (DKSM) und Kooperationspartner VAAO Deutschland und FK Frankfurt/Sachsenhausen. Datenbank und Promotions- und Forschungsgruppe genitale Sarkome, Greifswald 2016, www.medizin.uni-greifswald.de/gyn/dksm/

(66) Komdeur R, Klunder J, van der Graaf WT, van den Berg E, de Bont ES, Hoekstra HJ, Moleaar WM. Multidrug resistance proteins in rhabdomyosarcomas: comparison between children and adults. Cancer 2003; 97: 1999–2005

(67) Koscielniak E, Rodary C, Flamant F, Carli M, Treuner J, Pinkerton CR, Grotto P. Metastatic rhabdomyosarcoma and histologically similar tumors in childhood: a retrospective European multi-center analysis. Med Pediatr Oncol 1992; 20: 209–214

(68) Koukourakis GV, Kouloulias V, Zacharias G, Maravelis G, Papadimitriou C, Platoni K, Gouliamos A. Embryonal rhabdomyosarcoma of the uterine cervix. Clin Transl Oncol 2009; 11: 399–402

(69) Kriseman ML, Wang WL, Sullinger J, Schmeler KM, Ramirez PT, Herzog CE, Frumovitz M. Rhabdomyosarcoma of the cervix in adult women and younger patients. Gynecol Oncol 2012; 126: 351–356

(70) Leaphart C, Rodeberg D. Pediatric surgical oncology: management of rhabdomyosarcoma. Surg Oncol 2007; 16: 173–185

(71) Leitlinie der Gesellschaft für Pädiatrische Onkologie und Hämatologie Weichteilsarkome. www.awmf.org/uploads/tx_szleitlinien/025-007l_S1_Weichteilsarkome_01.pdf. 2011

(72) Li RF, Gupta M, McCluggage WG, Ronnett BM. Embryonal rhabdomyosarcoma (botryoid type) of the uterine corpus and cervix in adult women: report of a case series and review of the literature. Am J Surg Pathol 2013; 37: 344–355

(73) Magné N, Haie-Meder C. Brachytherapy for genital-tract rhabdomyosarcomas in girls: technical aspects, reports, and perspectives. Lancet Oncol 2007; 8: 725–729.

(74) Magné N, Oberlin O, Martelli H, Gerbaulet A, Chassagne D, Haie-Meder C. Vulval and vaginal rhabdomyosarcoma in children: update and reappraisal of Institut Gustave Roussy brachytherapy experience. Int J Radiat Oncol Biol Phys 2008; 72: 878–883

(75) Martelli H, Oberlin O, Rey A, Godzinski J, Spicer RD, Bouvet N, Haie-Meder C, Terrier-Lacombe MJ, Sanchez de Toledo J, Spooner D, Sommelet D, Flamant F, Stevens MC. Conservative treatment for girls with nonmetastatic rhabdomyosarcoma of the genital tract: a report from the Study Committee of the International Society of Pediatric Oncology. J Clin Oncol 1999; 17: 2117– 2122

(76) Mascarenhas L, Lyden ER, Breitfeld PP, Walterhouse DO, Donaldson SS, Paidas CN, Parham DM, Anderson JR, Meyer WH, Hawkins DS. Randomized phase II window trial of two schedules of irinotecan with vincristine in patients with first relapse or progression of rhabdomyosarcoma: A report from the Children's Oncology Group. J Clin Oncol 2010; 28: 4658–4663

(77) Maurer HM, Beltangady M, Gehan EA, Crist W, Hammond D, Hays DM, Heyn R, Lawrence W, Newton W, Ortega J, Ragab AH, Raney RB, Ruyman FB, Soule E, Teft M, Webber B, Wharam M, Vietti TJ. The Intergroup Rhabdomyosarcoma Study-I. A final report. Cancer 1988; 61: 209–220
(78) Mazzoleni S, Bisogno G, Garaventa A, Cecchetto G, Ferrari A, Sotti G, Donfrancesco A, Madon E, Casula L, Carli M. Outcomes and prognostic factors after recurrence in children and adolescents with nonmetastatic rhabdomyosarcoma. Cancer 2005; 104: 183–190
(79) McCluggage WG, Lioe TF, McClelland HR, Lamki H. Rhabdomyosarcoma of the uterus: report of two cases, including one of the spindle cell variant. Int J Gynecol Cancer 2002; 12: 128–132
(80) Merlino G, Helman LJ. Rhabdomyosarcoma—working out the pathways. Oncogene 1999; 18: 5340–5348
(81) Meza JL, Anderson J, Pappo AS, Meyer WH. Children's Oncology Group. Analysis of prognostic factors in patients with nonmetastatic rhabdomyosarcoma treated on intergroup rhabdomyosarcoma studies III and IV: The Children's Oncology Group. J Clin Oncol 2006; 24: 3844–3851
(82) Million L, Anderson J, Breneman J, Hawkins DS, Laurie F, Michalski J, Rodeberg D, Wharam M, Wolden S, Donaldson SS. Influence of noncompliance with radiation therapy protocol guidelines and operative bed recurrences for children with rhabdomyosarcoma and microscopic residual disease: A report from the Children's Oncology Group. Int J Radiat Oncol Biol Phys 2011; 80: 333–338.
(83) Missiaglia E, Williamson D, Chisholm J, Wirapati P, Pierron G, Petel F, Concordet JP, Thway K, Oberlin O, Pritchard-Jones K, Delattre O, Delorenzi M, Shipley J. PAX3/FOXO1 fusion gene status is the key prognostic molecular marker in rhabdomyosarcoma and significantly improves current risk stratification. J Clin Oncol 2012; 30: 1670–1677
(84) Miyamoto T, Shiozawa T, Nakamura T, Konishi I. Sarcoma botryoides of the uterine cervix in a 46-year-old woman: case report and literature review. Int J Gynecol Pathol 2004; 23: 78–82
(85) Moinfar F, Azodi M, Tavassoli FA. Uterine sarcomas. Pathology 2007; 39: 55–71
(86) Montag TW, D'ablaing G, Schlaerth JB, Gaddis O Jr, Morrow CP. Embryonal rhabdomyosarcoma of the uterine corpus and cervix. Gynecol Oncol 1986; 25: 171–194
(87) Moritake H, Kamimura S, Akiyoshi K, Nagatoshi Y, Chuman H, Okamura J. Prognostic significance of elevated lactate dehydrogenase and creatine kinase in patients with rhabdomyosarcoma. Med Pediatr Oncol 2003; 40: 187–188
(88) Morotti RA, Nicol KK, Parham DM, Teot LA, Moore J, Hayes J, Meyer W, Qualman SJ; Children's Oncology Group. An immunohistochemical algorithm to facilitate diagnosis and subtyping of rhabdomyosarcoma: The Children's Oncology Group experience. Am J Surg Pathol 2006; 30: 962–968
(89) Mousavi A, Akhavan S. Sarcoma botryoides (embryonal rhabdomyosarcoma) of the uterine cervix in sisters. J Gynecol Oncol 2010; 21: 273–275
(90) Mukherjee S, Sen S, Biswas P, Choudhuri M. Primary pleomorphic sarcoma of the ovary with rhabdomyosarcomatous differentiation. Indian J Pathol Microbiol 2009; 52: 217–218
(91) National Cancer Institute: PDQ® Childhood Rhabdomyosarcoma Treatment. Bethesda, MD: National Cancer Institute. Date last modified 10/29/2014. Available at: http://cancer.gov/cancertopics/pdq/treatment/childrhabdomyosarcoma/HealthProfessional
(92) National Comprehensive Cancer Network: NCCN Clinical Practice Guidelines in Oncology – Soft tissue sarcomas. Version 2.2016 www.nccn.org
(93) Ng TY, Loo KT, Leung TW, Lo SH, Yuen KK. Alveolar rhabdomyosarcoma of the cervix. Gynecol Oncol 2003; 91: 623–626
(94) Nielsen GP, Oliva E, Young RH, Rosenberg AE, Prat J, Scully RE. Primary ovarian rhabdomyosarcoma: A report of 13 cases. Int J Gynecol Pathol 1998; 17: 113–119

(95) Ogilvie CM, Crawford EA, Slotcavage RL, King JJ, Lackman RD, Hartner L, Staddon AP. Treatment of adult rhabdomyosarcoma. Am J Clin Oncol 2010; 33: 128–131

(96) Okada DH, Rowland JB, Petrovic LM. Uterine pleomorphic rhabdomyosarcoma in a patient receiving tamoxifen therapy. Gynecol Oncol 1999; 75: 509–513

(97) Oliva E, Caracangiu ML, Carinelli SG, Ip P, Loening T, Longacre TA, Nucci MR, Prat J, Zaloudek CJ. Tumours of the uterine corpus. Mesenchymal tumors. In: Kurman Rj, Carcangiu ML, Herrington CS, Young RH (eds.). WHO Classification of Tumors of Female Reproductive Organs. 4th edn. IARC: Lyon 2014, pp. 135–152

(98) Oliva E. Rhabdomyosarcoma, cervix. In: Nucci MR, Oliva E (eds). Diagnostic Pathology Gynaecological. Amirsys 2014; 3/180–3/96-97

(99) Ordi J, Stamatakos MD, Tavassoli FA. Pure pleomorphic rhabdomyosarcomas of the uterus. Int J Gynecol Pathol 1997; 16: 369–377

(100) Pappo AS, Lyden E, Breneman J, Wiener E, Teot L, Meza J, Crist W, Vietti T. Up-front window trial of topotecan in previously untreated children and adolescents with metastatic rhabdomyosarcoma: An intergroup rhabdomyosarcoma study. J Clin Oncol 2001; 19: 213–219

(101) Paulino AC, Okcu MF. Rhabdomyosarcoma. Curr Probl Cancer 2008: 32: 7–34

(102) Raney RB, Anderson JR, Barr FG, Donaldson SS, Pappo AS, Qualman SJ, Wiener ES, Maurer HM, Crist WM. Rhabdomyosarcoma and undifferentiated sarcoma in the first two decades of life: A selective review of intergroup rhabdomyosarcoma study group experience and rationale for Intergroup Rhabdomyosarcoma Study V. J Pediatr Hematol Oncol 2001, 23: 215–220

(103) Raney B, Stoner J, Anderson J, Andrassy R, Arndt C, Brown K, Crist W, Maurer H, Qualman S, Wharam M, Wiener E, Meyer W, Hayes-Jordan A. Impact of tumor viability at second-look procedures performed before completing treatment on the Intergroup Rhabdomyosarcoma Study Group protocol IRS-IV, 1991–1997: A report from the Children's Oncology Group. J Pediatr Surg 2010; 45: 2160–2168

(104) Raney RB, Anderson JR, Brown KL, Huh WW, Maurer HM, Meyer WH, Parham DM, Rodeberg DA, Wolden SL, Donaldson SS. Treatment results for patients with localized, completely resected (Group I) alveolar rhabdomyosarcoma on Intergroup Rhabdomyosarcoma Study Group (IRSG) protocols III and IV, 1984–1997: A report from the Children's Oncology Group. Pediatr Blood Cancer 2010; 55: 612–616

(105) Raney RB, Walterhouse DO, Meza JL, Andrassy RJ, Breneman JC, Crist WM, Maurer HM, Meyer WH, Parham DM, Anderson JR. Results of the Intergroup Rhabdomyosarcoma Study Group D9602 protocol, using vincristine and dactinomycin with or without cyclophosphamide and radiation therapy, for newly diagnosed patients with low-risk embryonal rhabdomyosarcoma: A report from the Soft Tissue Sarcoma Committee of the Children's Oncology Group. J Clin Oncol 2011; 29:1312–1318

(106) Regine WF, Fontanesi J, Kumar P, Ayers D, Bowman LC, Pappo AS, Coffey DH, Avery L, Rao BN, Kun LE. Local tumor control in rhabdomyosarcoma following low-dose irradiation: comparison of group II and select group III patients. Int J Radial Oncol Biol Phys 1995; 31: 485–491

(107) Riedlinger WF, Kozakewich HP, Vargas SO. Myogenic markers in the evaluation of embryonal botryoid rhabdomyosarcoma of the female genital tract. Pediatr Dev Pathol 2005; 8: 427–434

(108) Rodeberg DA, Garcia-Henriquez N, Lyden ER, Davicioni E, Parham DM, Skapek SX, Hayes-Jordan AA, Donaldson SS, Brown KL, Triche, TJ, Meyer WH, Hawkins DS. Prognostic significance and tumor biology of regional lymph node disease in patients with rhabdomyosarcoma: A report from the Children's Oncology Group. J Clin Oncol 2011; 29: 1304–1311

(109) Sahdev A, Sohaib SA, Jacobs I, Shepherd JH, Oram DH, Reznek RH. MR imaging of uterine sarcomas. Am J Roentgenol 2001; 177: 1307–1311

(110) Sanders MA, Gordinier M, Talwalkar SS, Moore GD. Embryonal rhabdomyosarcoma of the uterine cervix in a 41-year-old woman treated with radical hysterectomy and adjuvant chemotherapy. Gynecol Oncol 2008; 111: 561–563

(111) Saylors RL, Stine KC, Sullivan J, Kepner JL, Wall DA, Bernstein ML, Harris MB, Hayashi R, Vietti TJ. Pediatric Oncology Group. Cyclophosphamide plus topotecan in children with recurrent or refractory solid tumors: A Pediatric Oncology Group phase II study. J Clin Oncol 2001; 19: 3463–3469

(112) Schütte J, Hartmann JT, Reichardt P, Issels RD, Tunn PU, Budach V. Leitlinien Weichteilsarkome. www.dgho-onkopedia.de/de/onkopedia/leitlinien/weichteilsarkome/weichteilsarkome.pdf. 2011

(113) Shern JF, Chen L, Chmielecki J, Wei JS, Patidar R, Rosenberg M, Ambrogio L, Auclair D, Wang J, Song YK, Tolman C, Hurd L, Liao H, Zhang S, Bogen D, Brohl AS, Sindiri S, Catchpoole D, Badgett T, Getz G, Mora J, Anderson JR, Skapek SX, Barr FG, Meyerson M, Hawkins DS, Khan J. Comprehensive genomic analysis of rhabdomyosarcoma reveals a landscape of alterations affecting a common genetic axis in fusion-positive and fusion-negative tumors. Cancer Discov 2014; 4: 216–231

(114) Sorensen PH, Lynch JC, Qualman SJ, Tirabosco R, Lim JF, Maurer HM, Bridge JA, Crist WM, Triche TJ, Barr FG. PAX3-FKHR and PAX7-FKHR gene fusions are prognostic indicators in alveolar rhabdomyosarcoma: A report from the Children's Oncology Group. J Clin Oncol 2002; 20: 2672–2679

(115) Stegmaier S, Poremba C, Schaefer KL, Leuschner I, Kazanowska B, Békássy AN, Bielack SS, Klingebiel T, Koscielniak E. Prognostic value of PAX-FKHR fusion status in alveolar rhabdomyosarcoma: A report from the Cooperative Soft Tissue Sarcoma Study Group (CWS). Pediatr Blood Cancer 2011; 57: 406–414

(116) Sultan I, Qaddoumi I, Yaser S, Rodriguez-Galindo C, Ferrari A. Comparing adult and pediatric rhabdomyosarcoma in the surveillance, epidemiology and end results program, 1973 to 2005: An analysis of 2,600 patients. J Clin Oncol 2009; 27: 3391–3397

(117) Takano M, Kikuchi Y, Aida S, Sato K, Nagata I. Embryonal rhabdomyosarcoma of the uterine corpus in a 76-year-old patient. Gynecol Oncol 1999; 75: 490–494

(118) Tateishi U, Hosono A, Makimoto A, Nakamoto Y, Kaneta T, Fukuda H, Murakami K, Terauchi T, Suga T, Inoue T, Kim EE. Comparative study of FDG PET/CT and conventional imaging in the staging of rhabdomyosarcoma. Ann Nucl Med 2009; 23: 155–161

(119) Toro JR, Travis LB, Wu HJ, Zhu K, Fletcher CD, Devesa SS. Incidence patterns of soft tissue sarcomas, regardless of primary site, in the surveillance, epidemiology and end results program, 1978–2001: An analysis of 26,758 cases. Int J Cancer 2006; 119: 2922–2930

(120) Villella JA, Bogner PN, Jani-Sait SN, Block AM, Lele S. Rhabdomyosarcoma of the cervix in sisters with review of the literature. Gynecol Oncol 2005; 99: 742–748

(121) Völker T, Denecke T, Steffen I, Misch D, Schönberger S, Plotkin M, Ruf J, Furth C, Stöver B, Hautzel H, Henze G, Amthauer H. Positron emission tomography for staging of pediatric sarcoma patients: results of a prospective multicenter trial. J Clin Oncol 2007; 25: 5435–5441

(122) Walterhouse DO, Meza JL, Breneman JC, Donaldson SS, Hayes-Jordan A, Pappo AS, Arndt C, Raney RB, Meyer WH, Hawkins DS. Local control and outcome in children with localized vaginal rhabdomyosarcoma: A report from the Soft Tissue Sarcoma Committee of the Children's Oncology Group. Pediatr Blood Cancer 2011; 57: 76–83

(123) Walterhouse DO, Pappo AS, Meza JL, Breneman JC, Hayes-Jordan AA, Parham DM, Cripe TP, Anderson JR, Meyer WH, Hawkins DS. Shorter-duration therapy using vincristine, dactinomycin, and lower-dose cyclophosphamide with or without radiotherapy for patients with newly diagnosed low-risk rhabdomyosarcoma: A report from the Soft Tissue Sarcoma Committee of the Children's Oncology Group. J Clin Oncol. 2014; 32: 3547–3552

(124) Westhoff G, Dorigo O, Berek J, Karam A. Vaginal and vulvar sarcomas: a population based review of incidence, treatment and outcomes (2014 VAGO Abstr). Gynecol Oncol 2014; 135: 394–395
(125) Williamson D, Missiaglia E, de Reyniès A, Pierron G, Thuille B, Palenzuela G, Thway K, Orbach D, Laé M, Fréneaux P, Pritchard-Jones K, Oberlin O, Shipley J, Delattre O. Fusion gene-negative alveolar rhabdomyosarcoma is clinically and molecularly indistinguishable from embryonal rhabdomyosarcoma. J Clin Oncol 2010; 28: 2151–2158
(126) Wolden SL, Anderson JR, Crist WM, Breneman JC, Wharam MD Jr, Wiener ES, Qualman SJ, Donaldson SS. Indications for radiotherapy and chemotherapy after complete resection in rhabdomyosarcoma: A report from the Intergroup Rhabdomyosarcoma Studies I to III. J Clin Oncol 1999; 17: 3468–3475
(127) Yamada S, Harada Y, Noguchi H, Satoh N, Kimura S, Nakayama T, Tanimoto A. Embryonal rhabdomyosarcoma arising from the uterine corpus in a postmenopausal female: A surgical case challenging the genuine diagnosis on a cytology specimen. Diagn Pathol 2016;11: 3. DOI: 10.1186/s13000-016-0451-0
(128) Yang L, Takimoto T, Fujimoto J. Prognostic model for predicting overall survival in children and adolescents with rhabdomyosarcoma. BMC Cancer 2014; 14: 654. DOI: 10.1186/1471-2407-14-654
(129) Yeasmin S, Nakayama K, Oride A, Ishibashi M, Ishikawa N, Katagiri A, Iida K, Nakayama N, Miyazaki K. A case of extremely chemoresistant pure pleomorphic rhabdomyosarcoma of the uterus associated with a high serum LDH level. Eur J Gynaecol Oncol 2008; 29: 518–522
(130) Young RH, Scully RE. Alveolar rhabdomyosarcoma metastatic to the ovary. A report of two cases and a discussion of the differential diagnosis of small cell malignant tumors of the ovary. Cancer 1989; 64: 899–904
(131) Young RH, Kozakewich HP, Scully RE. Metastatic ovarian tumors in children: A report of 14 cases and review of the literature. Int J Gynecol Pathol 1993; 12: 8–19
(132) Zaloudek C, Hendrickson MR. Soslow RA. Mesenchymal tumors of the uterus. In: Kurman RJ, Ellenson RH, Ronnett M (eds.). Blaustein's Pathology Of The Female Tract. 6th edn. Springer 2011, pp. 453–527

Image references

Budihardjo-Welim H. Praxis für Pathologie Hemer, Hemer. Fig. 3.2.1 (B), (C)
Frericks B, Löhr G. DRK Kliniken Berlin | Westend, Radiologie, Berlin. Fig. 3.1.3 (A), (B)
Hartmann W. DRK-Kliniken Berlin Westend, Klinik für Gynäkologie und Geburtshilfe, Berlin. Figs. 3.1.1 (A); 3.1.2 (A)
Hoestermann C. Katharinen-Hospital, Gynäkologische Abteilung, Unna. Fig. 3.2.1 (A)
Hosten N, Hegenscheid K. Universitätsmedizin Greifswald, Institut für Diagnostische Radiologie und Neuroradiologie, Greifswald. Fig. 3.1.4 (B)
Klöppel R. Klinikum Chemnitz, Institut für bildgebende Diagnostik, Chemnitz. Fig. 3.1.5
Lampe B, Gröning T. Florence-Nightingale-Krankenhaus Kaiserswerther Diakonie, Zentrum für gynäkologische Chirurgie, Kaiserswerth. Fig. 3.1.2 (B)–(D)
Letzel M, Jäpelt Th. Gemeinschaftspraxis bildgebende Diagnostik, Nordhausen. Fig. 3.1.4 (A)
Radtke C. DRK Kliniken Berlin | Westend, Institut für Pathologie, Berlin. Fig. 3.1.1 (B), (C)

Günter Köhler, Katja Evert, Marek Zygmunt and Matthias Evert

4 Perivascular epithelioid cell tumor (PEComa)

4.1 PEComa of the uterus

4.1.1 General, epidemiology, etiology, pathogenesis, staging

The perivascular epithelioid cell tumor is a mesenchymal tumor that is more widely known under its acronym "PEComa". Current WHO Classification categorizes this type of tumor under "miscellaneous mesenchymal tumors" (32). Only very little is currently known in terms of its epidemiology, etiology and pathogenesis. PEComas more frequently occur in women (male–female ratio of 1 : 7) in a number of different organs and localizations, such as the lungs, the liver, the kidneys, the large and small intestines, and the bones (16). Compared to other localizations, PEComas are relatively frequently found in the uterus and the lesser pelvis, as around 40 % of PEComas in women arise in genital sites. Uterine PEComas can occur in the cervix and the corpus uteri. Patients are aged between 7 and 75 years (mean 45 years). Women with cervical primary involvement appear to be 10 years younger on average (9, 58). Median and mean age are 49 resp. 50 years when PEComas at extrauterine sites are included (41). The majority of women are thus premenopausal. About 15 % of affected women simultaneously present with tuberous sclerosis, an autosomal dominant hereditary disease that goes hand in hand with malformations and tumors of the brain. This clinical picture is associated with mutations of the tumor growth suppressor genes TSC1 and/or TSC2 (tuberous sclerosis 1 or 2 protein), the presence of which cannot, however, necessarily be verified in every case. The TSC1 gene encodes a growth suppression protein and, together with the TSC2 protein, serves to inhibit mTOR (mammalian Target of Rapamycin) – a protein that, among other effects, promotes cell proliferation as a protein kinase via different signaling pathways. Dysfunction of these genes can thus result in increased mTOR activity. At the end of its signaling pathway, overactive mTOR leads to a plethora of oncogenic effects, like e.g. proliferation, cell growth and angiogenesis. Activation of the mTOR pathway has also been verified in PEComas (25, 36). The presence of skin angiofibromas (typically in the central facial region), renal and extrarenal angiomyolipomas as well as lymphangioleiomyomas/lymphangioleiomyomatosis in the lung, the lesser pelvis or the uterus is another typical characteristic of PEComas. TFE3 translocation is an alternative molecular pathogenetic route that might be relevant for cases of malignant uterine PEComas. TSC gene mutations are absent in such cases, which could imply that mTOR inhibitors could be putatively ineffective (11). Clear cell tumors ("sugar tumors") of the lung and clear cell myomelanocytic tumors of the falciform ligament are further examples for PEComas. These neoplasms differ significantly in morphological terms and have already been known for many years. Conceptually, they have retained their names and are now members of the PEComa family (12). PEComas have also been observed to have arisen in polypoid adenomyoma (24). The mTOR pathway is overactivated in a large share of these cases (25, 29, 36).

Abdominopelvic sarcomas with perivascular epithelioid cells constitute another recently identified subgroup of tumors that was established together with the PEComa concept. Both uterine and extrauterine/pelvic PEComas belong to this subtype (12). Such tumors can also affect other organs than those previously stated, for example the heart, the gastrointestinal tract, the mesentery, and the thighs. What all of these tumors share in common is their immunoreactivity to the HMB-45 (Human Melanoma Black 45) AB-clone, combined with an expression of myogenic markers or even the presence of morphologically developed smooth muscle cells. Besides HMB-45, other melanocytic markers (e.g. AB against Melan-A or the S100 protein) can also be positive, albeit not as frequently. The tumor thus exhibits immunohistochemical features of both smooth muscle cells and melanocytes. In some cases, epithelioid LMS might possibly constitute a precursor of malignant PEComas. This assumption is supported by the fact that, occasionally, in addition to the myogenic filaments, melanocytic antigens also test positive in the metastases of primary LMS that are negative for S100 and HMB-45 (45). In a similar vein, it is thinkable that there could be a connection between benign or semi-malignant PEComa and epithelioid LM (cf. recurrences and metastases). Analogous to the uterine sarcomas, there is also an account of a PEComa arising after tamoxifen exposure (24).

Essentially, PEComas are defined as tumors with perivascular epithelioid cells that co-express smooth muscle and melanocytic markers (14). According to the WHO definition, PEComas are mesenchymal tumors with varying degrees of biological aggressiveness that typically contain epithelioid cells with clear to eosinophilic granular cytoplasm and that exhibit melanocytic and smooth muscle differentiations. The hypothesis that such tumors derive from so-called perivascular epithelioid cells (33) remains unproven to this day and is most likely incorrect.

There is no specific staging system or classification for malignant uterine PEComas (not all PEComas take a malignant clinical course!). In theory, one could draw on staging for uterine LMS, as the two groups of neoplasms share certain commonalities. Likewise, staging in accordance to that provided for STS would also be conceivable. The attending pathologist should always note which classification is being used. Based on the experiences made by the DKSM, pathologists usually only provide a description of the tumor's features and characteristics, without fully opting for a certain staging classification model.

Perivascular epithelioid cell tumors (PEComas) arise in numerous organs and localizations. Affected women are usually premenopausal, predominantly with primary uterine involvement. PEComas, like the tumors arising from or in the context of tuberous sclerosis, are frequently associated with overactivity of the protein kinase mTOR. PEComas exhibit features and characteristics of both smooth muscle cells and melanocytes, and are apparently related to both. PEComas can take a benign or a malignant clinical course. There is no specific staging system for uterine malignant PEComas.

4.1.2 Macroscopic and microscopic features

About 10 % of uterine PEComas are localized in the cervix. The majority arise as solitary tumors, though occasionally numerous nodules are found in the myometrium (58). As is also the case for LMS, a PEComa can occur simultaneously with numerous ordinary LM, which inevitably makes reaching the proper diagnosis more difficult. PEComas have a mean diameter of 6 cm, though sizes of up to 30 cm have also been reported. Outer inspection of the uterus usually reveals the same features and characteristics as those presented by LM (Fig. 4.1.1 (A)). PEComas are usually intramurally or subserously located and can be more or less clearly delineated from their surroundings, depending on whether they are malignant or benign. The surface is usually smooth and, like LM, appears to be encapsulated (Fig. 4.1.1 (B)), however without a real capsule actually being present. Uncut PEComa specimens can also bear strong resemblance to regular LM in terms of both their gross appearance and their consistency (58), but often appear to be soft and fleshy. Firm bands of collagen can give the tumor a multinodular appearance. It is also not uncommon for cystic structures to be present that are also noticeable in the results yielded from imaging diagnostics (Fig. 4.1.1 (B), (C)).

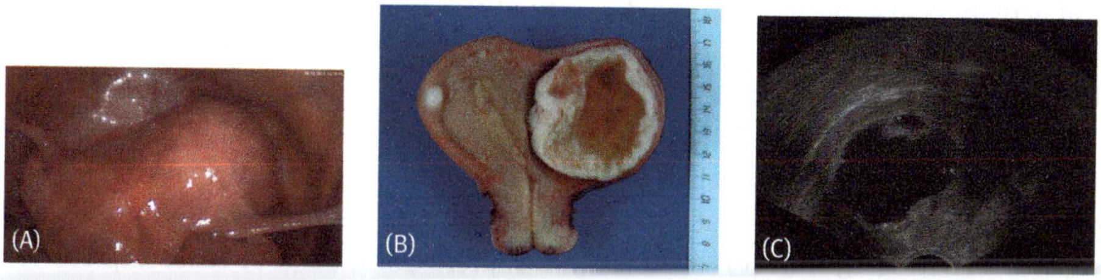

Fig. 4.1.1: PEComa – macroscopic appearance and sonography. (A) in endoscopic examination, the PEComa, localized in the anterior wall of the uterus, appears to be leiomyoma; its "softness" was already noticeable in clinical examination; (B) a large and a small cystic section are recognizable within the tumor on observation of the cut-open specimen. This benign PEComa was clearly/sharply delineated from the myometrium that formed a kind of "pseudo-capsule"; (C) vaginal sonography is predominated by a large cystic section, the smaller cyst is also clearly recognizable as can be seen in the cut-open specimen.

Broadly speaking, on the one hand, tumors within this subgroup can exhibit spindle cells containing eosinophilic-fibrillary cytoplasm and a fascicular growth pattern, and thus barely any clear cell proliferation. In such cases, reliable differentiation from conventional LM is barely possible. On the other hand, tumors can be predominantly epithelioid with eosinophilic clear cells. Such tumors usually exhibit distinct atypia and are reminiscent of clear cell epithelioid LMS (cf. below). PEComa cells generally have relatively uniform vesicular nuclei with coarse chromatin and distinct nucleoli (Fig. 4.1.2 (A), (B)). The nuclei of the epithelioid cells are predominantly round to oval, while in the spindle cells, they appear elongated in a fashion similar to LM. The tumor cells are arranged in short fascicles or nests that are compartmentalized by bands of collagen (Fig. 4.1.2 (B)) that, when as obvious as in Fig. 4.1.2 (B), (D), are a reliable indication that the tumor is a sclerosing PEComa. Though not always eye-catching, their focal perivascular arrangement around thin-walled, sometimes dilated vessels and a rich network of capillaries are typical features. The cells are often radially arranged around the vascular lumen, with the epithelioid cells usually located closer to the vessels, and the spindle cells located farther away from them. Larger accumulations of cells "mimicking" adipocytes or lipoblasts are often also found in lesser proximity to the blood vessels (16). Immunochemical staining serves to clearly highlight the perivascular accumulations of tumor cells, particularly those with partial melanocytic differentiation (Fig. 4.1.2 (H)).

The cells usually have low nuclear grading und exhibit few to no mitotic figures (Fig. 4.1.2 (C)), though nuclear polymorphism and higher grading are possible as well. Multinucleate giant cells are also a characteristic feature of PEComas. Independent of the aforementioned features, the tumors usually exhibit high cellularity, and mitotic activity of > 5 M/50 HPF with atypical mitoses are possible in cases of higher nuclear grading (41, 55). There are accounts of cases with extremely high MI ranging from 84 M/10 HPF to 395 M/50 HPF (25). The breadth of possible proliferative and cytological activity is also mirrored in the diversity of the biological behavior of PEComas. TCN are present in up to 50 % of cases, and can in fact take up 50 % of the tumor. Hyalinizations are common (sclerosing PEComa) (41).

The fact that a vast majority of PEComas expresses smooth muscle markers serves to firmly underline the close relationship PEComas share to smooth muscle cells – to epithelioid LM in particular, but also to epithelioid LMS. In fact, 49–100 % of PEComas express desmin (Fig. 4.1.2 (F)) and 73–93 % express SMA, 56 % of cases express vimentin and 92–100 % express caldesmon (13, 17, 41) (Fig. 4.1.2 (F)). Interestingly, there have been reports on three cases of uterine PEComa that tested entirely negative for h-Caldesmon, α-SMA, CD34, EMA and ER, but were positive for PGR and desmin (59). In another study, 25 % of cases were found to express CD10 (13).

Immunoreactivity to antibody clone HMB-45 is a key diagnostic characteristic expressed in 96–100 % of PEComas. The antibody clone HMB-45 typically stains cytoplasmic antibodies in melanocytes, which suggests that PEComas are related to such cells as well. Staining is often patchy and of intermediate intensity (29). The melanocytic antigen Melan-A can also be found in 72–88 % of PEComas (14, 29, 41), and around 2–30 % of tumors are also positive for the S100 protein (14, 41). The S100 protein is also traceable in melanocytes or melanocytic tumors. PEComas always express at least one of these melanocytic markers. Therefore, epithelioid tumors that are positive for the smooth muscle markers actin and desmin should be immunohistochemically examined via HMB-45 staining. If there is a positive reaction (Fig. 4.1.2 (G), (H)), the diagnosis must be "PEComa", as long as LMS can be ruled out (cf. DD). Cytokeratins, CD34 and CD117 are usually negative. CD117 positivity has been

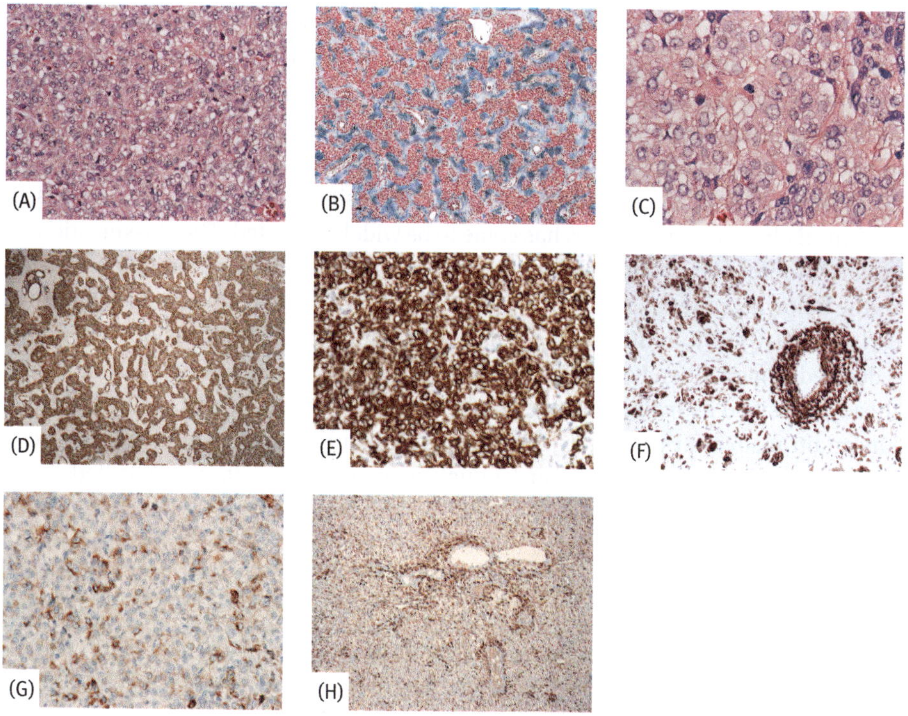

Fig. 4.1.2: PEComa – histological findings pertaining to an intraligamentarily located PEComa. (A) the cells are epithelioid throughout, sometimes clear celled and in part compartmentalized by bands of collagen fibers; (B) staining with azan clearly reveals the tumor cell nuclei in bright red, while the dense compartmentalizing collagen stains in blue (sclerosing PEComa); (C) blue enlarged nuclei with discernible nucleoli are visible in the epithelioid cells, necrosis is not present, mitotic density is low; (D)–(F) the tumor cells express various myogenic markers in both components, in this case smooth muscle actin (D), desmin (E) and caldesmon (F); in the past, such findings would have justified classification as epithelioid leiomyoma; (G), (H) expression of the melanocytic marker HMB45, strongest in the perivascularly located cells (H), makes classification of the lesion as PEComa mandatory.

documented in some cases, which, when present, can make discerning PEComa from a pelvic gastrointestinal stromal tumor more complicated (11).

There have been accounts of PEComas with glandular epithelial components or encapsulated endometrial glands (21, 29, 53). Most PEComas exhibit displacing growth into the myometrium or finger/tongue-like myometrial infiltrations that are reminiscent of LG-ESS (29). As already mentioned, PEComas could be categorizable into two morphologic groups, or subtypes (52). The first subtype consists of epithelioid cells with abundant eosinophilic cytoplasm, diffuse HMB-45 expression and only few positive smooth muscle markers, and demonstrates a finger-like growth pattern similar to that seen in LG-ESS. The other subtype consists of cells that are rather spindled than epithelioid, with less ample but clear cytoplasm. HMB-45 expression is lower, and smooth muscle marker expression is extensive. This latter subgroup might be more closely related to (epithelioid) smooth muscle tumors (44, 52). While PEComas and their metastases can be both ER and PGR negative (5), there have been numerous accounts of ER and PGR positivity (1, 28, 52, 58). ER expression tends to be stronger in some cases, but can also be entirely absent when PGR are positive (24).

Regarding the aggressiveness of PEComas, a classification system (4, 14, 16) based on clinical observational studies has come to be widely accepted. The classification in its current form (4) – a modified version of the original classification (14) – considers the following criteria: tumor size > 5 cm, high-grade nuclear atypia and cellularity, TCN, > 1 M/50 (!) HPF, infiltrative growth pattern, lymphovascular invasion. A PEComa is deemed benign when it fulfills < 2 factors and (!) is < 5 cm in size, while tumors are already classified as malignant when ≥ 2 factors are fulfilled. Tumors fall within the "uncertain malignant potential" risk category when they have a size that is ≥ 5 cm without other high risk features or (!) nuclear pleomorphism/multinucleated giant cells.

Tumors that fulfill four or more of the aforementioned features have a specificity and sensitivity of 100 % to be malignant PEComa (41).

PEComas arise in the myometrium in particular. They closely resemble leiomyoma in terms of their gross appearance and macroscopic features, but are usually fleshier. Necroses and hemorrhages can be present.

PEComas consist of epithelioid cells and/or spindle cells. The focal perivascular localization of the tumor cells around blood vessels is a prominent feature. The expression of smooth muscle markers suggests that PEComas are related to smooth muscle tumors. Immunoreactivity to melanocytic antigens, verified via antibody HMB-45 or Melan-A and S100, is a key diagnostic factor. PEComas are classified as benign, malignant or as tumors of uncertain malignant potential. Classification is made on the basis of the following factors: tumor size > 5 cm, high-grade-nuclear atypia, strong cellularity, tumor cell necrosis, > 1 M/50 (!) HPF, infiltrating/invasive margins, and lymphovascular invasion.

4.1.3 Clinical presentation, diagnostics, screening

Symptoms and clinical features correspond to those of regular LM. The diagnosis "PEComa" is thus usually only reached after surgery. AUB in form of heavy and prolonged menstrual bleedings, and dysmenorrhea are typical symptoms in pubescent women. Virtually all PEComas present with AUB and/or pelvic pain (41). Lower abdominal pains are suggestive of a rapidly growing lesion. The findings and features yielded from palpation also barely differ from those of regular LM. PEComas are usually solitary tumors. Identifying multiple lesions via palpation could be suggestive of multilocular PEComa or simultaneous LM. PEComas are usually softer than LM and have numerous clinical differential diagnostic alternatives. Simultaneous tuberous sclerosis or the presence of a tumor from the PEComa family, e.g. angiofibroma, angiomyolipoma or lymphangioleiomyoma, are factors strongly suggestive of a uterine PE-Coma.

Since a reliable diagnosis “PEComa” will only be possible prior to surgery in exceptional cases, the clinical diagnostic approach to be adopted corresponds to that for regular LM. As a matter of course, when there is the suspicion that a lesion is not regular LM, regardless of what it is thought to really be, diagnostics must be conducted with particular attentiveness, and the diagnostic flowchart presented in Chapter 6, Vol. 1 should be applied.

No particular screening has been established in practice for this extremely rare type of neoplasm. However, in some reported cases, cytological smears yielded findings suggestive of PEComa, including discohesiveness, epithelioid morphology with ample and pale to weakly eosinophilic cytoplasm, and low-grade nuclear atypia (48). The diagnosis as PEComa was later confirmed. Therefore, PEComa must be considered as a possibility whenever cytological smears/swabs contain corresponding cellular material.

The symptoms and clinical presentation of PEComas largely correspond to those of leiomyoma. However, PEComas usually appear to be softer in comparison. Joint occurrence with tumors associated with the tuberous sclerosis complex, such as angiofibroma, angiomyolipoma and lymphangioleiomyoma, is particularly suspicious. The diagnosis “PEComa” is reached postoperatively in the majority of cases. No particular screening methods have yet been established as standard practice, though cells suggestive of PEComa can occasionally be found in cytological swabs/smears.

4.1.4 Imaging

Literature pertaining to the imaging diagnostic features of uterine PEComas is sparse as corresponding cases are so rare. A PEComa should at least be considered as a possibility in cases in which assumed LM exhibit abnormal/suspicious features, and/or in which the patient has tuberous sclerosis, facial angiofibromas or otherwise localized angiomyolipomas. Performing imaging diagnostics on the lungs (CT) is worthwhile whenever a PEComa has been reliably diagnosed as such. Doing so not only serves to verify the absence of primary metastatic spread, but also helps rule out some tumors from the PEComa family (lymphangioleiomyomatosis for example) and thus to narrow down the precise variant of PEComa at hand.

Uterine and extrauterine PEComas produce a largely identical appearance in sonography. PEComas bear resemblance to LM in many cases, but it is not uncommon for them to be derounded and/or unclearly delineated and heterogeneously echogenic (50). Reports often describe the presence of irregularly circumscribed anechoic to hypoechoic sections that correlate to the macroscopically visible cystic structures or necroses (12, 43, 50) (Figs. 4.1.1 (C); 4.1.3 (A), (B)). As in CT, the walls of the cysts are usually thickened. It should be noted that these findings all also apply to STUMP,

LMS and LM degeneration and thus do not serve to rule them out from a differential diagnostics perspective. LM or LMS are thus also the most frequently made misdiagnoses in sonography, too (50). It happens on occasion that PEComas entirely resemble the features of a hemorrhage cyst in sonography, which can result in a misdiagnosis as a "chocolate cyst" or an endometrioma (56). Malignant variants of the PEComa family can show myometrial invasion or infiltration in the right conditions (50). These features notwithstanding, sonography is not suitable for specifying tumor types. The presence of these suspicious sonographic features should, however, give rise to further imaging diagnostic procedures (cf. Vol. 1, Chapter 6).

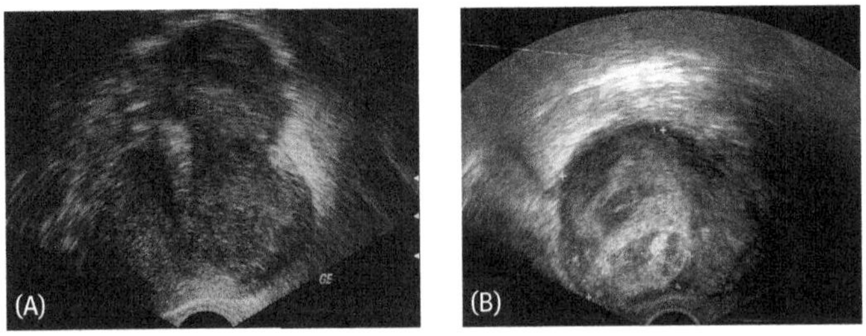

Fig. 4.1.3: Sonographic findings in PEComa. (A) A tumor with heterogeneous echogenicity that is predominantly hypoechoic containing hyperechoic as well as virtually anechoic spaces of varying size. Interestingly, pathologists diagnosed this tumor to be cellular leiomyoma at the time of primary diagnosis, as leiomyosarcoma at the time of initial recurrence, and finally as PEComa upon further relapse. The irregularly contoured margins in sonography already made a leiomyoma rather unlikely; (B) heterogeneous, predominantly hyperechoic tumor. The margins between the areas of differing echoicity are partly irregular, which is strongly suggestive of an irregular mesenchymal tumor.

CT is generally not an appropriate method for specifying tumor type, but it highly suitable for diagnosing extent and spread of disease, and as a means for monitoring palliative therapy (43). The features that uterine PEComas exhibit in CT and MRI correspond closely to those of their extrauterine/retroperitoneal counterparts and their metastases. The picture they emit is rather unspectacular, characterized in CT by a well-circumscribed, displacing solitary mass with heterogeneous density (26, 37). Other sources have described the tumor as being hypo- and isodense to the skeletal musculature (50). Hypodense sections usually correspond to necroses or cystic structures that do not enhance in CECT (43, 50) and that present as anechoic structures in sonography. The enhancement emitted is deemed significant and can be homogeneous and heterogeneous (50). According to some sources, enhancement is stronger at the margins of the tumor than at its center and higher in the venous phase than in the arterial phase (1, 22). Analogous to the clinical and sonographic findings, the features of PEComas in CT make such neoplasms very difficult to discern from LM. PEComas can even contain calcifications (37).

Analogous to uterine sarcomas, the malignant forms of PEComa, in particular, exhibit recognizable hemorrhages, cysts, necroses, and infiltrations in MRI (43). T1W reveals a hypointense tumor with hyperintense sections in hemorrhagic areas. In T2W images, the tumor has heterogeneous SI, containing hyperintense and hypointense regions with irregular and unclear margins (24, 50). Their heterogeneous enhancement in T1WC (50) makes PEComas almost impossible to discern from LMS. No appearances or features have yet been identified as being specific to PEComas, though MRI can largely serve to rule out regular LM. In MRI, PEComas can occasionally resemble the features of a hemorrhage cyst with an irregular, usually thickened wall (56).

In terms of PET-CT, the same criteria apply as for LMS.

In sonography, PEComas are characterized by exhibiting heterogeneous echogenicity across the entire tumor, often in combination with anechoic, occasionally larger cystic sections or necroses. While these features are suspicious, they do not serve to reliably discern PEComas from leiomyosarcomas.

CT is not suitable for reliably specifying tumor types. Nor can a specific diagnosis be reached via MRI. The imaging features that PEComas exhibit in MRI most closely resemble those of leiomyosarcoma, characterized in T2 weighted images by a tumor with heterogeneous signal intensity with hypointense and hyperintense areas with irregular and unclear margins.

4.1.5 Differential diagnostics

For rather soft tumors, the possible differential diagnostic alternatives are LM degeneration, an LMS, a CLM, a STUMP or an LG-ESS. Macroscopically discerning between the aforementioned types of neoplasms is often not even possible when observing the cut-open specimen (56).

Epithelioid LM and LMS are the most important DD at the microscopic level. Not only do these two tumor types have a similar morphologic appearance – they occasionally also express HMB-45 (focal expression in 36 % of LMS) and Melan-A (though the latter extremely rarely) (46, 51, 55). This is apparently an overlapping gray area in which the tumor types cannot reliably be discerned from each other, though it likely only involves very few cases in practice. However, tumors are very likely to be PEComas when there is clear staining for melanocytic markers, clear or mildly eosinophilic cytoplasm, round to oval nuclei, a prominent capillary network as well as multinucleated giant cells (52, 55). The difficulty of discerning PEComas from epithelioid LM can be somewhat alleviated by verifying the presence of a pronounced capillary network in the former, that cannot be found in the latter as such. Since differentiation is so challenging, it has been suggested that tumors that exhibit morphologic and immunohistochemical characteristics of LMS should be classified as such even when HMB-45 staining is positive, so long as no other features suggestive of PEComa are present. Tumors that do not exhibit the characteristics of LMS, but which do exhibit the morphologic criteria of PEComa and positive HMB-45 staining should be classified as PEComas, and subsequently categorized as benign, as having uncertain malignant potential, or as malignant depending on their further morphologic features (60). Notwithstanding, some also assume the stance that PEComas in fact only constitute a special form of epithelioid smooth muscle tumors that expresses melanocytic markers (44, 45, 51). This hypothesis questions the entire PEComa concept per se, since some PEComas, like angiomyolipoma of the liver for example, are certainly not variants of smooth muscle tumors. There is an interesting account of a case in which a PEComa was mistaken for LG-ESS of the uterus at primary diagnosis, and was only later identified as such on the basis of its metastases (10).

The expression of HMB-45, Melan-A, and the S100 protein makes it necessary to consider melanoma or metastases thereof as DD alternatives. Cervical melanomas are exceedingly rare, usually occur in postmenopausal patients, and – together with vaginal and vulvar melanomas, which occur five times as often – account for around 2 % of all malignant melanomas (38). Since melanomas test negative for smooth muscle markers, such findings serve to rule them out with a high degree of certainty. PEComas, in contrast to melanomas, only rarely express S100, and when they do, said expression is only very mild (41). Unlike most melanomas, PEComa cells virtually never form melanin pigment and thus do not have a noticeably dark macroscopic coloration. Cervical melanoma exhibits polypoid exophytic or ulcerous growth and spreads in the fashion of cervical carcinoma (38). Amelanotic cervical melanoma can be clinically mistaken for cervical carcinoma, and histologically mistaken for PEComa (Fig. 4.1.4). Cases in which PEComas have been misdiagnosed to this end have been recounted in the literature (6). The difficulties in differentiation are exacerbated by the fact that more than 50 % of cervical melanomas exhibit epithelioid or spindle-like cells.

The tongue- or finger-like growth pattern that infiltrating PEComas exhibit bears a strong microscopic resemblance to LG-ESS. LG-ESS and ESN can both contain ample epithelioid cells with eosinophilic cytoplasm (32). What both of these entities share in common with PEComas is that they can clinically and macroscopically "mimic" LM. The vessels in PEComas usually have thicker walls than those in LG-ESS. LG-ESS and ESN clearly exhibit stromal differentiation, have the typical spiral arterioles and usually have a CD10 positive and HMB-45 negative immune profile (55). However, CD10 expression can also be positive in PEComas (13).

Angiomyolipomas or lymphangioleiomyomatosis, both members of the PEComa tumor family, can occasionally be found in the uterus. The diagnosis "lymphangioleiomyomatosis" is usually histomorphologically footed, characterized by the presence of smooth muscle cells with flocculent eosinophilic cytoplasm in widened lymphatic vessels. Classic triphasic angiomyolipoma, in contrast, is a clinically recognizable benign tumor comprising atypical vessels, epithelioid smooth muscle cells, and fat. Both of these neoplasms express melanocytic markers by definition; HMB-45 positivity is particularly prominent (6). In principle, it can be assumed that present tuberous sclerosis or synchronous angiofibromas, epithelioid angiomyolipomas or

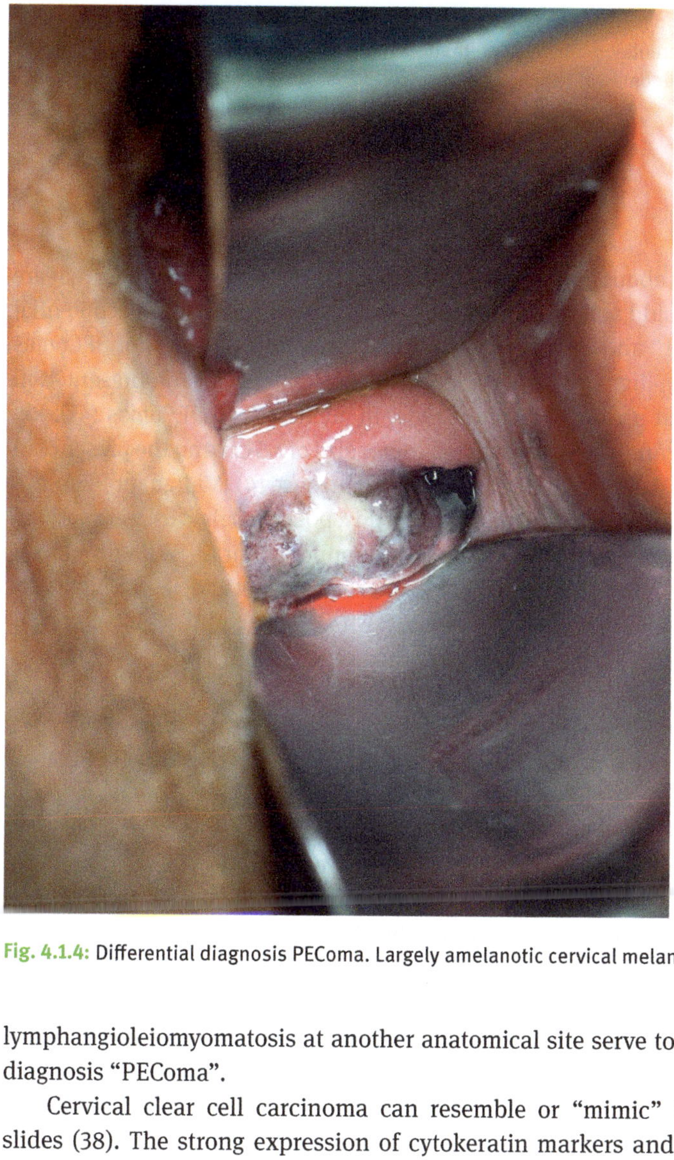

Fig. 4.1.4: Differential diagnosis PEComa. Largely amelanotic cervical melanoma.

lymphangioleiomyomatosis at another anatomical site serve to strongly support the diagnosis “PEComa”.

Cervical clear cell carcinoma can resemble or “mimic” PEComa in HE-stain slides (38). The strong expression of cytokeratin markers and the absence of verified melanocytic markers in carcinoma serve to resolve this diagnostic issue.

In summary, the key conclusion that can be drawn in the context of DD is that all mesenchymal tumors that contain epithelioid cells should be tested for HMB-45 expression.

Regular and degenerated leiomyoma, leiomyosarcoma, STUMP and low-grade endometrial stromal sarcoma constitute the most important macroscopic differential diagnoses for PEComa. Epithelioid smooth muscle tumors and melanomas (due to the expression of melanocytic markers, especially HMB-45) are the key differential diagnostic alternatives at the microscopic level. Synchronous or metachronous angiomyolipomas or lymphangioleiomyomatosis serve to sustainably support the diagnosis "PEComa".

4.1.6 Course, prognosis

Since so little is known about this family of neoplasms, even PEComa variants that are classified as benign should nonetheless be considered tumors with "very low potential for aggressive behavior" and be treated accordingly. Overall, up to 71 % of PEComas are said to fulfill the malignancy criteria (14). The malignancy criteria presented in the microscopic context are virtually always met in metastasized PEComas (41). Results from multivariate analysis suggest that a tumor size of > 5 cm and the presence of TCN are the factors most strongly associated with recurrence (4). Malignant PEComas can extend and spread beyond the uterus. In one study, positive pelvic LN were verified in 2 of 7 cases (41). However, 6 of the 7 patients who underwent LNE still developed metastatic disease. Tumors classified as malignant recur or metastasize within a median period of 21.6 mo (3–72 mo) (41). In one review (4), 29.6 % of the PEComas that had been classified as malignant had been advanced at the time of primary diagnosis or later developed recurrences or metastases.

The lungs, the liver, the kidneys and also the bones are the most important sites of metastatic involvement (14, 58). Accounts have been published in which PEComas were simultaneously present both in the uterus and in the lesser pelvis, the adnexa and/or the abdominal cavity (12, 58). The tumors exhibited criteria suggestive of a malignancy according to the classification presented earlier. The question remains unresolved whether or not the PEComas in question were synchronous or constituted/involved locoregional metastasization. Synchronicity should be assumed in cases of simultaneous tuberous sclerosis (12).

Generally speaking, PEComas that are classified as benign should nonetheless be treated as tumors with "very low potential for aggressive behavior". Tumor sizes > 5 cm and TCN are the factors most strongly associated with disease recurrence. Metastatic spread is to the lungs, the liver, the kidneys and the bones in the majority of cases.

4.1.7 Primary surgery

THE without injuring the uterus or the tumor is the therapeutic method of choice for PEComas, not least due to the difficulties involved in ascertaining whether or not they are malignant. Like for LG-ESS, STUMP and LMS, the main problem with PEComas is that they are usually not detected as such on the basis of their clinical behavior and symptoms and are subsequently subjected to surgical treatment under the assumption of LM. Such cases have also been encountered in the advisory work of the DKSM. No standards exist in terms of surgical management (4, 41). The current NCCN Guidelines on uterine tumors and soft tissue sarcomas provide no recommendations (30, 31). Until valid, reliable data have been published, malignant PEComas should be surgically treated analogous to LMS, while PEComas with uncertain malignant potential should be subjected to surgery analogous to that for STUMP (cf. variants of LM and LMS Vol. 1, Chapters 1 and 2). This applies equally to conservative or uterus-sparing surgical procedures. A 24-year-old patient with uterine PEComa who underwent primary tumor extirpation twice developed a cervical recurrence, both of which were subsequently resected. The patient was without further relapse for 12 mo thereafter (end of follow-up) (56). Morcellation must be regarded as contraindicated for PEComas as well. Details in this regard are provided in the chapters on STUMP, LMS, and LG-ESS (cf. Vol. 1, Chapters 1, 2, 4 and 6). There are currently no data which suggest that performing RAH, BSO, LNE, or omentectomy on tumors that are confined to the uterus has an impact on OS or PFS. Among 7 patients with malignant PEComas (2 of whom had positive LN) who underwent LNE, 6 nonetheless developed metastatic disease or local recurrences (4, 25).

For advanced PEComas that extend beyond the uterus, reference should be made to the respective provisions for LMS.

Total hysterectomy without injuring the uterus or the tumor must currently be regarded as the therapeutic method of choice. Overall, reference can be taken to the specifications made for STUMP and leiomyosarcoma, depending on degree of malignancy. The same applies to conservative and additional surgical measures.

4.1.8 Adjuvant and additive radio-, chemo- and hormone therapy

There is currently no evidence to even remotely justify subjecting patients with malignant PEComas to postoperative RT. It must be assumed that, analogous to pure uterine sarcomas, postoperative ERT will not have a favorable impact on survival. Nor are any data available regarding the RFI of local recurrence. It currently remains unclear whether VBT serves to reduce the rate of vaginal stump recurrence in malignant uterine PEComas.

There are also no data that could give any insight into whether or not subjecting R0 resected malignant and semi-malignant PEComas to adjuvant CHT yields beneficial results (4, 41). The NCCN Guidelines Uterine Sarcomas and Soft Tissue Sarcomas (30, 31) do not consider PEComas in this context. The same applies to the RX situations that so regularly arise following morcellation or tumor enucleation. Nor are there any data which verify that adjuvant CHT improves PFI or OS in asymptomatic R1 resected patients. In one study, all 4 women with malignant PEComas who received CHT developed metastatic disease (41). According to one review, adjuvant therapy was even associated with higher recurrence and mortality rates, though selection bias might possibly have had a role to play (4).

MTOR inhibitors might be suitably applied in the adjuvant context (see recurrences and metastases), though the literature does not provide any reliable data to this end. There have been isolated accounts of treatment with everolimus, though no effects on RFI or OS can be concluded from the results (29). There is consensus in the available literature that there is currently no indication for administering adjuvant CHT to patients whose disease has been R0 resected. One study recounts a case in which a patient with pelvic PEComa in the posterior cul de sac was suboptimally debulked (R2 resection) in initial surgery. Upon 12 cycles of subsequent additive therapy using temsirolimus (25 mg IV weekly) there was no evidence of remaining disease (7).

While some PEComas express steroid receptors, no data are available that pertain to the application of adjuvant HT. Drawing on what is known for HR positive LMS, adjuvant HT currently cannot be deemed indicated for HR positive PEComas, regardless of whether R0, RX or R1/2 resection margins have been achieved.

There is currently no discernible indication for postoperative radiotherapy. In general, the standards and provisions pertaining to leiomyosarcoma can also be adhered to in cases of PEComa. Likewise, there is currently no indication for subjecting R0 and RX resected PEComas to adjuvant chemotherapy. Additive therapy that antagonizes mTOR (e.g. temsirolimus) might be a useful option when there are postoperative tumor residuals. Nor is there an indication for adjuvant and additive hormone therapy.

4.1.9 Primary radio-, chemo- and hormone therapy, approach in cases of general inoperability

Only insufficient data are available on the application of neoadjuvant RT, for achieving operability. Therapy attempts using radiotherapy could be considered in cases of general inoperability, though nothing is known about what the benefits of doing so might be.

Regarding neoadjuvant CHT, there is one case report of a soft tissue PEComa in which administering a combination of doxorubicin and ifosfamide achieved an 80 % tumor shrinkage (35). Bearing in mind the tumor's pathogenesis, treatment with an mTOR inhibitor might be plausible. In one DKSM case (27), treating a patient with primarily inoperable metastases and extensive recurrence with everolimus effected dramatic tumor shrinkage that rendered disease accessible for R0 resection (Fig. 4.1.6 (A)–(E)). In this case, mTOR overexpression had been verified prior to the onset of CHT (cf. recurrences and metastases). These results allow the conclusion to be drawn that neoadjuvant or even primary systemic therapy with an mTOR inhibitor could be possible in cases of PEComas that are extensive or inoperable at primary diagnosis. In another case, dramatic tumor shrinkage was achieved under temsirolimus, though the PFI was only 5 mo. One study recounts a case in which a patient with pelvic PEComa in the posterior cul de sac was suboptimally debulked (R2 resection) in initial surgery, and who showed a CR upon undergoing additive therapy using temsirolimus (7). No experiences have yet been published in terms of what the benefits would actually be of subjecting patients who have undergone successful neoadjuvant therapy to subsequent surgery. Administering mTOR inhibitors (off-label use) could serve to achieve temporary remission in generally inoperable patients. Whenever possible, mTOR activation in the tumor tissue should be immunohistochemically measured and verified.

No data are available regarding the application of primary or neoadjuvant HT to PEComa patients. Neoadjuvant or adjuvant therapy with GnRH analogues is apparently ineffective (56). Postmenopausal patients with inoperable HR positive tumors could undergo HT with AI (cf. palliative HT).

There is no indication for administering primary/neoadjuvant radiotherapy. Regarding primary/neoadjuvant chemotherapy, there are only insufficient data. Therapy with mTOR inhibitors (e.g. temsirolimus) is the most likely to achieve an effect. Primary/neoadjuvant hormone therapy is not indicated. Nor are there standards that pertain to cases of general inoperability. Systemic treatment with mTOR inhibitors, or in case of hormone receptor positive tumors with aromatase inhibitors could be conceivable.

4.1.10 Aftercare, recurrences, metastases

Aftercare for cases of malignant PEComas and PEComas with uncertain malignant potential should be designed in accordance with the approach adopted for LMS and STUMP, respectively. More details are presented in the corresponding Chapters 1 and 2 of Volume 1. TVS constitutes an essential element of PEComa follow-up, not least because it is very effective at identifying pelvic recurrences. The sonographic features essentially correspond to those of the primary tumor. They typically include numerous anechoic to weakly echoic spaces that correspond to cysts and necroses in particular, though this finding is not specific to PEComas (Fig. 4.1.5).

Any lesion that is assumed to be a metastasis of a primary uterine PEComa could theoretically in fact constitute a primary extrauterine PEComa. This is especially the case when disease is associated with tuberous sclerosis, not least because multilocular tumors can also arise in that context.

For malignant PEComas, aftercare and follow-up should be designed in accordance with the approach adopted for leiomyosarcomas, while for PEComas with uncertain malignant potential, reference should be taken to STUMP. The general suspicion must apply that any lesion assumed to be a metastasis of uterine PEComa could in fact be primary extrauterine PEComa.

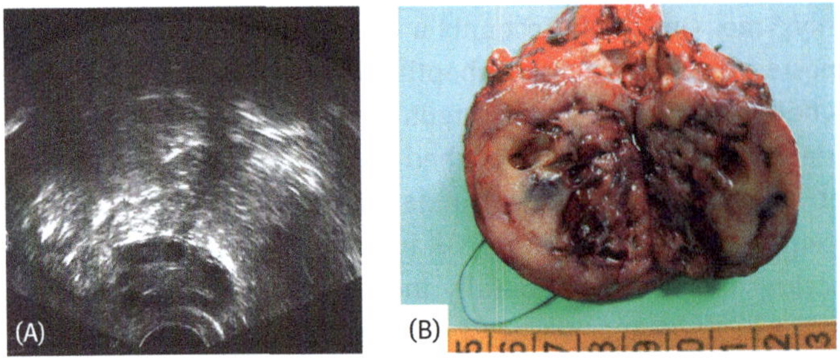

Fig. 4.1.5: Sonography and macroscopy of a pelvic PEComa recurrence. (A) Sonography reveals a tumor with heterogeneous echogenicity with numerous anechoic voids that correspond to cysts or necroses; (B) the macroscopic specimen serves to confirm the sonographic diagnosis.

4.1.11 Surgical management and postoperative additive treatment for recurrences and metastatic disease

In general, R0 resection is regarded as the measure of choice for recurrences and metastases (4, 10, 34). Overall, the data situation is very weak as only very few corresponding cases have been covered in the literature. In principle, reference can be made to the data that pertain to LMS (cf. Vol. 1, Chapter 2). Likewise analogous to LMS, early recurrences need to be reckoned with.

There have been no experiences to date that suggest that R0 resecting recurrences and metastases in asymptomatic women yields any benefits in terms of PFI and OS (4, 41). Nor are there sufficient data concerning the effects of targeted RT. Administering temsirolimus achieved a CR of residual tumor in a patient with advanced primary PEComa (7). However, there is also a report of PD following R2 resection of a colonic PEComa (40). Generally speaking, treatment with mTOR inhibitors can be considered, though it remains unproven that doing so has an effect on OS in asymptomatic patients. Symptomatic tumor residuals should be treated analogous to the palliative context.

Experiences to date suggest that R0 resection is the method of choice for recurrences and metastases. In general, reference can be made to the data and approach presented for leiomyosarcoma in this context.

It has yet to be proven that performing any form of postoperative additive therapy on patients who have undergone R0 resection of recurrences and metastases offers any benefits. Treatment with mTOR inhibitors can be considered when there is residual disease, though doing so has not yet been proven to improve survival.

4.1.12 Palliative radio-, chemo- and hormone therapy, therapy with small molecules, supportive therapy

Only isolated case studies have been published on palliative RT and PEComas. These sources suggest that RT has largely no effect on metastases or disease recurrences (8, 28). Targeted RT could conceivably serve to achieve short-term symptom control in isolated cases. Reference can be made to the criteria for LMS in this regard as well.

Palliative CHT has been the subject of only few retrospective studies and sporadic case studies on PEComa. In one case, application of liposomal doxorubicin resulted in PD (28). Combinations of carboplatin plus paclitaxel and gemcitabine plus docetaxel appear to be equally ineffective (8, 20, 40), as does the highly toxic combination of ifosfamide, vincristine and actinomycin D (34). "Positive" experiences with doxorubicin plus ifosfamide are currently limited to one case in which SD was achieved for 9 mo (23, 40).

Building on the mTOR signal pathway and its potential role in the etiology and pathogenesis of PEComas (cf. etiology and pathogenesis), the recent literature has included case studies on the targeted application of mTOR inhibitors (sirolimus/rapamycin, everolimus, temsirolimus). Within a sample of 10 patients, temsirolimus achieved a PR in 50 % and SD in 10 % of cases (3). In a recent literature review covering a total of 22 advanced cases treated with sirolimus or temsirolimus, a CR was achieved in 18 %, and a PR was achieved in 63 % of cases (RR: 81 %) (19). Besides lasting remissions, PFI was otherwise between 2–37 mo. Other sources report significant PR and a corresponding PFI of 2–22 mo for a total of 6 cases with IHC verified mTOR overactivation (one case without verification) (18, 23, 54). In a DKSM case, a patient with primarily extensive, inoperable pelvic and retroperitoneal recurrence with IHC verified mTOR overactivation was given everolimus (3 mg oral daily). The patient underwent R0 resection after 4 mo of treatment. The pulmonary metastases present vanished completely (Fig. 4.1.6 (A)–(E)) (27).

In two further case studies, mTOR inhibitors administered either alone or in combination with topotecan achieved no responses, though elevated mTOR activity had not been immunohistochemically verified prior (40, 47). The recently reported cases of TFE3 translocation-associated PEComas that lack TSC mutations (42), but that do not putatively exhibit mTOR overactivation, could well serve to explain why therapies that aims to antagonize against mTOR are ineffective. Overall, it might be sensible to expand the spectrum of predictive molecular diagnostics for individualized treatment. Overall, it would likely be sensible to verify mTOR overactivation prior to administering mTOR inhibitors. This can be achieved by presentation of mTOR target structures via IHC testing for overexpression of phospho-ribosomal protein S6, or of phosphorylated binding protein-1 of eukaryotic indication factor 4E (p-4EBP1). Since recently, the current NCCN Guidelines Soft Tissue Sarcomas have recommended the application of the mTOR inhibitors sirolimus and everolimus as a means for treating PEComa patients (30). The TKI imatinib is apparently ineffective (8).

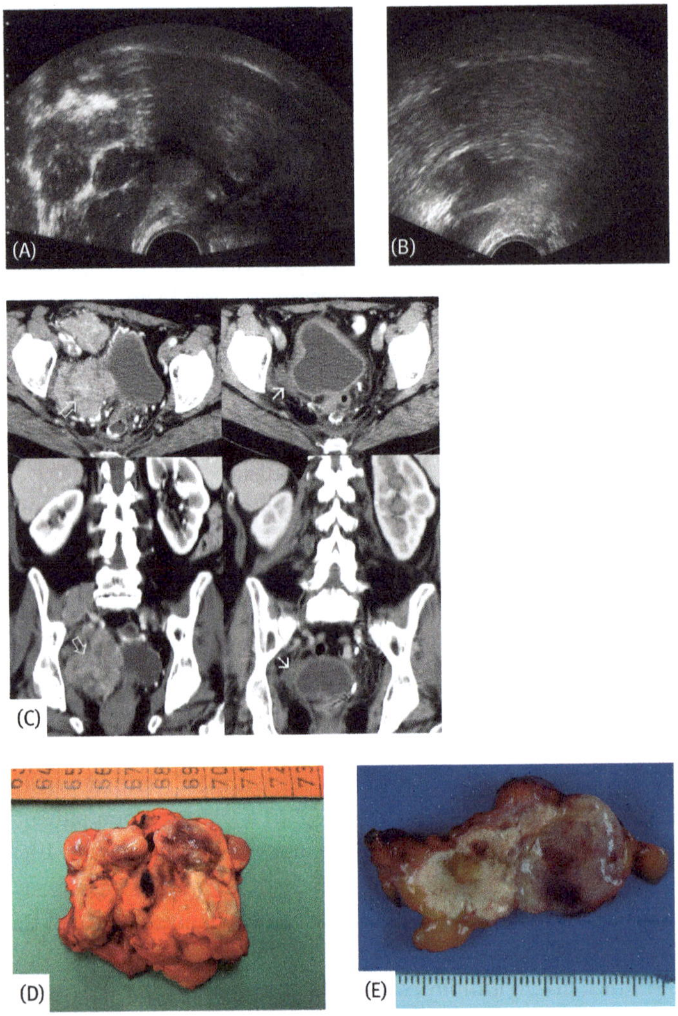

Fig. 4.1.6: Clear partial remission of an extensive PEComa recurrence treated with everolimus for 3 months, imaging and macroscopy. (A) Pre-therapeutic vaginal sonography of the recurrent lesion with numerous necroses and cysts which correspond to the anechoic spaces; (B) post-therapeutic sonography reveals substantial tumor shrinkage; (C) axial CECT confirms the findings in (A) (upper left, open arrow); coronal CECT clearly reveals that the tumor extends beyond the lesser pelvis (bottom left, open arrow), and has irregularly defined cystic and necrotic areas. Axial and coronal CECT (top and bottom right, thin arrows) after everolimus therapy show that massive tumor shrinkage has occurred; (D), (E) the remaining, subsequently resected and opened residual tumors; (D) the cystic structures and macroscopically yellow necroses correspond to the sonographic findings; (E) histology revealed necroses in the yellow areas, while the hyaline part still contained vital tumor cells, a fact that serves to confirm that remission was only partial.)

Therapy proposal

mTOR inhibitor	Everolimus	3 × 1 mg daily oral

While PEComas also express HR, no data are currently available regarding the application of palliative HT to patients with uterine PEComas. One publication reports a case of a postmenopausal patient with a massive chemo- and radio-resistant retroperitoneal PEComa with positive ER and PGR. The patient showed a lasting (at the time of publication of the report) PR and a significant reduction of symptoms after 12 wk of treatment with AI (letrozole 2.5 mg daily) (28). HT with AI thus appears to be effective in tumors with positive HR. Therefore, a therapy attempt using AI can be considered in corresponding cases. There are currently no data which suggest that the application of GnRH analogues in premenopausal women has any potential benefits. As already stated, analogous to breast cancer, combining HT with an mTOR inhibitor as a therapy attempt could be a conceivable option.

Regarding supportive therapy, the same criteria apply as for uterine sarcomas.

Palliative radiotherapy appears to be ineffective. There are no known cases of complete remission being achieved under palliative chemotherapy. Short-term partial remissions are possible under a regimen of anthracyclines and ifosfamide. When there is mTOR overactivation, applying mTOR inhibitors is the measure most likely to achieve positive results, with remission rates of up to 81 %. A hormone therapy attempt using aromatase inhibitors, possibly in combination with an mTOR inhibitor, can exceptionally be considered for tumors with positive hormone receptors.

4.2 Extrauterine and extragenital PEComas

4.2.1 General, pathogenesis, pathologic-anatomical features

The extrauterine variants should be classified as soft tissue PEComas. Patients aged as young as 8 years can be affected (34). Since the uterus is the most common site of PEComas in women, it must be considered in every case of extrauterine PEComa that there might well be a primary tumor in the uterus, and corresponding diagnostic steps should be initiated. Medical histories in such cases often reveal a STUMP or a uterine LMS that had not been recognized as a PEComa at primary diagnosis (27). Re-evaluation and re-examination of the initial specimen is sensible in any case.

There have only been isolated reports of PEComas arising in the ovaries, the vagina, the vulva, the ligamentum teres and the ligamentum latum (29, 34, 37, 55). Tumors in the wall of the bladder are reported to reach sizes of up to 9 cm. Growth is usually predominantly extravesical. PEComas of the bladder as well as tumors between the posterior vaginal wall and the anterior wall of the rectum (11) are difficult to clinically discern from uterine or vaginal PEComas. The few known cases of vesical PEComa were not recognizably associated with tuberous sclerosis (32, 47). Overall, any solid tumor within the female pelvis that bears clinical resemblance to an LM could in fact be a PEComa. The presence of further tumors from the PEComa family must always be deemed suggestive of the presence of extrauterine PEComa (see etiology and pathogenesis).

Extrauterine PEComas can occur both in genital and extragenital sites. Patients with extrauterine PEComas frequently have a past medical history of uterine PEComa that has been misdiagnosed as STUMP or leiomyosarcoma.

The uterine and extrauterine variants of PEComa do not differ in terms of macroscopic appearance, microscopic features and IHC. These tumors all appear to be more or less well encapsulated in terms of gross appearance (22, 48), with a shape and consistency that are reminiscent of LM. Positive ER have also been verified in retroperitoneal PEComas without uterine involvement (28, 57). Classification and assessment of malignancy and prognosis occurs in accordance to the criteria described for uterine PEComas.

The macroscopic and microscopic features and the assessment of the degree of malignancy of extrauterine PEComas do not differ from those of their uterine counterparts.

4.2.2 Clinical presentation, diagnostics, imaging, differential diagnostics

Extrauterine genital and pelvic PEComas are usually incidentally discovered during gynecologic examinations. Depending on their exact localization in the lesser pelvis, they can compress the ureter and sometimes the intestines and subsequently become evident via examinations conducted in the respective medical disciplines. Features in palpatory examination generally correspond to those of LM. The presence of cystic structures and/or necrosis can let the tumor appear softer. The outer surface can be smooth or occasionally (like LM) have a more nodular appearance. There are no known tumor markers, nor are there any specific or suggestive paraclinical features. Overall, for extrauterine PEComas too, present tuberous sclerosis or synchronous angiofibromas, epithelioid angiomyolipomas or lymphangioleiomyomatosis at another site serve to strongly support the diagnosis “PEComa”.

Further clarification must be sought via imaging and/or diagnostic LSC. Since benign extrauterine LM are also rather the exception, the possibility of a benign, semimalignant or malignant tumor should always be considered when palpatory and imaging examinations are suggestive of LM. Corresponding tumors should thus always be R0 resected for histologic examination. Wedge and other biopsies must always be avoided in such cases, regardless of access route. RX situations are an automatic consequence of such measures, for which an elevated risk of recurrence needs to be reckoned with.

Extrauterine PEComas can emit a strong clinical impression of ovarian tumors or other extrauterine benign and malignant soft tissue tumors.

Extrauterine PEComas barely differ from uterine PEComas in terms of their imaging features. Their extrauterine origin is usually recognizable in CT. Imaging often also reveals evidence of micturition problems in PEComas of the bladder (22).

The features and characteristics that extrauterine PEComas exhibit in imaging diagnostics do not differ from those of uterine PEComas.

Clinically speaking, extrauterine and pelvic PEComas are most likely to be mistaken for an ovarian tumor or a smooth muscle tumor of the respective site. Sonography or CT/MRI are generally capable of determining the organ of origin or whether the tumor has an extraperitoneal origin. LMS, other STS and GIST need to be considered as well whenever an extraovarian and/or retroperitoneal lesion exhibits rapid growth. While a lesion cannot be reliably diagnosed as PEComa on the basis of clinical, biochemical and imaging-based methods, PEComa is a possibility that should nonetheless be considered.

GIST can exhibit features and characteristics of PEComa, for example epithelioid cells and spindle cells or multinucleate giant cells, which can occasionally make these entities difficult to discern from each other histologically. Melanocytic markers (HMB-45, S100) as well as CD34, DOG1 and CD117 facilitate microscopic differentiation between these entities, though in GIST, the former is negative and the latter are positive (cave: CD117 positivity exceptional in PEComa) (11).

Alveolar STS constitutes another important histologic DD (41). Alveolar STS account for only 1 % of all STS and only exceptionally arise in the female genital tract (39); they also lack the joint expression of actin and melanocytic markers (15). Clear cell sarcoma is also a melanin-producing STS in younger women that expresses S100 and HMB-45, but does not express muscular markers. In principle, vaginal clear cell carcinoma can also first be mistaken with PEComa in HE-stained histological samples. The diffuse expression of cytokeratins and the lack of melanocytic markers in such carcinomas are the key suggestive factors that help to differentiate between these two types of neoplasm. Amelanotic vulvar melanoma is a differential diagnostic option for the extremely rare vulvar PEComa (Fig. 4.2.1)

Malignant PEComas in female patients that are located extragenitally and/or in the bones could in fact constitute metastatic lesions from a primary uterine tumor that subsequently needs to be searched for (58). Such PEComas in the lower extremity are more likely to be primarily localized in the bone (58).

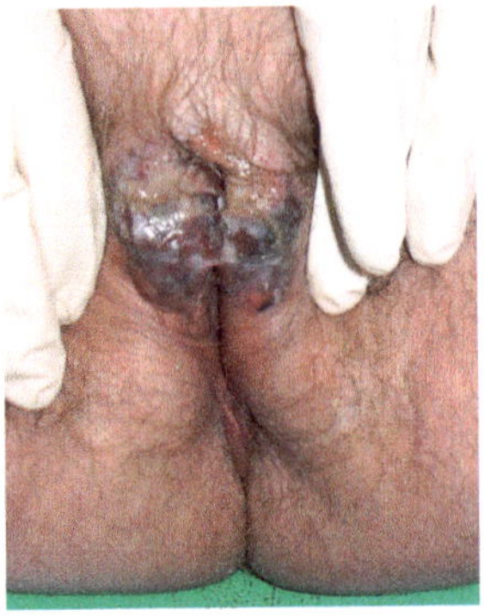

Fig. 4.2.1: Amelanotic vulvar melanoma.

GIST, alveolar soft tissue sarcoma, abdominopelvic sarcoma and clear cell sarcoma all share numerous histologic commonalities with PEComas. Successful differentiation requires intensive immunohistochemical testing with a particular focus on melanocytic markers.

4.2.3 Course, prognosis, operative, systemic and radiogenic therapy

Course and prognosis of extrauterine PEComas correspond to those of their uterine counterparts. Excision with wide clear resection margins is currently regarded as the therapeutic method of choice (2, 22, 29, 34). No data have been published to date that pertain to the potential benefits of performing LNE and other forms of farther reaching surgery. Regarding adjuvant treatment, the surgical management of advanced tumors, recurrences and metastasis, and systemic therapy, reference should be made to the uterine forms of PEComa. One study recounts a case in which a patient with pelvic PEComa in the posterior cul de sac was suboptimally debulked (R2 resection) in initial surgery. Upon 12 cycles of subsequent additive therapy using temsirolimus (25 mg IV weekly) there was no evidence of remaining disease (7). Therefore, additive therapy with an mTOR inhibitor should be considered in cases in which only R1/2 resection has been achieved in primary surgery (for details see uterine PEComas). Another publication reports a case of a patient with a massive chemo- and radio-resistant retroperitoneal PEComa with positive ER and PGR. The patient showed a lasting (at the time of publication of the report) PR and a significant reduction of symptoms after 12 wk of treatment with AI (letrozole 2.5 mg daily) (28). HT with AI thus appears to be effective in tumors with positive HR. Combining HT with an mTOR inhibitor could be possible as a “therapy attempt”.

R0 resection constitutes the therapeutic method of choice for treating extrauterine PEComas. Otherwise, the same criteria apply as for uterine PEComas.

References

(1) Armah HB, Parwani AV. Malignant perivascular epithelioid cell tumor (PEComa) of the uterus with late renal and pulmonary metastases: A case report with review of the literature. Diagnostic Pathology 2007; 2: 45 DOI: 10.1186/1746-1596-2-45

(2) Armah HB, Parwani AV. Perivascular epithelioid cell tumor. Arch Pathol Lab Med 2009; 133: 648–654

(3) Benson C, Vitfell-Rasmussen J, Maruzzo M, Fisher C, Tunariu N, Mitchell S, Al-Muderis O, Thway K, Larkin J, Judson I. A retrospective study of patients with malignant PEComa receiving treatment with sirolimus or temsirolimus: The Royal Marsden Hospital experience. Anticancer Res 2014; 34: 3663–3668

(4) Bleeker JS, Quevedo JF, Folpe AL. "Malignant" perivascular epithelioid cell neoplasm: risk stratification and treatment strategies. Sarcoma 2012; Article ID 541626, 12 pages. DOI: 10.1155/2012/541626

(5) Bonetti F, Martignoni G, Colato C, Manfrin E, Gambacorta M, Faleri M, Bacchi C, Sin VC, Wong NL, Coady M, Chan JK. Abdominopelvic sarcoma of perivascular epithelioid cells. Report of four cases in young women, one with tuberous sclerosis. Mod Pathol 2002; 15: 87–90

(6) Bradshaw MJ, Folpe AL, Croghan GA. Perivascular epithelioid cell neoplasm of the uterine cervix: An unusual tumor in an unusual location. Rare Tumors 2010; 2: e56. DOI: 10.4081/rt.2010.e56

(7) Bunch K, Sunde J. Fertility sparing treatment of a malignant uterine perivascular epithelioid cell tumor: A case report. Gynecol Oncol Case Rep 2014; 8: 14–16

(8) Ciarallo A, Makis W, Hickeson M, Derbekyan V. Malignant perivascular epithelioid cell tumor (PEComa) of the uterus: serial imaging with F-18 FDG PET/CT for surveillance of recurrence and evaluation of response to therapy. Clin Nucl Med 2011; 36: e16–19

(9) Clement PB, Young RH. Atlas of Gynaecologic Surgical Pathology. Elsevier Saunders 2014

(10) Dimmler A, Seitz G, Hohenberger W, KirchnerT, Faller G. Late pulmonary metastasis in uterine PEComa. J Clin Pathol 2003; 56: 627–628

(11) Evert M, Wardelmann E, Nestler G, Schulz HU, Roessner A, Röcken C. Abdominopelvic perivascular epithelioid cell sarcoma (malignant PEComa) mimicking gastrointestinal stromal tumour of the rectum. Histopathology 2005; 46:115–117

(12) Fadare O, Parkash V, Yilmaz Y, Mariappan MR, Ma L, Hileeto D, Qumsiyeh MB, Hui P. Perivascular epithelioid cell tumor (PEComa) of the uterine cervix associated with intraabdominal "PEComatosis": A clinicopathological study with comparative genomic hybridization analysis. World J Surg Oncol 2004; 2: 35

(13) Fadare O. Perivascular epithelioid cell tumor (PEComa) of the uterus: An outcome-based clinicopathologic analysis of 41 reported cases. Adv Anat Pathol 2008; 15: 63–75

(14) Folpe AL, Mentzel T, Lehr HA, Fisher C, Balzer BL, Weiss SW.: Perivascular epithelioid cell neoplasms of soft tissue and gynecologic origin: A clinicopathologic study of 26 cases and review of the literature. Am J Surg Pathol 2005; 29: 1558–1575

(15) Folpe AL, Deyrup AT. Alveolar soft-part sarcoma: A review and update J Clin Pathol 2006; 59: 1127–1132

(16) Folpe AL, Kwiatkowski DJ. Perivascular epithelioid cell neoplasms: pathology and pathogenesis. Hum Pathol 2010; 41: 1–15

(17) Fukunaga M. Perivascular epithelioid cell tumor of the uterus: report of four cases. Int J Gynecol Pathol 2005; 24: 341–346

(18) Gennatas C, Michalaki V, Kairi PV, Kondi-Paphiti A, Voros D. Successful treatment with the mTOR inhibitor everolimus in a patient with perivascular epithelioid cell tumor. World J Surg Oncol 2012; 10: 181

(19) Ghosh I, Arun I, Sen S, Mishra L. Metastatic perivascular epithelioid cell tumor responding to mammalian target of rapamycin inhibition. Indian J Med Paediatr Oncol 2014; 35: 99–102

(20) Greene LA, Mount SL, Schned AR. Recurrent perivascular epithelioid cell tumour of the uterus (PEComa): An immunohistochemical study and review of the literature. Gynecol Oncol 2003; 90: 677–681

(21) Horn LC, Einenkel J. Uterine perivascular epitheloid cell tumor (PEComa) with CD117 and PNL2 positivity and entrapped endometriotic glands, mimicking sex-cordlike differentiation. Ann Diagn Pathol 2011; 15: 216–218

(22) Huang Y, Lu G, Quan J, Sun H, Li H, Hu H, Guo J. Primary perivascular epithelioid cell tumor of the bladder. Ann Diagn Pathol 2011; 15: 427–430

(23) Italiano A, Delcambre C, Hostein I, Cazeau AL, Marty M, Avril A, Coindre JM, Bui B. Treatment with the mTOR inhibitor temsirolimus in patients with malignant PEComa. Ann Oncol 2010; 21: 1135–1137

(24) Ishibashi T, Nakayama K, Nakayama N, Katagiri H, Ishikawa N, Miyazaki K. Perivascular epithelial cell tumor arising from polypoid adenomyoma: A case report. Eur J Gynaecol Oncol 2013; 34: 104–106

(25) Kenerson H, Folpe AL, Takayama TK, Yeung RS: Activation of the mTOR pathway in sporadic angiomyolipomas and other perivascular epithelioid cell neoplasms. Hum Pathol 2007; 38: 1361–1371

(26) Koenig AM, Quaas A, Ries T, Yekebas EF, Gawad KA, Vashist YK, Burdelski C, Mann O, Izbicki JR, Erbersdobler A. Perivascular epitheloid cell tumour (PEComa) of the retroperitoneum – a rare tumor with uncertain malignant behaviour: A case report. J Med Case Reports 2009; 16: 629

(27) Köhler G, Belau, A, Dennis K, Evert K, Evert M, Hesse J, Hegenscheid K, Köller M, Krichbaum J, Kühnast M, Lehnhoff H, Lehr A, Linke L, Marcinek A, Müller S, Riechmann C, Schalitz S, Simon J, Spring P, Schädler, J, Ständer C, Trojnarska D, Wilcke S, Witte N, Zygmunt M.; Deutsches klinisches Kompetenzzentrum für genitale Sarkome und Mischtumoren an der Universitätsmedizin Greifswald (DKSM) und Kooperationspartner VAAO Deutschland und FK Frankfurt/Sachsenhausen. Datenbank und Promotions- und Forschungsgruppe genitale Sarkome, Greifswald 2016, www.medizin.uni-greifswald.de/gyn/dksm/

(28) Le P, Garg A, Brandao G, Abu-Sanad A, Panascl L. Hormonal manipulation with letrozole in the treatment of metastatic malignant PEComa. Curr Oncol 2014; 21: e518–20.

(29) Martignoni G, Pea M, Reghellin D, Zamboni G, Bonetti F. PEComas: The past, the present and the future. Virchows Arch 2008; 452: 119–132

(30) National Comprehensive Cancer Network: NCCN Practice Guidelines in Oncology – Soft Tissue Sarcoma – Version 2.2016. www.nccn.org

(31) National Comprehensive Cancer Network: NCCN Practice Guidelines in Oncology – Uterine Tumors – Version 2.2016. www.nccn.org

(32) Oliva E, Clement PB, Young RH. Epithelioid endometrial and endometrioid stromal tumors: A report of four cases emphasizing their distinction from epithelioid smooth muscle tumors and other oxyphilic uterine and extrauterine tumors. Int J Gynecol Pathol 2002; 21: 48–55

(33) Oliva E, Caracangiu ML, Carinelli SG, Ip P, Loening T, Longacre TA, Nucci MR, Prat J, Zaloudek CJ. Mesenchymal tumors. In: Kurman Rj, Carcangiu ML, Herrington CS, Young RH (eds.): WHO Classification of Tumors of Female Reproductive Organs. 4th ed. IARC: Lyon 2014, 135–152

(34) Ong LY, Hwang WS, Wong A, Chan MY, Chui CH. Perivascular epithelioid cell tumour of the vagina in an 8 year old girl. J Pediatr Surg 2007; 42: 564–566

(35) Osei DA1, Alvandi F, Brooks JS, Ogilvie CM. PEComa of the upper extremity: A unique case and description of an initial response to neoadjuvant chemotherapy. Sarcoma. 2007; 2007:53056. DOI: 10.1155/2007/53056

(36) Pan CC, Chung MY, Ng KF, Liu CY, Wang JS, Chai CY, Huang SH, Chen PC, Ho DM. Constant allelic alteration on chromosome 16p (TSC2 gene) in perivascular epithelioid cell tumour (PEComa): genetic evidence for the relationship of PEComa with angiomyolipoma. J Pathol 2008; 214: 387–393

(37) Pattamapaspong N, Khunamornpong S, Phongnarisorn C, Pojchamarnwiputh S. Malignant perivascular epithelioid cell tumour of the round ligament mimics leiomyoma on computed tomography. Singapore Med J 2009; 50: e239–42

(38) Pusceddu S, Bajetta E, Carcangiu ML, Formisano B, Ducceschi, M Buzzoni R. A literature overview of primary cervical malignant melanoma: An exceedingly rare cancer. Crit Rev Oncol Hematol 2012; 81: 85–95

(39) Roma AA, Yang B, Senior ME, Goldblum JR. TFE3 immunoreactivity in alveolar soft part sarcoma of the uterine cervix: Case report. Int J Gynecol Pathol 2005; 24: 131–135

(40) Scheppach W, Reissmann N, Sprinz T, Schippers E, Schoettker B, Mueller JG. PEComa of the colon resistant to sirolimus but responsive to doxorubicin/ifosfamide. World J Gastroenterol 2013; 19: 1657–1660

(41) Schoolmeester JK, Howitt BE, Hirsch MS, Dal Cin P, Quade BJ, Nucci MR. Perivascular epithelioid cell neoplasm (PEComa) of the gynecologic tract: clinicopathologic and immunohistochemical characterization of 16 cases. Am J Surg Pathol 2014; 38: 176–188

(42) Schoolmeester JK1, Dao LN, Sukov WR, Wang L, Park KJ, Murali R, Hameed MR, Soslow RA. TFE3 translocation-associated perivascular epithelioid cell neoplasm (PEComa) of the gynecologic tract: morphology, immunophenotype, differential diagnosis. Am J Surg Pathol 2015; 39: 394–404

(43) Shah SH, Jagannathan JP, Krajewski K, O'Regan KN, George S, Ramaiya NH. Uterine sarcomas: then and now. AJR Am J Roentgenol 2012; 199: 213–223

(44) Silva EG, Deavers MT, Bodurka DC, Malpica A. Uterine epithelioid leiomyosarcomas with clear cells: reactivity with HMB-45 and the concept of PEComa. Am J Surg Pathol 2004; 28: 244–249

(45) Silva EG, Bodurka DC, Scouros MA, Ayala A. A uterine leiomyosarcoma that became positive for HMB45 in the metastasis. Ann Diagn Pathol 2005; 9: 43–45

(46) Simpson KW, Albores-Saavedra J. HMB-45 reactivity in conventional uterine leiomyosarcomas. Am J Surg Pathol 2007; 31: 95–98

(47) Subbiah V, Trent JC, Kurzrock R. Resistance to mammalian target of rapamycin inhibitor therapy in perivascular epithelioid cell tumors. J Clin Oncol 2010; 28: e415

(48) Sukov WR, Cheville JC, Amin MB, Gupta R, Folpe AL. Perivascular epithelioid cell tumor (PEComa) of the urinary bladder: report of 3 cases and review of the literature Am J Surg Pathol 2009; 33: 304–308

(49) Tajima S, Koda K. Perivascular epithelioid cell tumor of the uterine cervix identified on a conventional cervical smear. Diagn Cytopathol 2015; 43: 1011–1016

(50) Tirumani SH, Shinagare AB, Hargreaves J, Jagannathan JP, Hornick JL, Wagner AJ, Ramaiya NH. Imaging features of primary and metastatic malignant perivascular epithelioid cell tumors. Am J Roentgenol. 2014; 202: 252–258

(51) Toledo G, Oliva E. Smooth muscle tumors of the uterus: A practical approach. Arch Pathol Lab Med 2008; 132: 595–605

(52) Vang R, Kempson RL. Perivascular epithelioid cell tumor ('PEComa') of the uterus: A subset of HMB-45-positive epithelioid mesenchymal neoplasms with an uncertain relationship to pure smooth muscle tumors. Am J Surg Pathol 2002; 26: 1–13

(53) Vega RB, Camino FV, Fernández MDCV, Segura GQ, González JMM, González-Tejero C. The PEComa tumor: could it be considered an independent neoplasmic entity? J Gynecol Surg 2005; 21: 161–166

(54) Wagner AJ, Malinowska-Kolodziej I, Morgan JA, Qin W, Fletcher CD, Vena N, Ligon AH, Antonescu CR, Ramaiya NH, Demetri GD, Kwiatkowski DJ, Maki RG. Clinical activity of mTOR inhibition with sirolimus in malignant perivascular epithelioid cell tumors: targeting the pathogenic activation of mTORC1 in tumors. J Clin Oncol 2010; 28: 835–840
(55) Weiss SW, Goldblum JR. (eds.) Enzinger and Weiss's Soft Tissue Tumors. 5th edn. Mosby Elsevier, Philadelphia 2008
(56) Yamamoto E, Ino K, Sakurai M, Takigawa S, Iwase A, Kikkawa F. Fertility-sparing operation for recurrence of uterine cervical perivascular epithelioid cell tumor. Rare Tumors 2010; 2: e26
(57) Yamashita K, Fletcher CD. PEComa presenting in bone: clinicopathologic analysis of 6 cases and literature review. Am J Sur g Pathol 2010; 34: 1622–16299
(58) Yang W, Li G, Wei-qiang Z. Multifocal PEComa (PEComatosis) of the female genital tract and pelvis: A case report and review of the literature. Diagn Pathol 2012; 7: 23 DOI: 10.1186/1746-1596-7-23
(59) Yu Y, Shi HY, Huang HF. Uterine perivascular epitheliod cell tumor. J Obstet Gynaecol 2014; 34: 519–522
(60) Zaloudek CJ, Hendrikson MR, Soslow RA. Mesenchymal tumors of the uterus. In: Kurman RJ, Ellenson LH, Ronnet BM (eds). Blaustein's Pathology of the Female Genital Tract. Springer Science+Business Media 2011, pp. 453–527

Image references

Arndt D. Überörtliche Gemeinschaftspraxis Arndt/Nikschick, Anklam – Greifswald. Fig. 4.1.1 (A), (C)

Evert M, Evert K. Universitätsmedizin Greifswald, Institut für Pathologie, Greifswald. Figs. 4.1.1 (B); 4.1.2 (A)–(H); 4.1.6 (E)

Horsch-Wutschel E. Frauenärztinnen am Wilhelm-Platz, Dortmund. Fig. 4.1.3 (A)

Hosten N, Hegenscheid K. Universitätsmedizin Greifswald, Institut für Diagnostische Radiologie und Neuroradiologie, Greifswald. Fig. 4.1.6 (C)

Köhler G, Zygmunt M. Universitätsmedizin Greifswald, Klinik Frauenheilkunde und Geburtshilfe, Greifswald. Figs. 4.1.4; 4.2.1

Köhler G, Mustea A. Universitätsmedizin Greifswald, Klinik Frauenheilkunde und Geburtshilfe, Greifswald. Figs. 4.1.5 (B); 4.1.6 (D)

Mustea A. Universitätsmedizin Greifswald, Klinik Frauenheilkunde und Geburtshilfe, Greifswald. Figs. 4.1.5 (A); 4.1.6 (A), (B)

Niesel A, Klinik Preetz, Abt. Gynäkologie, Preetz. Fig. 4.1.3 (B)

Günter Köhler, Katja Evert, Marek Zygmunt and Matthias Evert

5 Adenofibroma

Genital AF belongs to the group of benign genital mesodermal mixed tumors. Adenomyoma is a further benign entity.

5.1 Uterine adenofibroma

5.1.1 General, pathogenesis, pathologico-anatomical features

Uterine AF is a rare benign epithelial-mesenchymal mixed tumor (benign mixed Müllerian tumor) of the uterus that consists of a benign epithelial and a benign mesenchymal fibroma-like component. Malignant transformation of only the epithelial component results in a carcinofibroma, in which the tumorous fibrous matrix remains in the form of ample fibromatous tissue, however without losing its benign features. Carcinofibroma is generally not officially recognized as an individual or independent tumor entity, and its particularities pertaining to clinic and therapy correspond to those of EC. Malignant transformation of only the mesenchymal component of an AF creates an AS. It has long been known that an AS can develop from an AF in this manner (Fig. 5.1.2 (A), (B)) (8, 14, 15, 19), and the boundaries between these two neoplasms in terms of their features and characteristics are gradual rather than abruptly different. Patients with AS often have a prior medical history of cervical or corporal polyps. It is likely that AS or AF were primarily misdiagnosed as such or missed in these cases.

If both the epithelial and the mesenchymal matrix are malignant, the tumor in question is a CS. AS and CS are two typical examples for malignant mixed tumors. At the very least, AF is histologically located between the three aforementioned types of neoplasm.

Barely any data are available regarding the prevalence, epidemiology and etiology of AF. Such tumors are estimated to account for less than 5 % of all uterine mixed Müllerian tumors. AF usually originate in the uterine corpus, while the cervix is the primary site of disease in only around 10 % of cases. Benign biphasic AF are predominantly found in postmenopausal patients with a median age of 68 years (38), though there are also known accounts of younger patients as well (3, 32). AF can coexist with adenomyosis and endometriosis (30). As is also the case for uterine sarcomas, there have been multiple reports of a connection with previous or ongoing exposure to tamoxifen (16, 28, 30). In one case (30), a tamoxifen-associated AF continued to grow under toremifene therapy, while in another (8), an AF developed into an AS during toremifene treatment. It occasionally occurs that AF develop simultaneously in both the uterus and the ovary while subjected to ongoing tamoxifen therapy (30).

Uterine adenofibroma belongs to the group of malignant mixed Müllerian tumors and predominantly occurs in postmenopausal women. Histologically, adenofibroma is located between adenosarcoma, carcinofibroma, and carcinosarcoma, and constitutes a potential antecedent of adenosarcoma. Multiple publications report an association between adenosarcoma and exposure to tamoxifen.

The macroscopic similarities between AF and AS are striking. AF usually originate from a broad-based stem, often fill the entire uterine cavum (Fig. 5.1.1), and can cause the uterus to become irregularly enlarged (37). Tumors are known to reach sizes in excess of 15 cm and to weigh up to 800 g. When the connective tissue accounts for a large share of overall lesion volume, the mass can appear relatively solid or elastic with a grayish to whitish color, characteristics that become clearly visible when the uterus has been cut open, and that allow the assumption that the mass is an AF. It is also not uncommon for AF to have a yellowish to brownish, spongy, partly grape-like or honeycomb-like aspect caused by ample larger and smaller cysts and numerous clefts (Fig. 5.1.1). Consequently, AF are macroscopically similar to AS in this regard.

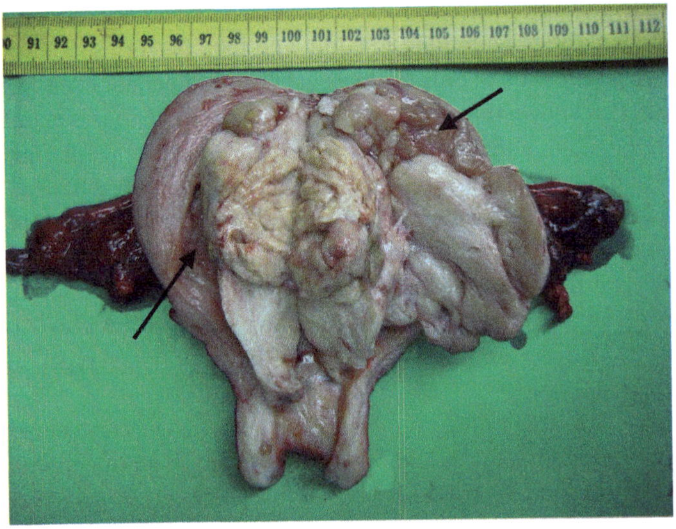

Fig. 5.1.1: Large adenofibroma with predominantly fibrous, white solid sections and centrally located areas with a sponge-like structure. This sponge-like structure causes the typical black sponge appearance in T2W-MRI. An endometrial carcinoma (arrows) was also incidentally detected that possibly developed from the adenofibroma.

In terms of their prominent microscopic features, AF exhibit papillary structures and leaf-like (phylloid) contours. The entire fibrous stroma is covered by the epithelium (Fig. 5.1.2), which also fills the gaps and voids between the papillary and phylloid contours and the intrastromal cysts, which constitute dilated glands.

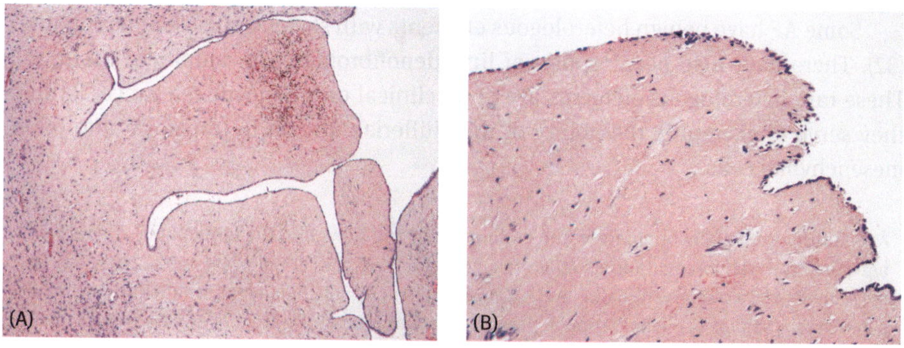

Fig. 5.1.2: (A) on low magnification, adenofibroma exhibit a leaf-like, phylloid growth pattern. The diagnostic criteria "no cellular atypia" (especially regarding the stromal cells) and "no ample mitotic activity" serve to distinguish adenofibromas from adenosarcomas. Therefore, only very few tumors, usually with a high amount of collagen fibers and low cellularity, can be classified as adenofibromas; (B) the tumor depicted here is in fact the adenofibroma component of the adenosarcoma shown in Fig. 6.1.4 (A), (B) and was its precursor (see adenosarcoma below).

Individual glandular systems can be entirely trapped/surrounded by the stroma. The epithelium is sometimes hyperplastic and can bear close resemblance to that of the endometrium, the cervix, and the fallopian tube. It can also exhibit irregular proliferations (24). The epithelium can be squamous, though this occurs only very rarely. Epithelia of various different origins can be simultaneously present within the same tumor (38). The epithelial component largely corresponds to that of AS (11). The fibrous stroma typically has a higher level of cellularity than usual and is normally fibroblastic. AF typically do not exhibit the periglandular condensation of the stromal cells that is so characteristically observable in AS. The MI is low and does not exceed 2 M/10 HPF. Atypia are not present bar for a few mild variants (11). As a general rule, a lesion should not be diagnosed as AF if the MI exceeds 2 M/HPF (37). Tumors with an MI of 2 M/HPF or more, mild atypia, moderate hypercellularity, and focal periglandular cuffs consisting of cell-rich stroma are very difficult to discern from AS. Such lesions do not yet fulfil the microscopic criteria that would allow the diagnosis "AS". They do, however, constitute a kind of "transitional entity", not least due to their immunohistochemical commonalities, e.g. in terms of Ki-67 index and p53 expression (14, 34). Unfortunately, there are no clear histopathological criteria for reliably distinguishing AF from AS (14). It is probable that tumors that are currently classified as AF due to their low mitotic counts and the absence of nuclear atypia are in fact well-differentiated AS (14).

Generally, the base of the AF is well delineated from the myometrium and is almost exclusively limited to the endometrium. Invasion of the cervical stroma and the myometrium is observed in rare individual cases (11). There are also accounts in which invasion reached almost to the serosa, with worm-like tumor plugs extending into the veins. Such cases demand thorough diagnostic effort in order to be able to reliably rule out AS (10).

Some AF have benign heterologous elements with skeletal muscle differentiation (32). There have also been reports of lipoadenofibromas with ample fat tissue (2). These rare heterologous elements are of no clinical or prognostic relevance. Rather, they serve to exemplify the ability of the Müllerian stroma to transform into other mesenchymal cells.

Adenofibromas usually originate in the endometrium and grow into the cavum uteri. Tumors are typically brownish in color and usually present with clearly discernible cysts and clefts. The tumor consists of a benign epithelial and a benign mesenchymal component. Adenofibromas have a noticeable papillary, phylloid growth pattern with ample cystic spaces. The cysts and papillary structures are lined by the epithelium, which in turn usually bears resemblance to the endometrial epithelium. High cellularity, hypercellular stromal cell condensations around the glands, atypia and a mitotic index of 2 M/10 HPF or above are features suggestive of adenosarcoma.

5.1.2 Clinical presentation, diagnostics, imaging, differential diagnostics, screening

AUB in form of intermenstrual bleedings or postmenopausal bleeding are the typical symptoms. Speculum examination quite often reveals a tumor bulging from the cervical canal. Palpation often reveals irregular uterine enlargement. Growth and cervical dilation cause lower abdominal pains. Uterine growth in postmenopausal women is a significant reason to seek help. Since all symptoms and features are also typical for uterine sarcomas, diagnostics are frequently performed under the assumption of that diagnosis. Anamnesis frequently reveals a history of polyps, in the context of which the AF might not have been recognized as such or missed. The many cysts are often clearly hysteroscopically recognizable, and give the tumor its grape-like surface structure.

Further diagnostic features pertaining to AF are identical to those of AS and LG-ESS and are elaborated in more detail in the respective chapters (cf. Chapter 6 and Vol. 1, Chapter 4). The diagnosis "AF" cannot be reached with a sufficient degree of certainty on the basis of curettage specimens alone (9, 14, 26).

No particular screening methods are applied for this rare disease in practice, and screenings in general would be uneconomic. The absence of cytological atypia makes it almost impossible to detect and correctly diagnose AF as such early on. However, such tumors can be detected in routine clinical examinations and in sonography.

Abnormal uterine bleedings are the most typical symptom of adenofibromas. They usually present with the clinical features of polyps, and often have a grape-like appearance. No specific screening methods are available for adenofibroma.

In accordance with the aforementioned gross and histologic features, sonography reveals intrauterine echoic tumor masses with well-defined margins and the quintessential ample presence of small cysts, in part reminiscent of a honeycomb structure (17, 21, 25, 30). Furthermore, the RI is low (25). One study has reported cases in which there was a lack of central vascularity (30). The overall sonographic appearance and features of AF closely resemble those of AS (cf. Chapter 6).

AF show heterogeneous enhancement in CECT, though attenuation is lower than that of the myometrium. The cystic sections can be visualized very well (21, 23, 31). CT is not a viable means for reliably discerning AF from other types of neoplasms.

In T2W-MRI, AF show up as tumor masses with heterogeneous high SI (16, 21, 23, 28, 31). Myometrial invasion, when present, can be visible in T2W images under certain circumstances (15). AF are characterized by heterogeneous low SI in T1W. Smaller sections with high SI usually represent hemorrhages (23, 31). In T1WC, the enhancement in the solid tumor sections and/or the septa between the many non-enhancing cysts is clearly visible (23, 31). The cysts show no enhancement (21) and thus give the tumor its characteristic appearance. Overall, there are barely any differences between AF and AS in terms of their MRI-related features. As also applies to AS, AF typically originate from the endometrium with a broad base and more or less fill the entire cavum uteri. Further detail is provided in the chapter on AS.

There are no data pertaining to PET-CT and AF.

> In sonography, adenofibroma usually presents as an echoic tumor within the uterine cavity with ample cysts of differing sizes. Adenofibroma and adenosarcoma cannot be differentiated from each other via CT or MRI.

Uterine polyps are the most important clinical DD for AF. AF can bear resemblance to common or necrotic pedunculated polyps, or necrotic myoma in statu nascendi. Compared to AF, necrotic myoma in statu nascendi (when not necrotic) are smooth, less fissured and jagged, and are usually more or less clearly pedunculated. Atypical polypoid adenomyoma needs to be considered as a possibility especially during pubescence. Such adenomyoma typically develop in the lower segment of the uterus and, like AF and uterine sarcomas, can protrude from the cervical canal. At the microscopic level, adenomyomas are characterized by cellular myofibroblastic stroma. The endometrial glands exhibit mitotic activity and varying degrees of cytological atypia. The smooth muscle or myofibroblastic components can occasionally contain mild to moderate atypia. ESN, the pure uterine sarcomas (LMS, LG-ESS, HG-ESS, UUS cf. Vol. 1, Chapters 2, 4, 5), and CS (cf. Chapter 7) are further differential diagnostic options to be considered when diagnosing broad-based tumor masses that are protruding from the cervix. Depending on the extent and share of their fibroblastic component, AF have a noticeably more solid, harder consistency compared to the aforementioned malignancies. Cystic structures, when present, constitute a further pivotal clinical feature that helps to distinguish AF from those malignancies, with the exception of AS. Reliably differentiating an AF from an AS on the basis of gross examination of the cut-open uterus alone is thus virtually impossible.

Endometrial polyps are also the most important DD at the microscopic level, though they are usually more glandular and have a lower degree of cellularity in the stromal part than in AF. Endometrial polyps usually lack the papillary, phylloid growth pattern. AS and carcinofibromas are further DD in this regard. In this regard, it must be borne in mind that the transition of a lesion from an AF to an AS is a gradual, flowing one that is far from abrupt (Figs. 5.1.2 (A), (B); 6.1.4 (A), (B)), which can make differentiation very difficult (14). An MI of 2 M/10 HPF and above, cellular and nuclear atypia and diffuse periglandular cuffs consisting of cell-rich stroma are factors that serve to exclude AF from the list of possible options. It happens again and again that AF need to be reclassified as AS upon closer examination and assessment (14). Curettage specimens alone are insufficient for reliably diagnosing an AF as such and thus for safely distinguishing AF from AS. Therefore, from a pathologico-anatomical perspective, reliably reaching the proper diagnosis requires that the entire tumor be present for examination and assessment (26).

Uterine polyps and adenosarcomas are the key clinical and pathologico-anatomical differential diagnostic options for adenofibromas. The diagnosis "adenofibroma" cannot be reliably and safely reached on the basis of tissue specimens retrieved via curettage alone.

5.1.3 Course, prognosis, operative, systemic and radiogenic therapy

AF are benign tumors as a general rule. What makes them so significant is their ability and potential for malignant transformation into an AS, a CS and an EC (carcinofibroma). One publication has presented an account in which a serous carcinoma and an endometrial intraepithelial carcinoma developed within an AF (35). Furthermore, patients with AF occasionally develop local recurrence. In one larger review, 12 % of patients developed local recurrences within 3–96 mo of primary surgery on the primary tumor (7). A risk of recurrence is essentially only present in cases in which uterus-sparing surgery has been performed. The risk of developing recurrent disease is however at its highest when patients are subjected to curettage alone. In actual fact, the majority of recurrences are reported for patients who have only been subjected to curettage without careful hysteroscopic R0 resection at the base of the tumor (1). Repeated conservative operations can be accompanied by repeated recurrences (29). Due to the lack of relevant data caused by the rarity of these neoplasms, it is unknown whether morcellation increases the risk of relapse and thus has adverse effects on the prognosis for AF patients, as it does for STUMP (cf. Chapter 1, Vol. 1) patients. There have been no known cases of death resulting from local disease recurrence, not least because all known cases of recurrence were subjected to THE without exception. These findings notwithstanding, malignant courses with distant metastasis have also been observed in AF with < 2 M/10 HPF, moderate cellularity, mild nuclear atypia and focal periglandular cuffs consisting of cell-rich stroma. These tumors will most probably have been AS that were misdiagnosed or not microscopically diagnosable as such (14). In summary, epithelial-mesenchymal mixed tumors with mild nuclear atypia and negligible mitotic activity, though still classified as AF, can nonetheless be associated with aggressive courses and behavior. AF could possibly also constitute a form of low-grade AS (3) or a kind of "borderline tumor" (7). AF is nonetheless classified as a benign neoplasm. Accordingly, pathologists must precisely adhere to the very strict criteria for diagnostically distinguishing AF from AS so as to prevent underdiagnosis.

In principle, adenofibromas are benign tumors. Recurrences virtually only occur following uterus-sparing surgical procedures. Analogous to STUMP, conservative surgery and/or morcellation must be considered as having adverse effects on patient prognosis. The key problem lies in the difficulty of histologically distinguishing adenofibromas from adenosarcomas, and the potential of the former to transform into adenosarcoma, carcinosarcoma or carcinofibroma.

The potential for AF to transform into an AS, a CS, and/or a carcinofibroma as well as the increased risk of recurrence that said transformation entails, make it imperative that diagnosed AF be subjected to surgical treatment. In postmenopausal patients and patients without a desire to preserve their fertility, performing THE without injuring or damaging the tumor is the therapeutic method of choice. No data are available pertaining to whether or not a BSO should be performed. Accordingly, performing a BSO (or not) will depend on the will of the patient, her menopausal status, or whether or not there is an independent indication for doing so. There is no indication for subjecting patients to BSO ex post.

Should the patient desire fertility-preserving surgery, R0 tumor resection or hysteroscopic removal via "polypectomy" can be considered. Due to the danger of developing recurrences, the tumor must be separated away at its base leaving verifiable R0 (disease-free) resection margins (24). The pathologist will not be able to safely and reliable exclude AS from the equation if the tumor is not removed in its entirety. Patients should be reresected if need be. THE is insistently recommended from a pathologico-anatomical perspective (26, 38). The same recommendation applies to patients who have undergone tumor extirpation if they no longer wish to preserve their childbearing abilities.

The tumor tissue must be completely removed via maximal cytoreductive surgery in cases of extrauterine extension.

Total hysterectomy without damaging or injuring the uterus is the therapeutic method of choice. R0 resection can be considered in cases in which patients wish to preserve their fertility. Hysterectomy should then be performed ex post. Morcellation is associated with an elevated risk of relapse and should thus not be resorted to.

Adjuvant RT, CHT and HT are neither indicated nor effective for AF.

There is no indication for subjecting operable AF to primary and neoadjuvant RT and/or CHT.

The fact that there are no data specific to AF notwithstanding, analogous to AS, progestins can be administered to patients with advanced disease as a therapeutic attempt (cf. AS) with a view to achieving tumor shrinkage. Generally inoperable patients with an intact uterus or with tumor residuals can be subjected to clinical and sonographic observation in an oncologic and clinical symptom-oriented follow-up strategy. Patients who test positively for HR can alternatively be directed to therapy with progestins, though there are no data available which would reliably support such an approach.

There are no indications for administering adjuvant therapy of any type or form. It is also not indicated that adenofibroma patients be given primary radio- or chemotherapy. For generally inoperable patients, a therapy attempt using progestins can be considered.

5.1.4 Aftercare, recurrences, metastases and their treatment

Patients with benign AF need only undergo clinical follow-up. Examinations should be scheduled in three month intervals during the first two years and should also include TVS. The intervals and the TVS are rooted in the elevated risk of recurrence in patients who have undergone uterus-sparing surgery or morcellations, as well as the fact that an AS might have been overlooked at primary diagnosis. Analogous to the procedure for STUMP, in these cases, a laparoscopic follow-up examination can be performed within six months. Within the same time period, patients who have only been primarily subjected to curettage or resection via HSC could undergo a hysteroscopic follow-up examination. Later examination intervals correspond to those for gynecologic malignancies.

There are currently no hard data against giving HRT when an AF has been reliably and safely diagnosed as such or when an AS or an LG-ESS have been reliably and correctly ruled out. At the same time, it cannot be ruled out to any degree of certainty that the development of AF may also be hormonally influenced. Therefore, when hormones are administered, it should be done with restraint. Since tamoxifen is very likely pathogenetically involved in the genesis of AF, administering tamoxifen as a form of therapy is to be deemed contraindicated. Where tamoxifen therapy is indicated as treatment for simultaneous or metachronous breast cancer, aromatase inhibitors can be given in standard dosages, as can GnRH analogues in cases of young women.

There have been isolated cases in which patients with AF developed distant metastatic disease. However, it is likely that they were in fact a result of a misdiagnosed or overlooked AS. Treatment should therefore be designed analogous to that for AS (cf. Chapter 6). Local recurrence at the site of primary disease occurs in 12 % of AF patients, almost exclusively in patients who underwent uterus-sparing primary surgical procedures (29).

No follow-up or aftercare is necessary in cases in which the adenofibroma has been removed via total hysterectomy. For patients who have undergone uterus-sparing surgery, it is sensible to design follow-up in accordance with the approach adopted for malignant tumors. Analogous to the practice for STUMP, an endoscopic follow-up examination within 6 months should be considered in such cases. There are no data that speak against hormone replacement therapy. Tamoxifen therapy is regarded as contraindicated. Recurrences of adenofibromas are virtually always locoregional or confined to the remaining uterus.

Surgical removal is the only available method for treating recurrent AF. The same principles apply as do for primary surgical treatment. THE should be performed urgently, if it has not been already, when disease recurs within the uterus. There are no data pertaining to postoperative additive therapy, so that administering such therapy is not indicated.

R0 resection is the therapeutic method of choice for treating recurrent disease. Total hysterectomy should be performed if not already done. There are no additive therapeutic methods or strategies that could be regarded as standard practice.

It essentially does not occur in practice that an AF develops distant metastatic disease that requires palliative therapy. Accordingly, there are no data on this issue. Progestin therapy would be a justifiable option when HR are positive.

Palliative contexts basically never arise in adenofibroma patients. Progestin therapy can be considered in cases in which the tumor tests positive for hormone receptors.

5.2 Extrauterine adenofibromas

5.2.1 Adenofibromas of the ovary and the fallopian tube

There exists an assumption that the development of ovarian AF is associated with endometriosis. In many such cases, the AF was also associated with a sarcoma or carcinoma of the ovaries (4). Ovarian AF are also referred to as cystadenofibromas when ample cysts are present (Fig. 5.2.1).

An AF can also be referred to as “ovarian endometrial AF” when the epithelium is of endometrial origin, and it is these cases in particular that are more frequently associated with an endometriosis (30). Otherwise, AF can also be serous, clear celled or mucinous, depending on the (non-endometrial) origin of the epithelium (20). AF of the ovaries have to be distinguished from borderline tumors that exhibit an atypical epithelial proliferation (purely epithelial papillae, mild cellular atypia). Differentiat-

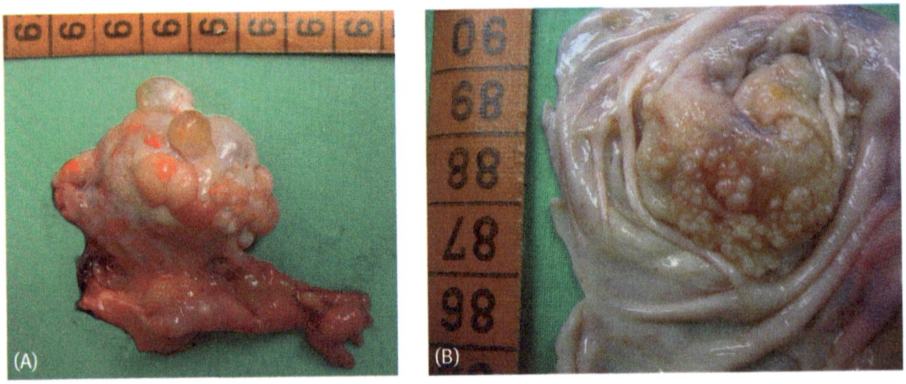

Fig. 5.2.1: Intact and opened ovary with a cystadenofibroma. (A) the epithelial cysts are already clearly grossly discernible within and alongside the fibroblastic nodules on the surface of the ovary; (B) the very solid, fibrous structure of the adenofibroma is both palpable and visualized nicely at the base of the otherwise smooth intraovarian cysts.

ing between harmless and atypical cells is particularly challenging for the clear celled types and is often subjective.

Sonography reveals solid tumors in which the (usually multilocular) cysts stand out as anechoic sections, especially in cystadenofibromas. Other sources have described a sonographic appearance that is identical to that of uterine AF (30). Doppler sonography shows a strong degree of vascularity in 50 % of cases, though it can also be entirely absent (30).

Calcifications can sometimes be found in CT, and the solid and cystic components of the tumor exhibit a heterogeneous enhancement in CECT (6).

In T2W images, the solid sections have very low SI, which is typical for fibroblastic tissue (22, 18, 27). Accordingly, ample small cysts with high SI are usually clearly visible within the very dark solid sections. These features combined serve to generate the characteristic aspect of a black sponge in T2W images. The septa of the cysts (high SI) also have low SI and are thus discernible. The cysts can compress the solid components of the tumor to narrow bands or seams (18). Ovarian AF are homogeneously isointense to the musculature in T1W (22). Enhancement is relatively low in T1WC and is weaker than that of the myometrium, and the cysts do not enhance at all (22, 18, 27). The combination of these characteristics and features, when found in the ovary, quickly results in a diagnosis of AF or cystadenofibroma. However, it should be noted that, in some cases, no cystic structures can be found at all.

AF can also occur in or on the fallopian tube. Such tumors are usually incidental findings and rarely exceed 1 cm in diameter. They almost exclusively develop in the vicinity of the fimbriae, can arise bilaterally and as multiple rather than only as solitary lesions. The epithelium in these tumors corresponds to that of endosalpingeal differentiation. Tubal and ovarian AF are difficult to discern from one another, and might in fact be identical tumors merely with differing localizations (5). In one case in which a patient had had a positive pregnancy test, a cystic tumor in the tube with embryo-like solid structures was initially mistaken for a tubal pregnancy. Salpingectomy revealed the solid mass to be an AF. The embryo was later discovered in the uterus, and the pregnancy ended with the birth of a mature child (13).

Ovarian AF are deemed to be benign neoplasms. However, relatively recent findings do suggest that clear cell OC can develop from clear cell AF (36). Ovarectomy is the therapeutic method of choice. Smaller, well-circumscribed, primarily solid tumors can be removed via organ-sparing R0 resection. There is an account of a patient who carried three subsequent pregnancies to full term after having undergone organ-sparing AF resections on both ovaries (12).

> Adenofibromas of the ovary and the fallopian tube are usually incidental findings with a favorable prognosis. T2W-MRI shows numerous cysts with high signal intensity and solid components with low signal intensity, within which yet more smaller cysts with high signal intensity can be found. R0 resection is the therapeutic method of choice.

References

(1) Agarwal PK, Husain N, Chandrawati. Adenofibroma of uterus and endocervix. Histopathology 1991; 18: 79–80

(2) Akbulut M, Zekioglu O, Terek MC, Ozdemir N. Lipoadenofibroma of the endometrium: A rare variant of benign mullerian mixed tumor. Arch Gynecol Obstet 2008; 278: 283–286

(3) Bettaieb I, Mekni, A, Bellil K, Haouet S, Bellil S, Kchir N, Chelly H, Zitouna M. Endometrial adenofibroma: A rare entity. Arch Gynecol Obstet 2007; 275: 191–93

(4) Boruban MC, Jaishuen A, Sirisabya N, Li Y, Zheng HG, Deavers MT, Kavanagh JJ. Ovarian endometriosis associated with carcinoma and sarcoma: case report. Eur J Gynaecol Oncol 2008;29: 393–396

(5) Bossuyt V, Medeiros F, Drapkin R, Folkins AK, Crum CP, Nucci MR. Adenofibroma of the fimbria: A common entity that is indistinguishable from ovarian adenofibroma. Int J Gynecol Pathol. 2008l; 27: 390–397

(6) Castro-Aragon I. Adenofibroma. In: Hricak HH, Akin O, Sala E, Ascher SM, Levine D, Reinhold C (eds.) Diagnostic Imaging Gynecology. Amirsys 2007, 7/32–7/33

(7) Chen XD, Shi HY, Zhang XF. Clinicopathologic analysis of 102 cases of mixed epithelial and mesenchymal tumors of the uterus. Zonghua Fu Chan Ke Za Zhi 2007; 42; 219–221

(8) Chung YW, Bae HS, Han SI, Song JY, Kim IS, Kang JS. Endometrial mullerian adenosarcoma after toremifene treatment in breast cancer patients: A case report. J Gynecol Oncol 2010; 21:269–272

(9) Clement P, Scully R. Mullerian adenosarcoma of the uterus: A clinico-pathologic analysis of 100 cases with a review of the literature. Hum Pathol 1990; 21: 363–381

(10) Clement PB, Scully RE. Müllerian adenofibroma of the uterus with invasion of myometrium and pelvic veins. Int J Gynecol Pathol 1990; 9: 363–371

(11) Clement PB, Young RH. Atlas of Gynaecologic Surgical Pathology. Elsevier Saunders 2014

(12) Ewing TL, Suh-Burgmann B. Preservation of fertility after partial resection of bilateral ovarian cystadenofibromas: A case report. J Reprod Med 2011; 56: 364–365

(13) Fukushima A, Shoji T, Tanaka S, Sugiyama T. A case of fallopian tube adenofibroma: difficulties associated with differentiation from ectopic pregnancy. Clin Med Insights Case Rep. 2014; 7:135–137.
(14) Gallardo A, Prat J. Mullerian adenosarcoma: A clinicopathologic and immunohistochemical study of 55 cases challenging the existence of adenofibroma. Am J Surg Pathol 2009; 33: 278–288
(15) Haque TL, Togashi K, Koyama T. Fujii S, Konishi J. An unusual presentation of endometrial polyp. Eur Radiol 2002; 12: 2906–2909
(16) Hayasaka K, Morita K, Saitoh T, Tanaka Y. Uterine adenofibroma and endometrial stromal sarcoma associated with tamoxifen therapy: MR findings. Comput Med Imaging Graph 2006; 30: 315–318
(17) Huang KT, Chen CA, Cheng WF, Wu CC, Jou HJ, Hsieh CY, Lin GJ, Hsieh FJ. Sonographic characteristics of adenofibroma of the endometrium following tamoxifen therapy for breast cancer: two case reports. Ultrasound Obstet Gynecol 1996; 7: 363–366
(18) Jung DC, Kim SH, Kim SH. MR imaging findings of ovarian cystadenofibroma and cystadenocarcinofibroma: clues for the differential diagnosis. Korean J Radiol 2006; 7: 199–204
(19) Kaku T, Silverberg SG, Major FJ, Miller A, Fetter B, Brady MF. Adenosarcoma of the uterus: A Gynecologic Oncology Group clinicopathologic study of 31 cases. Int J Gynecol Pathol 1992; 11: 75–88
(20) Köbel M, Gilks CB. Endometrioid Adenofibroma/cystadeomfibroma. In: Nucci MR, Oliva E (eds.). Diagnostic Pathology Gynecological. Amirsys 2014, 4/46–4/47
(21) Konishi Y, Sato H, Fujimoto T, Tanaka H, Takahashi O, Tanaka T. Adenofibroma of the endometrium protruding into the vaginal cavity: findings on transvaginal ultrasonography, MRI and CT. J Obstet Gynaecol Res 2006; 32: 623–627
(22) Kozawa E, Inoue K, Takahashi M, Kato T, Yasuda M, Kimura F. Diffusion-weighted MR imaging findings of ovarian adenocarcinofibromas and adenofibromas. Clin Imaging 2014; 38: 483–489
(23) Lee HK, Kim SH, Cho JY, Yeon KM. Clinical Image. Uterine adenofibroma and adenosarcoma: CT and MR findings. J Comput Assist Tomog 1998; 22: 314–316
(24) Löning T. Funktionelle Morphologie und Pathologie des Myometriums. In: Löning T, Riethdorf L (eds.). Pathologie der weiblichen Genitalorgane III – Pathologie des Uterus der Vagina und Vulva. Springer, Berlin – Heidelberg – New York 2001, pp. 652–704
(25) Maciel R, Carvalho S, Teixeira M, Areias MJ. Adenofibroma in a young patient: A rare entity in an uncommon age. Case Rep Obstet Gynecol. 2013;2 013:308464. DOI: 10.1155/2013/308464
(26) McCluggae WG. Benign diseases of the endometrium. In: Kurman RJ, Ellenson LH, Ronnet M (eds.). Blaustein's Pathology of the Female Tract. Sixth edn. Springer 2011, pp. 305–358
(27) Montoriol PF, Mons A, Da Ines D, Bourdel N, Tixier L, Garcier JM. Fibrous tumours of the ovary: aetiologies and MRI features. Clin Radiol 2013; 68: 1276–83.
(28) Oshima H, Miyagawa H, Sato Y, Satake M, Shiraki N, Nishikawa H, Arakawa A, Ogino H, Hara M. Adenofibroma of the endometrium after tamoxifen therapy for breast cancer: MR findings. Abdom Imaging 2002; 27: 592–594
(29) Seltzer VL, Levine A, Spiegel G, Rosenfeld D, Coffey EL. Adenofibroma of the uterus: multiple recurrences following wide local excision. Gynecol Oncol 1990; 37: 427–431
(30) Shi H, Chen X, Lv B, Zhang X. Concurrent tamoxifen-related Müllerian adenofibromas in uterus and ovary. Int J Clin Exp Pathol 2015; 8: 15381–15385
(31) Shin YR, Rha SE. Miscellaneous tumors of the uterus. In: Kim SH (ed.). Radiology Illustrated Gynecologic Imaging. Sec. edn. Springer 2012, pp. 249–297
(32) Sinkre P, Mille, DS, Milchgrub S, Hameed A. Adenomyofibroma of the endometrium with skeletal muscle differentiation. Int J Gynecol Pathol 2000; 19: 280–283

(33) Sölder E, Huter O, Müller-Holzner E, Brezinka C. Adenofibrom und Adenosarkom des Uterus bei jungen Frauen. Geburtshilfe Frauenheilkd. 1995; 55: 118–120

(34) Soslow RA, Ali A, Oliva E. Mullerian adenosarcomas: An immunophenotypic analysis of 35 cases. Am J Surg Pathol 2008; 32: 1013–1021

(35) Venkatraman L, Elliott H, Steele EK, McClelland HR, McCluggage WG. Serous carcinoma arising in an adenofibroma of the endometrium. Int J Gynecol Pathol 2003; 22: 194–197

(36) Yamamoto S, Tsuda H, Takano M, Hase K, Tamai S, Matsubara O. Clear-cell adenofibroma can be a clonal precursor for clear-cell adenocarcinoma of the ovary: A possible alternative ovarian clear-cell carcinogenic pathway. J Pathol 2008; 216: 103–110

(37) Zaloudek CJ, Norris HJ. Adenofibroma and adenosarcoma of the uterus: A clinicopathologic study of 35 cases. Cancer 1981; 15: 354–366

(38) Zaloudek C, Hendrickson MR, Soslow RA. Mesenchymal tumors of the uterus. In: Kurman RJ, Ellenson LH, Ronnet M (eds.). Blaustein's Pathology of the Female Tract. Sixth edn. Springer 2011, pp. 453–527

Image references

Evert M, Evert K. Universitätsmedizin Greifswald, Institut für Pathologie, Greifswald. Fig. 5.1.2 (A), (B)

Köhler G. Universitätsmedizin Greifswald, Klinik Frauenheilkunde und Geburtshilfe, Greifswald. Figs. 5.1.1; 5.2.1 (A), (B)

Günter Köhler, Katja Evert, Marek Zygmunt and Matthias Evert

6 Adenosarcoma

AS is a typical mixed tumor consisting of a benign epithelial and a malignant mesenchymal component. In the USA, AS is also referred to as "Müllerian adenosarcoma". AF (see Chapter on AF) is the respective benign variant. There are no "evidence-based" therapeutic standards for AS due to the rarity of this type of neoplasm. AS receives no mention in the NCCN Guidelines for uterine sarcomas. Without exception, studies pertaining to AS are retrospective case studies that usually cover relatively small samples.

6.1 Uterine adenosarcoma

6.1.1 General, epidemiology, etiology, pathogenesis, staging

In one study, AS accounted for only 5.5 % of all uterine sarcomas (1). In the DKSM materials database, only 5.7 % of all sarcomas including CS were AS. Their share is slightly larger (8.9 %) when CS are excluded (54). More precise prevalence data are not available. The majority of patients with AS are aged between 50 and 70 years, with a median age of 54–58 years (14). According to the DKSM data, women with AS are between 22 and 82 years old (mean 54.6 years, median age 56 years), and 61.9 % of them are postmenopausal (54). AS with and without SO (see below) do also occur in adolescents from the age of 10 onwards (13, 14, 16, 19, 30, 34, 37, 49, 72, 96). AS can also primarily originate in the cervix (63). They have been reported to account for 20.7 % of all cervical sarcomas (median age 45 years) (9). In adolescents, the cervix appears to be more frequently affected than the uterine corpus. One meta-analysis and two further casuistics report on a total of 18 cervical tumors in patients aged between 10 and 19 years (13, 26, 34). There are clear and noticeable differences between AS with and without SO in terms of patient age. A review of the literature reveals a median age of 58 years (29–87 years) among patient with AS without SO (see below), while the median age of women with AS with SO (see below) is 67 years (38–94 years) (9). Respective median ages in the DKSM material database are 56 and 55 years. There is a known account of a 14-year-old patient with AS with SO (72). AS primarily originate in the uterine corpus in 71–77 % of cases, while 10–22 % have primarily developed in the cervix, 8–15 % in the ovary and 6–12 % in other structures of the lesser pelvis, including the vagina and the intestines (37, 97, 111, 113). Over 90 % of uterine AS develop in the endometrium, a feature that serves to distinguish this type of neoplasm from LG-ESS, which primarily originates in the myometrium in the majority of cases. AS in the myometrium have likely developed out of an adenomyosis (38, 71). In this regard, the potential impact of an estrogeneous environment has also been discussed (19).

As is also the case for CS and pure uterine sarcomas, a look at the medical history of AS patients occasionally reveals previous subjection to pelvic irradiation (19). For more than a decade, however, reports have been amassing that point to AS arising within 5 mo to 8 years after exposure to tamoxifen (8, 17, 20, 32, 45). One study has also reported on a patient who developed an AF that subsequently transformed into an AS under toremifene treatment (18).

The possibility that an AF can transform into an AS (cf. Chapter 5) has been known for some time (Fig. 6.1.4 (A)–(D)). Patients with AS often have a prior medical history of cervical or corporal polyps. It is likely that AS or AF had not been initially correctly recognized as such in these cases. Malignant transformation of the epithelial component can cause an AS to develop into a CS. Furthermore, an AS and an EC can grow into each other to form a CS (collision tumor) (91). Accordingly, both an EC and an AS can develop and be simultaneously present in the uterus. Such cases are likely to be incidental findings, not least because more recent data point out that AS and CS are unlikely to be closely related lesions (77). The respective studies (77) have found that the mesenchymal, but not the epithelial components of AS harbor clonal somatic genetic alterations. It is thus assumed that, similar to fibroepithelial breast tumors, the somatic alterations would be restricted to the mesenchymal component and absent in the epithelium. These findings provide evidence that AS are mesenchymal neoplasms, and that the epithelium is independent and clonally unrelated to the mesenchymal component. The presence of the non-neoplastic epithelium may be the result of the almost invariable polypoid growth of AS. The authors hypothesize (77) that the neoplastic sarcomatous component arises within the endometrial stromal compartment, and as the stromal component grows it may eventually result in entrapment of non-neoplastic endometrium. With tumor progression, interactions with the mesenchymal neoplastic component may promote the expansion of the non-neoplastic endometrium, and the non-neoplastic endometrium itself may also elicit factors that stabilize the relationship between the epithelium and the neoplastic mesenchymal component, or even support the growth of the latter. The repertoire of somatic genetic alterations found in CS (47) was significantly less in AS. These findings are consistent with the notion that AS and CS are unrelated entities.

An overexpression of Her-2/neu has not yet been found in AS (4, 101).

Since 2009, new binding FIGO staging and UICC classifications (33, 95) have been in place for AS, that differ from those provided for pure uterine sarcomas (Tab. 6.1.1). They take into account that AS generally originate in the endometrium. One problem lies in the fact that, in the old staging system, stage II included AS that are confined to the uterus but extend to the cervix. The current stage II, by contrast, refers to disease that has spread beyond the uterus yet only to the pelvis. Stage III has experienced a dramatic adaptation. AS that now belong to stage III had previously been categorized as stage IV. Therapeutic recommendations that had in the past applied to stages II and III can thus not simply be adopted for current FIGO stage II and III.

Tab. 6.1.1: FIGO staging for adenosarcoma.

I	**Tumor limited to uterus**
IA	Tumor limited to endometrium/endocervix with no myometrial invasion
IB	Less than or equal to half myometrial invasion
IC	More than half myometrial invasion
II	**Tumor extends to the pelvis**
IIA	Adnexal involvement
IIB	Tumor extends to extrauterine pelvic tissue
III	**Tumor invades abdominal tissues**
IIIA	One site/organ
IIIB	> One site/organ
IIIC	Metastasis to pelvic and/or para-aortic lymph nodes
IV	**Tumor invades bladder and/or rectum and/or distant metastasis**
IVA	Tumor invades bladder and/or rectum
IVB	Distant metastasis

Uterine adenosarcomas are predominantly found in postmenopausal patients and most frequently develop in the endometrium, and occasionally in the cervix. Adenosarcoma can develop from an adenofibroma. Uterine adenosarcoma has its own staging that takes into consideration the fact that it predominantly arises in the endometrium, and this staging differs from staging for endometrial carcinoma.

6.1.2 Macroscopic and microscopic features

AS are usually polypoid or papillary, often broad-based pedunculated masses that frequently fill the endometrial cavity. Over 90 % of AS originate in the endometrium (Fig. 6.1.1 (A), (B)), which is causative for its early intracavitary expansion.

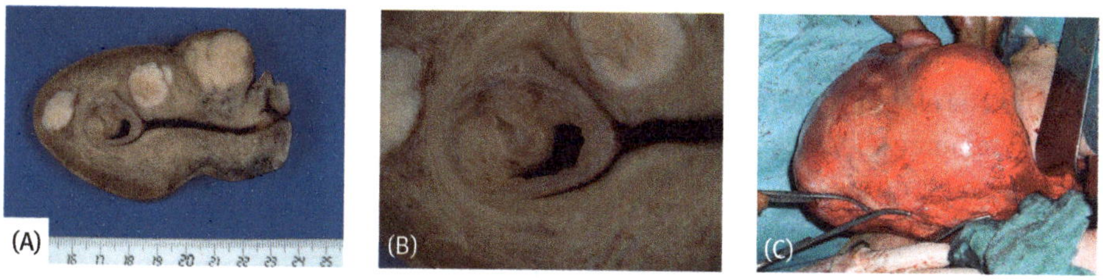

Fig. 6.1.1: Adenosarcoma – macroscopic appearance. (A) an AS alongside several LM in the fundus of the uterus; (B) it becomes apparent upon magnification that the AS developed from the endometrium and subsequently advanced into the cavum like a broad-based polyp. Numerous smaller and larger cysts are recognizable within the tumor. They usually correspond to dilated endometrial glands; (C) Adenosarcomas without sarcomatous overgrowth can also reach a substantial size.

AS can grow to a considerable size (Fig. 6.1.1 (C)). Diameters of up to 20 cm have been described in the literature (37). The tumor forces the myometrium far apart; however myometrial infiltration only rarely occurs in cases of AS without SO. AS contain epithelial cysts that vary in size and that effect a spongy appearance on the cut surface. Grape-shaped tumor masses are also typical in this context ("botryoidal" appearance) (Fig. 6.1.2 (A)–(C)).

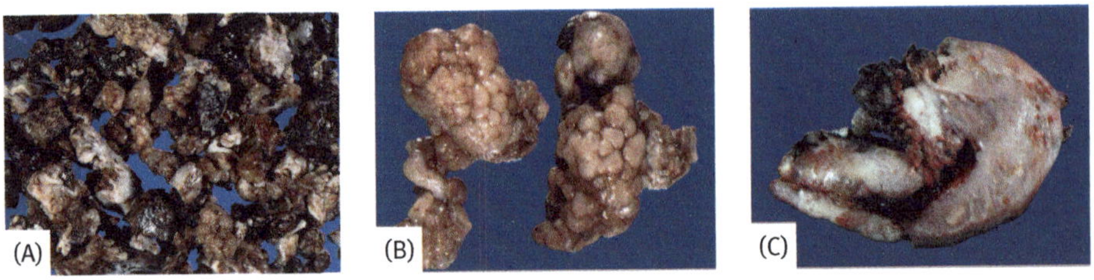

Fig. 6.1.2: Adenosarcoma without sarcomatous overgrowth – macroscopic appearance. (A), (B) the AS specimens obtained via curettage have a noticeable grape-like appearance that becomes even more apparent when magnified (B); (C) corresponding hysterectomy specimen, the uterus was perforated during curettage causing bleeding (bottom of image). The polypoid residual tumor is visible in the cavum uteri.

The cysts also constitute the pivotal feature of AS in imaging diagnostic procedures (see below). Their content can be mucinous, serous, gelatinous or hemorrhagic. The fact that AS are closely related to AF is also obvious on gross observation. The yellowish to brownish, pink or white to gray tumor is usually also macroscopically well differentiated from the myometrium. Outside the cystic areas, the tumor can be of a solid or fleshy, but also a soft and gelatinous consistency. Grossly visible necroses and hemorrhages can be observed in roughly one quarter of all cases.

AS generally originate in the endometrium. They consist of a benign epithelial component (endometrial glands) and a mesenchymal sarcomatous component. Therefore, from a purely morphologic perspective, AS lies between AF and CS. However, more recent studies (77) have shown that AS and CS are unlikely to be related.

An AS is classified as homologous when the sarcomatous component is of uterine origin (endometrial stroma, myometrium, connective tissue, vessels). Said component is comprised of an LG-ESS, an HG-ESS, an UUS, or an LMS in the majority of such cases. FS structures are additionally detected in up to 9 % of cases. There have also been rare accounts of foci of UTROSCT being found within the LG-ESS component (100). Roughly 75–80 % of AS are homologous tumors (19, 37).

By contrast, an AS is heterologous if the sarcomatous component derives from extrauterine tissue. In those cases, the mesenchymal component usually consists of RMS, chondrosarcoma, osteosarcoma, LS, or another form of sarcoma in rarer cases. Focal and entirely heterologous sarcomatous components can be found in about 45 % of AS.

Heterologous AS can also contain homologous components.

Classification of AS into tumors with or without SO is of considerable clinical and prognostic importance. An AS is classified as having SO (AS with sarcomatous expansion) when more than 25 % (61) of the tumor volume is composed of pure (i.e. epithelium-free) sarcoma. Tumors with an epithelium-free volume share below 25 % are referred to as AS without SO.

AS without SO is regarded as the "classical" or "typical" variant of AS. Unfortunately, numerous studies and publications make no precise distinction between these two AS variants. While some authors take the term AS to generally imply AS without SO, others include AS both with and without SO under that nomenclature. A look at the histological appearance of AS reveals an eye-catching phylloid, leaf-like, or papillary growth pattern. Epithelium-lined clefts and cysts of varying size, combined with papillary protrusions of cellular stroma into these cysts, serve to generate this appearance (Figs. 6.1.1 (B), 6.1.2 (A)–(C), 6.1.3 (A)–(D)).

The benign epithelial layer can be immunohistochemically visualized using cytokeratins, while the endometrial stromal cells can be highlighted by administrating an AB that targets CD10. These findings clearly show that the growth pressure that is responsible for the development of the plump protrusions is of a stromal origin. The epithelium is distributed across the entire tumor, usually in the form of benign

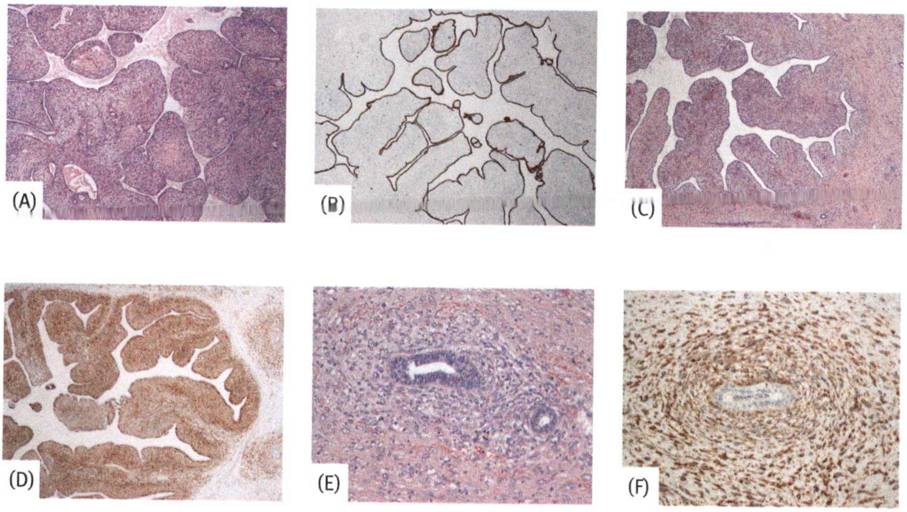

Fig. 6.1.3: Adenosarcoma – microscopic findings. (A) adenosarcoma with the typical phylloid histologic growth pattern; (B) the plump protrusions are merely covered by the flat, cytokeratine positive epithelium; (C), (D) the protrusions grow from a stromal component consisting of low-grade endometrial stromal sarcoma ((C) HE-stain, (D) CD10, serial sections); (E), (F) the hypercellularity of the subepithelial stroma, an important diagnostic feature, can also be found around the benign glands that the tumor has entrapped, a feature that can be accentuated by visualizing CD10 (F) and that led to the coining of the term "cuffing".

glandular isles (exception: AS with SO!), however without fostering an impression of infiltration. In most cases, the epithelium is atrophic/inactive or resembles the normal phase of proliferation. Like AF, AS can contain different types of Müllerian cells (endometrioid, tubal, cervical), but also metaplastic squamous and clear cells, as well as glandular hyperplasia. Complex atypical hyperplasia can occur and are usually focal. The presence of malignant epithelial cells is indicative of CS. Microscopically distinguishing AS from CS can be very difficult.

The characteristic abounding, collar-like growth of stroma cells around the benign glands (Fig. 6.1.3 (E), (F)) has resulted in the coining of the term "cuffing", a phenomenon that is strongly suggestive of an AS both in diagnostics and DD.

The fact that AS are closely related to AF is also more than apparent at the microscopic level. The case depicted in (Fig. 6.1.4 (A)–(D)) is an example for an AS that has developed from an AF.

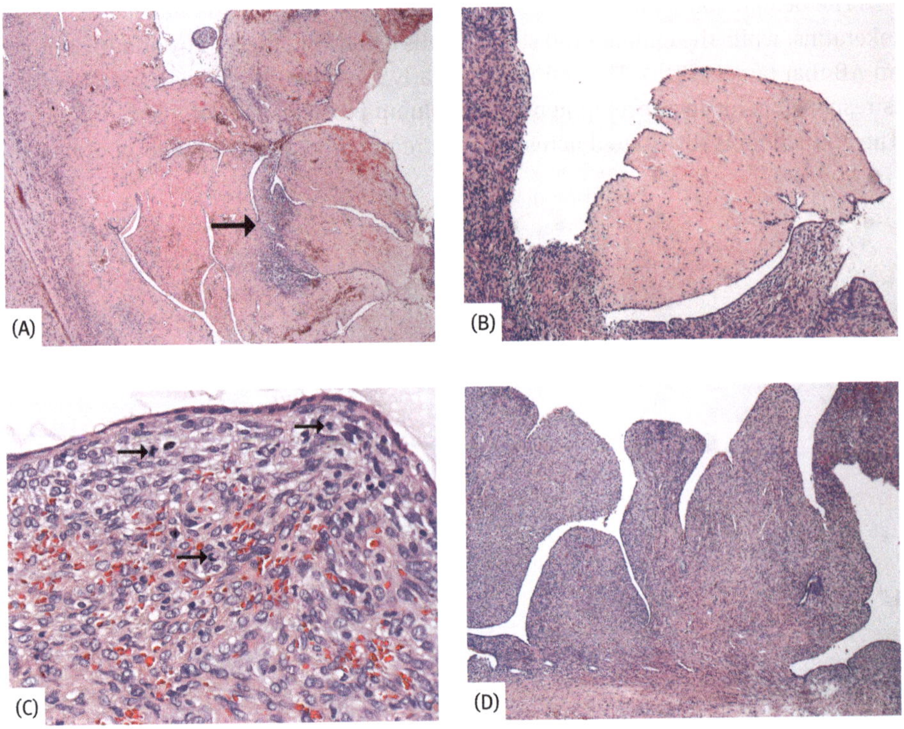

Fig. 6.1.4: Adenosarcoma – development from an adenofibroma. (A) infiltration of the adenofibroma portions by the sarcoma (arrow); (B) only small parts of the adenofibroma remain; (C) mitotic count is the decisive feature for discerning adenofibromas from adenosarcomas – in this case, 3 mitoses in one field of vision (arrows); (D) typically, this tumor exhibits no significant myometrial invasion (bottom of image).

Prime criteria for distinguishing AS from AF are: an MI ≥ 2 M/10 HPF (Fig. 6.1.4 (C)), marked stromal hypercellularity with periglandular or subepithelial stroma cell congestions (collar, cuff), and significant stromal cell atypia. The mitotic rate is usually between 2–4 M/10 HPF. However, the mean mitotic rate across the whole tumor is only 2.2 M/10 HPF (97). Occasionally, between 9 and 40 M/10 HPF have been measured in the so-called mitotic hot spots. Nuclear atypia are predominantly mild to moderate. In practice, biphasic tumors with cellular atypical stroma and periglandular cell accumulations should be classified as AS even when no mitoses are measured (19, 21, 91). The majority of AS without SO are confined to the cavity of the uterus or to the endometrium. Non-destructive myometrial invasions are rare, occurring in roughly 20 % (16–42 %) of cases, and usually reach only a few millimeters deep (19, 37) (Fig. 6.1.4 (D)). LVI is reported in only 7 % of cases (49).

Analogous to LG-ESS, AS without SO are characterized by high levels of HR expression: in one study, ER resp. PGR positivity were measured in the epithelial component of 85 resp. 65 % of AS without SO, while the stromal component was ER resp. PGR positive in 80 resp. 60 % of cases. Both ER and PGR positivity were detected in 90 % of cases (2). Seventy-seven and 81 % of the tumors covered in a further study were ER and PGR positive, respectively, while 37 % exhibited AR positivity (97). In yet another study, 33 % of AS exhibited ER positivity regardless of whether or not SO was present (44). Analogous to LG-ESS, CD10 expression tests positively in 81–100 % of AS without SO (Fig. 6.1.3 (D), (F)). Moreover, IHC testing has verified a myogenic differentiation in numerous cases (smooth muscle actin, desmin) (2, 65, 97). With levels around 5 %, the Ki-67 index is typically low (37, 97). Overall, AS without SO and LG-ESS share numerous morphological and immunophenotypical commonalities. Contrary to LG-ESS, c-Kit is only rarely expressed (up to 5 % of cases) (97).

AS with SO (Fig. 6.1.5) differ from the aforementioned "typical or classic" AS in numerous aspects. The literature suggests a rather wide range of frequency, from 8 to 60 % of all AS. The majority of studies narrow their share down to 20 % (19, 37, 49, 61, 90, 97, 106). More recent studies (14) revealed a share of 48 %, and 35.1 % of all AS in the DKSM materials exhibited SO (54). While no significant differences between AS with and without SO are discernible in the epithelial component of the tumor, the sarcomatous component of AS with SO usually consists of an HG-ESS, an UUS, or another high-grade sarcoma, for instance RMS or ANS, predominantly with severe nuclear atypia.

With an MI of up to 115 M/10 HPF and a mean MI of 13.5 M/10 HPF, the number of mitoses is significantly higher in AS with SO compared to AS without SO (19, 37, 97). Myometrial invasion is observed in 53–60 % of cases (19, 37) and often borders on the serosa. LVI is verified in up to 24 % of cases. Hemorrhaging, TCN, and heterologous components are much more frequent in this neoplasm than in its counterpart without SO (48). Analogous to HG-ESS and UUS, and in contrast to LG-ESS, ER and PGR expression are very low or non-existent. The epithelial component has shown ER and PGR positivity in 50 % resp. 25 % of cases, while the stromal component has shown ER

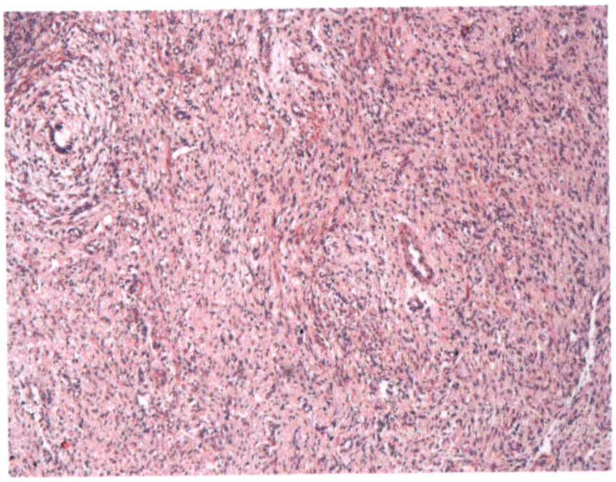

Fig. 6.1.5: Adenosarcoma with sarcomatous overgrowth. Histological analysis reveals that about 50 % of the biphasic tumor (epithelial glands and sarcoma) has been overgrown by the sarcoma. The tumor thus had to be classified as adenosarcoma with sarcomatous overgrowth, even though in this case, quite unusually, there was no histologic transformation into an undifferentiated sarcoma (small epithelium residual with "cuffing" at top left).

positivity in 0 % and PGR positivity in only 0–12 % of cases (3, 37). Seventy-seven and 14 % of the tumors covered in a further study were ER and PGR positive, respectively, while 71 % exhibited AR positivity. Malignant mesenchymoma was the only type of neoplasm in which ER and PGR expression were noticeably rarer (4 and 28 %, respectively) (97). CD10 expression tests positive in the sarcomatous component of no more than 28 % of AS with SO (2, 37, 97). Compared to "classical AS", AS with SO have a significantly higher Ki-67 and noticeably higher levels of p53 and EGFR expression (37, 97). Overall, AS with SO and HG-ESS and UUS share numerous morphologic and immunophenotypic commonalities (97). An AS can also consist of two clearly distinct areas, one with and one without SO, that can already be easily discerned from each other on gross observation. The part with SO has noticeable necroses, hemorrhages and a pleomorphic macroscopic appearance. Diagnoses can be incorrect when made on the basis of curettage specimens.

Only up to 5 % of AS with SO express c-Kit. SO can also develop as a result of an extensive UTROCST component within the sarcomatous LG-ESS (100).

The majority of adenosarcomas are localized in the uterine cavity and can prolapse into and protrude from the cervix when growth is continuous. Due to the presence of numerous cysts, adenosarcomas typically have a spongy, grape-like macroscopic appearance.

In terms of histology, adenosarcomas consist of a benign epithelial and a malignant mesenchymal (sarcomatous) component. The latter can be homologous or heterologous. Marked stromal hypercellularity with periglandular or subepithelial stromal cell accumulations are highly characteristic features. Dilated benign glands result in numerous cysts and effect a phylloid pattern. An adenosarcoma has sarcomatous overgrowth if the sarcomatous (epithelium-free) component accounts for more than 25 % of the total tumor volume. Adenosarcomas with sarcomatous overgrowth usually contain a high-grade sarcomatous component, while the sarcomatous component is usually low-grade in tumors without overgrowth. The latter usually also test positive for steroid hormone expression.

6.1.3 Clinical presentation, diagnostics, screening

Since AS originate in the endometrium or the cervix, AUB in form of intermenstrual bleedings or postmenopausal bleeding are the most common presenting symptoms. Overall, the symptoms correspond to those of EC. Palpatory examination reveals an enlarged uterus in up to 40 % of cases. Analogous to the other uterine sarcomas, a broad-based, usually polypoid tumor protruding from the cervix that can fill the entire vagina is a commonly reported finding (Fig. 6.1.6 (A)). Especially in very young patients, such tumors usually turn out to be cervical AS. Lower abdominal pain is a frequent symptom resulting from rapid tumor growth, which in turn causes the uterus to expand and/or the cervix to dilate. AS with SO can exhibit rapid growth in some cases, and can even cause the uterus to spontaneously rupture and subsequent intraperitoneal hemorrhaging (72). Anamnesis very frequently reveals a history of recurring polyps that are likely to have been primarily overlooked AF or AS (21).

Performing an HSC and/or fractional curettage is indicated when patients present with AUB or postmenopausal bleeding. AS can primarily originate in the myometrium; however, this is only rarely known to have occurred. Notwithstanding, in such cases, the AS might not be traceable in tissue specimens retrieved via curettage. The tumor can thus be missed or overlooked when patients are subjected to HSC and/or curettage. Further imaging diagnostic procedures, such as Doppler sonography or MRI, should be performed when there are obvious contradictions or differences between the histological findings yielded via curettage and the clinical and/or sonographic findings (cf. Vol. 1, Chapter 6). Overall, though, HSC and curettage are generally adequate measures for diagnosing AS. The grape-like structure encountered in imaging and microscopy is occasionally already recognizable during HSC, and is sometimes described as “cloudy” or “cloud-like” by clinicians. It is also not uncommon for such tumors to be smooth and bulging into the cavum (Fig. 6.1.6 (B), (D)). It is conceivable that the tumor depicted in Fig. 6.1.1 (A) could come to exhibit such an appearance upon further progression. In cases in which tumor masses are protruding from the cervix, measures should be limited to performing a respective biopsy. It is vital that sufficient tissue is taken during biopsy, as failing to do so increases the likelihood of a misdiagnosis as pure uterine sarcoma (cf. differential diagnostics).

Analogous to LMS, some advanced AS have been observed that exhibited elevated LDH levels, that in turn receded following cytoreductive surgery in one case and following effective CHT in another (62, 111).

AF are not suitable for a cytological screening as they lack cellular atypia. Cytological intrauterine swabs are known to have returned negative results for AS (104). Reference should be made to the screening data and information presented for LG-ESS. There are currently no adequate clinical tumor markers, the fact that elevated LDH values have been observed in some cases of AS notwithstanding (62, 111).

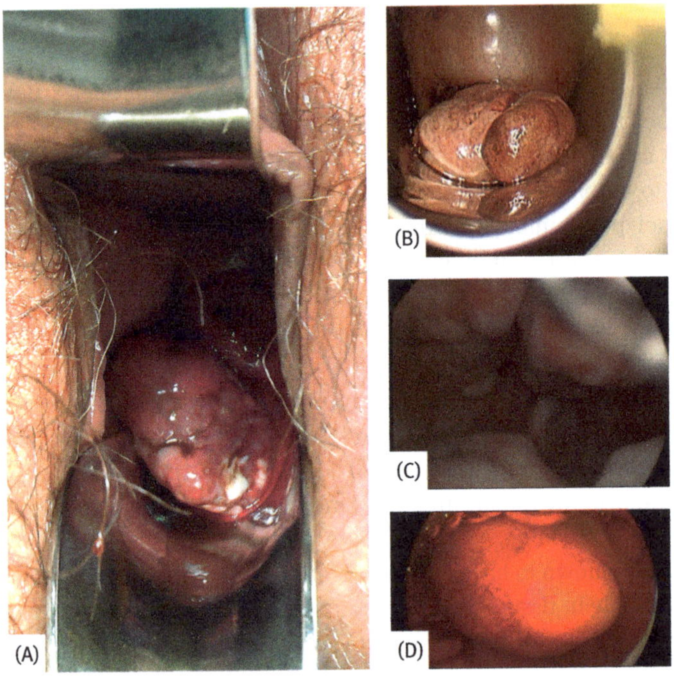

Fig. 6.1.6: Adenosarcoma – clinical appearance. (A) adenosarcoma without sarcomatous overgrowth that has prolapsed into the vagina. The cystic polypoid structure is only barely recognizable; (B) two polyps removed via hysteroscopic resection that turned out to actually be adenosarcoma with sarcomatous overgrowth. Small cystic glands are just barely visible and are an important diagnostic pointer; (C) typical HSC image with numerous grape-like tumors in a 21-year-old patient; (D) hysteroscopic findings of a relatively smooth intracavitary adenosaroma with sarcomatoeus overgrowth, the gross appearance of which had not aroused any suspicion of adenosarcoma.

Abnormal vaginal bleeding is the central symptom of adenosarcoma. The uterus is usually enlarged, and it is not uncommon for tumors to protrude from the cervix. Hysteroscopy and curettage are the key diagnostic procedures and must be accompanied by sonographic examination. No specific or adequate screening methods have yet been established in practice.

6.1.4 Imaging

Since more than 90 % of AS originate in the endometrium, in almost all imaging methods, the characteristic and typical structures of AS are virtually always only to be found in the endometrial region, or to originate from that region. The cavity is often completely filled and subsequently substantially expanded by the tumor, which can also prolapse into or originate from the cervix. In contrast to polyps, which constitute a central differential diagnostic alternative, imaging reveals a broad-based connection with the endometrium almost without exception. Narrow, stem or stalk-like connections are very rare. AS that originate from an adenomyosis can also be largely localized within the myometrium (84). The presence of extensive adenomyosis is thus also an important differential diagnostic pitfall in the imaging context. Adenomyosis usually affects the posterior uterine wall and originates from a clearly widened junctional zone. Other tumorous diseases that originate from the endometrium, like adenomatous polyps, atypical polypoid adenomyoma, EC and CS, are further imaging-related differential diagnostic options.

In contrast to LG-ESS and LMS, AS appear to be confined to the endometrium or predominantly centrally localized in sonography. AS express a heterogeneous echogenicity in the majority of cases (104) and largely correspond to the echogenic texture of the endometrium (17). Tumors have a higher echogenicity than the surrounding myometrium and can thus be easily discerned from it. Sonography typically reveals a polypoid tumor mass that fills the cavum, displaces the myometrium, and that has a broad connection to the thickened, heterogeneous endometrium from which it originates. Such findings are, however, apparently not consistently made (Fig. 6.1.7 (A)–(C)). Analogous to the macroscopic and microscopic features characterized by cystically dilated glands, sonography, too, reveals an internal structure that comprises numerous anechoic areas that represent said glands (17). These anechoic areas could theoretically also resemble vessels, which can be easily verified in Doppler sonography (Figs. 6.1.7 (C), (D); 6.1.8 (A), (B)). The usually ample presence of anechoic spaces or cysts is a key diagnostic feature. The presence of large numbers of dilated glands can also generate a honeycomb-like appearance that can often also be found in CT and MRI (Fig. 6.1.8 (C)). The phylloid growth pattern can also be clearly recognized in fortunate cases (Fig. 6.1.7 (A)–(C)). In AS with SO, gland-associated anechoic voids are noticeably rarer, because the number of endometrial glands is significantly lower in such tumors, as can already be clearly seen on gross observation (Fig. 6.1.6 (B)). Invasions of the myometrium can occasionally also be visible. AS can also exhibit features in sonography that are characteristic and typical of uterine sarcomas (cf. Vol. 1, Chapter 2 and 6).

AF can barely be discerned from AS in sonography. The localization of these tumors within the cavity and their predominantly hyperechoic texture often make them undiscernible from CS and EC.

Doppler sonographic criteria correspond to those of stromal sarcomas, characterized in particular by strong irregular central vascularity (see also Chapter LG-ESS and LMS, Vol. 1, Chapter 2 and 4). One marked difference, however, lies in the fact that, in AS, the numerous differently sized cysts are easily recognizable alongside the visible vessels (Fig. 6.1.7 (D); 6.1.8 (B)). One or multiple larger vessels can often be seen to originate from the endometrium into the tumor (17, 84).

CT frequently reveals an uncharacteristically enlarged uterus and a tumor that is isodense to soft tissue, with areas of necroses particularly in AS with SO. While these necrotic areas are suggestive of sarcoma, their presence alone is not specific enough to allow a particular tumor type to be reliably deduced. AS have clearly lower atten-

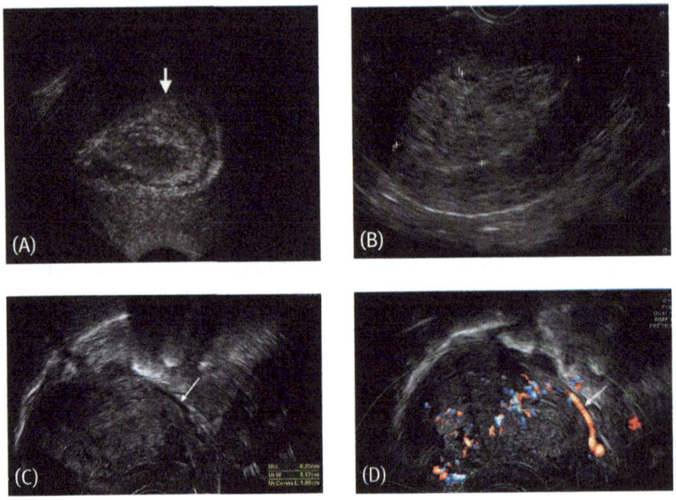

Fig. 6.1.7: Sonography – adenosarcoma. (A) hyperechoic adenosarcoma with sarcomatous overgrowth with recognizable broad origination from the posterior uterine wall (arrow); (B) sonographic examination of the tumor covered in Fig. 6.1.6 (C). The tumor is largely echogenic and contains numerous anechoic voids that correlate to the dilated endometrial glands and the phylloid growth pattern, (C) the presented image shows a polypoid adenosarcoma that fills the entire cavum. Numerous anechoic voids/areas are visible in the tumor. They correspond to the often substantially dilated glands and form a correlate to the phylloid growth patterns revealed by histologic examination, as can be seen here; (D) however, in color Doppler sonography, ample echo-free areas can also be caused by dilated vessels (arrow in (C) and (D)), the presence of which was extensive in the case at hand.

uation than that of the surrounding myometrium. In AS without SO, numerous cysts can be visible that are isodense to water and that correspond to dilated glands. The same applies to CECT, which reveals a heterogeneous enhancement alongside non-enhancing necrotic tissue. In AS without SO, the ample dilated glands can present as non-enhancing cysts. This, together with the sonographic findings, is indeed reminiscent of AS without SO (Fig. 6.1.8 (C)). Therefore, they constitute a factor strongly suggestive of AS in CT as well. Interruptions of the continuously strong, light myometrial signal in CECT are reliable evidence for myometrial invasion.

AS have heterogeneous SI in T2W images, with hypointense, intermediate, and hyperintense areas. The multitudinous hyperintense regions represent the cystic components, while the areas of low to intermediate SI correspond to the solid components of the tumor (102, 104, 105, 110). The tumor usually has an SI that is higher than that of normal myometrium. Interestingly, like LG-ESS, the tumor is surrounded by a hypointense margin (Fig. 6.1.8 (D), (E)). Clusters of cystic components with high SI correspond to the ample presence of dilated glands (in AS with SO in particular), and are a finding strongly suggestive of AS (Fig. 6.1.8 (D), (E)). T1W MRI reveals a heterogeneous tumor with an SI that is intermediate and usually isointense to the myometrium.

Focal hemorrhages exhibit high SI, while cysts are characterized by low SI (17, 116). The tumor components that are hypointense in T2W images show a strong enhancement in T1WC images (102). There are accounts of cases in which the myometrium has a stronger enhancement than the tumor, making tumor invasions easy to recognize. There are, however, also tumors with an SI that appears isointense compared to the myometrium (116). The enhancing solid tumor components, as well as the enhancing septa between the non-enhancing cystic areas, often serve to create a lattice-, truss-, honeycomb-like overall visual impression (Fig. 6.1.8 (F)) (17, 105, 116). The junctional zone has low SI and is clearly recognizable, and is not interrupted when there is no myometrial invasion. An "intact" junctional zone is therefore regarded as the most important factor suggestive of an AS that is confined to the endometrium.

There is currently no evidence that would justify the use of PET-CT for primary diagnostics (81). FES-PET-CT is indicated for cases in which difficulties are encountered trying to assess the HR in recurrent tumors or metastases, as the presence of HR can be accurately verified using this method (112). FDG-PET-CT has a high sensitivity, specificity and accuracy in detecting recurrences (80–92.1 %, 96.2–100 % and 83.3 %). According to the results from a comparative trial, FDG-PET-CT offered no benefits compared to CT (83, 93). In cases in which recurrences and/or metastases are suspected, PET-CT can, however, be helpful for deciding on further therapeutic steps and for monitoring the efficacy of palliative treatment (90). False-positive findings, in the form of miliary tumor deposits on the bowel, need to be reckoned with.

Since distant metastasis is frequently already present in patients with SO at the time of primary presentation, such cases must be subjected to imaging-based staging of the pelvis, the abdomen and the thorax via MRI and/or CT. There is currently no scientific justification for administering primary PET (79).

For adenosarcomas, sonography typically reveals tumor masses with heterogeneous echogenicity within the uterine cavum. The presence of numerous large anechoic voids or spaces, that correspond to dilated endometrial glands, are a key diagnostic sonographic feature. CT is largely only suitable for assessing spread and extent of disease, but can on occasion also provide information pertaining to diagnosis. In CECT, the non-enhancing cysts are a key diagnostic feature.

In MRI, T1 weighted images show a heterogeneous, intermediately intense to isointense tumor. Hyperintense sections represent areas of hemorrhage. In T2 weighted images, the solid tumor components have a noticeably heterogeneous hypo- to isointense (and sometimes also hyperintense) SI. The numerous cysts are hyperintense in T2W and do not enhance in contrast MRI, making them a clear indication of adenosarcoma.

If not achievable by other means, FES-PET-CT can be helpful in assessing hormone receptors in recurrent tumors and metastases.

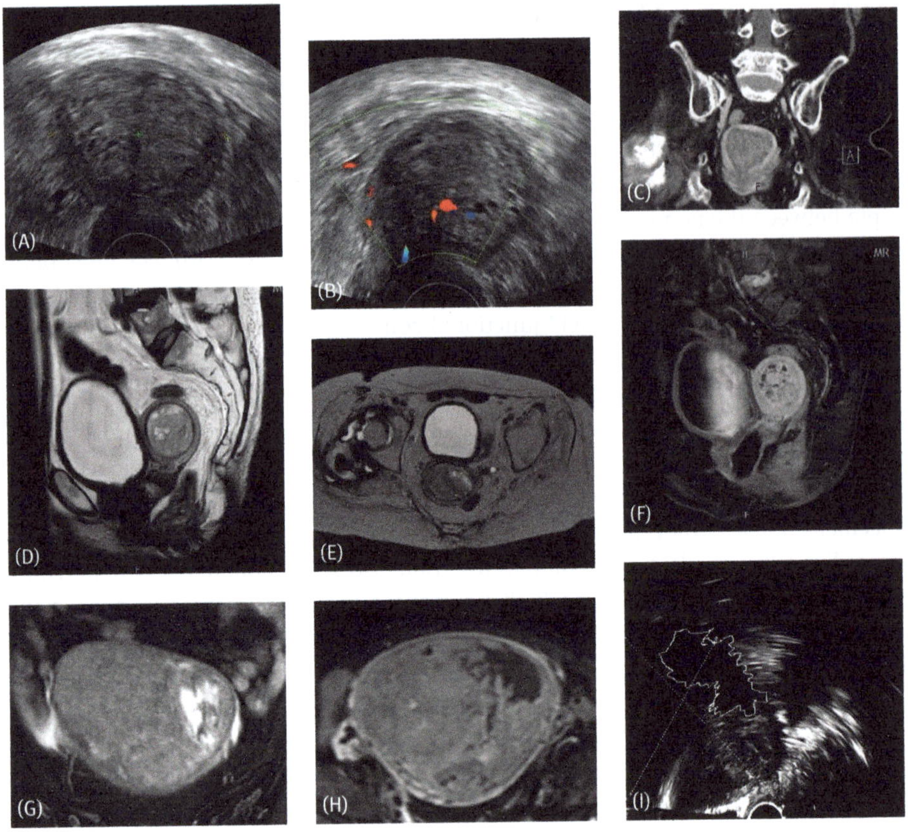

Fig. 6.1.8: Sonography, CT and MRI of one identical patient with adenosarcoma without sarcomatous overgrowth and MRI of a patient with an adenosarcoma with sarcomatous overgrowth. (A) in axial gray scale sonography the uterine cavum is distended. As exemplified in the following CT (C) and MRI (D–F) images, the surrounding myometrium is rather visible, at least in the immediate vicinity of the transducer. The tumor has heterogeneous echogenicity. The margins between the areas with differing echogenicities are only barely visible, and appear to be irregular to bizarre. In this plane, the echo voids most likely correspond to central vessels with a visible narrow hyperechoic border margin; (B) Doppler sonography reveals dilated vessels alongside anechoic voids, that most likely resemble dilated glands; (C) in contrast CT, the tumor generally shows a strong enhancement, but also contains areas with lower attenuation. The overall picture corresponds to the "lattice-" or "truss"-like structure described in the literature; (D), (E) the tumor is hyperintense to the myometrium in sagittal (D) and axial (E) T2W, and exhibits numerous areas of even greater SI that correlate to dilated glands; (F) the dilated glands do not enhance in contrast-MRI, thus serving to help secure a reliable diagnosis. All images clearly show that the margin or border to the myometrium is irregular, best exemplified by the fact that the hypointense margin is repeatedly interrupted in the MR images. The tumor has infiltrated the myometrium in these areas. Additionally, the protrusion of the tumor into the cervix is visible in (C) and (F); (G) in a case with sarcomatous overgrowth the tumor is heterogeneous hyperintense in T2W-MRI with a greater and only some small regions of high SI; (H) the greater and some small hyperintense regions do not enhance in contrast MRI. The large area corresponds to a necrosis, while the smaller sections correspond to glands; (I) in the corresponding sonography the outlined necrosis is also visible. In contrast to the findings in (C)–(E), in (G)–(I) the sarcoma share typically consists of a high-grade sarcoma with very few glands but extensive necrosis.

6.1.5 Differential diagnostics

Grossly differentiating AS from EC, CS, AF, stromal sarcomas as well as from large necrotic endometrial polyps solely on the basis of the macroscopic appearance of incidental findings in the resected and opened uterus is barely possible. The same applies to tumor masses protruding from the cervix. Real polyps usually have a tapered, gradually narrowing stem and a generally smooth appearance. AS, by contrast, usually have a broad-based connection to the corpus or the cervix. RMS should also be considered as a possible option in pediatric and adolescent patients with polypoid cervical tumors, as RMS share numerous microscopic and macroscopic commonalities with AS (97) (cf. Chapter 3), including entrapped endometrial glands at the periphery of the RMS with periglandular cuffing in same cases. This also makes discerning such RMS from heterologous AS with an RMS component particularly challenging. In postmenopausal women, but also in adolescents (72), a rapidly growing uterus or a myoma can in fact be caused by or constitute a number of other types of neoplasms, such as sarcomas and mixed tumors, including AS.

AF constitutes the most difficult and challenging DD, since the histological transition from AF to AS is a continuous, gradual one (19, 37). Accordingly, it is not the exception for primary AF to be reclassified as AS upon reassessment. There is a possibility that AF is in fact "merely" a mild form of AS and that it thus does not constitute an independent entity of neoplasm (37). Diagnostically differentiating AS from AF is discussed in the chapter on AF in greater detail. At the microscopic level, discerning AS from endometrial polyps with atypical stroma cells, or polyps with periglandular stromal cell aggregations without mitotic activity, can be a complicated endeavor. However, polyps lack the phylloid structure, and their stroma largely corresponds to that of the neighboring endometrium. Similarly, an atypical polypoid adenomyoma could be wrongly classified as AS, especially if the cellular smooth muscle or myofibroblastic stroma with atypia is mistaken for a sarcomatous component. However, the periglandular aggregations of stromal cells, the intraglandular stromal papillae, and the phylloid structure are all absent in atypical polypoid adenomyoma.

Accounts have also been reported in which intra- and extrauterine AS have been misdiagnosed as endometriosis (43, 64). It can in fact occur that an AS "imitates" the features of an endometriosis (Fig. 6.1.9) and is subsequently overlooked when both are present in the same specimen.

Glands from surrounding normal endometrium can be "captured" or "entrapped" up to 2 mm deep in the edge margins of LG-ESS (cf. Vol. 1, Chapter 4) (19, 91). The latter can thus appear to resemble AS in curettage specimens. Very recently, there have been accounts of intrauterine and extrauterine LG-ESS with endometrial glands that are either focal or distributed across the entire tumor (LG-ESS with extensive endometrioid glandular differentiation). Making this distinction is indeed challenging, as most recent studies have revealed that the epithelial parts of the AS are probably "trapped" endometrial glands (77). Compared to AS, however, LG-ESS lack stromal protrusions

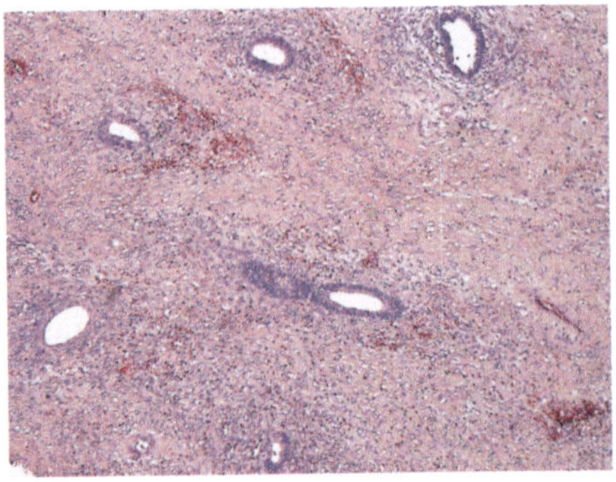

Fig. 6.1.9: Differential diagnosis endometriosis – adenosarcoma. Under weak magnification, the areas of the tumor that are farther away from the surface can barely be discerned from banal endometriosis. The key to reaching the proper diagnosis lies in macroscopic appearance, histological findings and the atypia in the stromal cuffs.

into the glands, and the periglandular stromal cuffs are less pronounced or entirely absent. Since LG-ESS and AS are largely morphologically and immunophenotypically identical, distinguishing these two types of neoplasm from each other can be difficult to impossible (64, 97). It should be noted that LG-ESS most usually arise in the region of the myometrium, while AS originate in the endometrial stroma in a majority of cases.

ANS, too, can still contain endometrial glands in areas of endometrial invasion and thus be mistaken for AS. Particular scrutiny must thus be applied when examining AS with a sarcomatous component that appears to be ANS, though testing for CD31 and/or ERG serves to quickly resolve this diagnostic question mark (cf. Chapter 1).

Assessing frozen sections or tissue specimens yielded from curettage is associated with numerous challenges and much room for misinterpretations. For instance, if too small an amount of tissue is available for analysis, the areas containing the epithelial isles can be missing entirely from the specimens or overlooked in them, which facilitates a misdiagnosis as pure sarcoma. In the DKSM database, 17.6 % of AS were initially diagnosed as a pure homologous or heterologous sarcoma on the basis of tissue specimens taken via curettage (LG-ESS, HG-ESS, UUS, LMS, RMS) (54). Seventeen point seven percent were each diagnosed as LM or endometrial polyps via curettage, i.e. curettage only revealed that the tumors were not malignancies in those cases (52). Because AS sometimes express myogenic markers, they can also be microscopically mistaken for CLM. Verifying the presence of CD10 and caldesmon expression can be helpful in such cases. CD10 is usually not so strongly expressed in CLM, while AS generally do not express caldesmon. Due to the substantial differential diagnostic difficulties, more than one third of AS are primarily misdiagnosed on the basis of histological examination (19, 94). Correct final diagnosis is frequently only reached upon examination of the surgical specimen. Therefore, tissue samples obtained from curettage are not appropriate for reliably correctly diagnosing different types and entities of sarcoma.

Metastases of primary AS are purely sarcomatous in up to 70–100 % of cases (11, 19), while local recurrences usually also contain epithelial components (91). AS that are deemed homologous at primary diagnosis can develop heterologous metastases (103). It cannot be ruled out in these cases that the heterologous component had been overlooked in the primary tumor. There have been cases in which transformation into a CS has been observed in metastases (19). Here, too, it cannot be ruled out that the primary tumor had in fact been CS. The primary tumor can, therefore, not be accurately or reliably identified or verified on the basis of the metastases alone. This state of affairs generally applies to all malignant mixed tumors of the female genital tract. The simultaneous presence of AS in the uterus and in the ovary need not automatically imply that they are in some way connected, as they could also be independent synchronous tumors. Metastatic spread of AS to the ovaries is extraordinarily rare.

Endometrial polyps, endometrial carcinomas and the other uterine sarcomas are the most important macroscopic differential diagnostic options. Adenofibroma, endometrial polyps, atypical polypoid adenomyoma, stromal sarcomas, angiosarcoma, and – occasionally – carcinosarcoma and rhabdomyosarcoma are the most important differential diagnoses in the microscopic context. Correctly and reliably diagnosing adenosarcoma as such on the basis of tissue specimens obtained via curettage is often not possible.

6.1.6 Course, prognosis

The few studies on AS that have been published often make no differentiation between AS with SO and such without SO, even though these two tumor types differ substantially in terms of their clinical features and prognosis. Most of the few available data pertaining to survival are essentially “mixed calculations” that do not allow individual assessments to be made for the two different variants of AS. These problems notwithstanding, they do indeed also share a number of common features. Generally speaking, stage of disease is the most important prognostic factor for AS as well (1). There is apparently no correlation between MI levels and rates of recurrence (49). There are accounts of metastasized AS with an MI of < 2 M/10 HPF, but also of recurrence-free tumors with 40 M/10 HPF (19, 37). Deep myometrial invasion and LVI are regarded as predictors of recurrence and metastasis (37, 49). Compared to early invasion, the rate of recurrence is 5.3 times higher in cases in which invasion has already reached the outer two-thirds of the myometrium. Opinions going in the other direction have also been voiced, namely that myometrial invasion has no significant influence on the rate of recurrence (113). A further study reported a recurrence rate of 60 % in AS patients presenting with LVI (49).

According to the DKSM database and the majority of other studies, metastatic spread to the ovaries is not observed at the time of primary diagnosis (7, 11, 54, 106). One further study reported ovarian involvement at the time of primary therapy in 8 % of cases. Metastases were not visible on gross observation in 2 of 5 cases (14). There are (albeit weak) data which suggest that leaving the adnexa in situ in premenopausal women with HR positive uterine sarcomas could impact negatively on prognosis and increase the risk of relapse (5, 10, 39, 58). In contrast, more recent reports (albeit with numerous biases) have stated that DFS and OS are identical for patients who have and who have not undergone BSO. According to extensive SEER analyses, leaving the ovaries in situ in premenopausal women has no adverse effects on OS (92). These findings notwithstanding, the SEER data, too, feature numerous inherent biases.

Only limited data are available pertaining to the rate to which LN test positive in cases of AS with and without SO. In one study covering 262 cases of AS, nodal metastases were found in only 3.1 % of cases of AS (all stages) with and without SO (7). A further, smaller study determined that 3.4 % of AS that are confined to the uterus had positive LN (113). In yet another study, pelvic and para-aortic sampling revealed no nodal involvement in 14 AS without SO. Among 17 tumors with SO, 2 were found to have positive LN (11 %), while only 3 % of cervical AS exhibited LN involvement (9). A more recent study (14) found positive LN in only one case of AS with SO, however with simultaneous further extrauterine spread. Within the DKSM materials, LN metastases could be verified for 33 % of AS with SO and 11 % of AS without SO. Interestingly, recurrences only occurred in patients with negative LN. Twenty-five percent of distant metastases occurred in patients with positive LN, while the LN of the remaining 75 % of patients who developed distant metastatic disease tested negative (54). Accordingly, the prognostic value of verifying LN positivity is indeed questionable. Moreover, it has yet to be scientifically proven to any degree that performing LNE has favorable effects on OS.

The typical (classical) AS variant – AS without SO – is associated with a relatively favorable prognosis (analogous to LG-ESS) and is often cited as a tumor with low malignant potential (37, 49, 78, 88). In actual fact, up to 96 % of AS patients initially present with stage I disease (11). Tumor growth is relatively slow and recurrences usually occur in the form of late recurrences in the vagina, the lesser pelvis (Fig. 6.1.10 (A)), and the abdomen. Reported rates of recurrence range from 7–14 % (11, 19, 49, 106). Distant metastasis is reported to have been found in up to 50 % of cases (11). It is assumed that this indolent behavior is caused by the fact that myometrial invasion is both rare and usually not particularly deep. However, just because myometrial invasion is minor, it does not rule distant metastasis out per se (37). AS without SO, too, can biologically progress during metastasization, i.e. dedifferentiation with complete or partial loss of HR, as is impressively shown in Fig. 6.1.10 (B), (C).

The presence of SO is statistically significantly associated with less favorable OS and is regarded as an independent prognostic determinant per se (13, 37, 113). Thirty to forty percent of AS with SO are already at an advanced stage of disease at the time

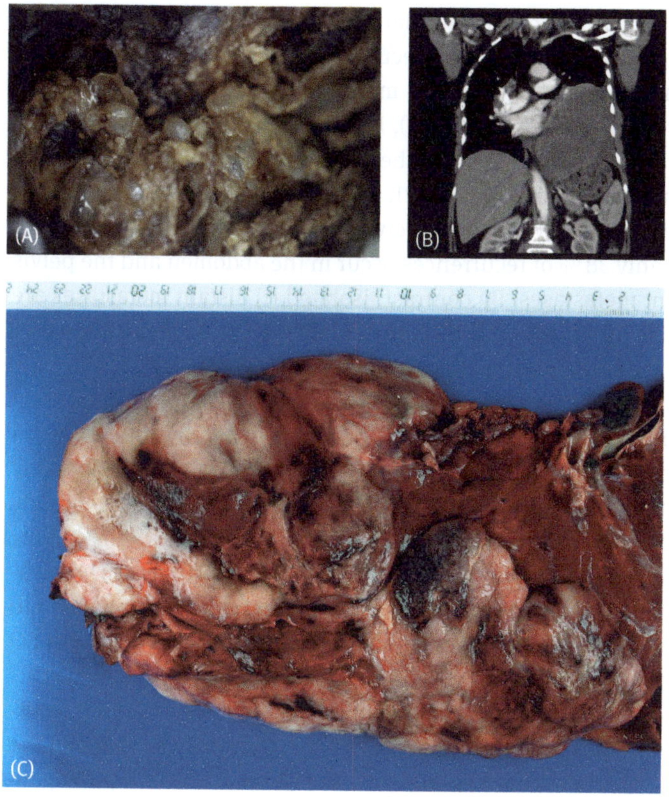

Fig. 6.1.10: Recurrences and metastases of adenosarcomas. (A) late pelvic recurrence of an adenosarcoma without sarcomatous overgrowth 24 years after initial treatment that continues to exhibit the typical macroscopic appearance characterized by ample cysts; (B), (C) CT and surgical specimen of massive metastatic involvement of the lungs in a patient with primary adenosarcoma without sarcomatous overgrowth, the metastatic mass only consists of a largely undifferentiated sarcoma with epithelial components and has lost its estrogen receptors.

of initial diagnosis (11, 56). Overall, rapid tumor growth and early recurrence and/or metastasization should be expected when SO is present. Reported recurrence rates for AS with SO have ranged from 44–80 % (11, 19, 49, 106) and distant metastases occur in up to 90 % of cases (11). In 30 % of cases overall, pulmonary metastases arise without local recurrences or abdominal cavitary metastases (11). The risk of recurrence is roughly 3.2 times higher than for classic AS (49). The simultaneous presence of SO and deep myometrial invasion is a particularly unfavorable constellation. Such cases have a recurrence rate of 70 %. That rate continuously improves when only one (46 %) or neither (12.7 %) of the two aforementioned factors can be verified. Metastases with SO can also originate from an AS without primary SO. According to one publication, it has no bearing on prognosis if the SO is the result of an extensive UTROCST component within a sarcomatous LG-ESS component of the AS (103).

Overall, the presence of SO and/or myometrial invasion as well as LVI are regarded as the most reliable histological predictors for recurrence of AS (14, 39, 97). According to a recent publication, "TCN" is the strongest multivariate and "cell atypia" is the strongest univariate prognostic factor for AS (1). Five-year OS for AS with and without necroses was 92 % and 43 %, respectively. The malignant potential of AS with SO reportedly corresponds to that of CS and LMS (21, 56).

Isolated recurrences in the vagina and the pelvis are observed in 33 % and 28 % of cases, respectively. Roughly 38 % of recurrences occur in the abdomen and the pelvis with and without distant metastases. By contrast, isolated (!) distant metastases are observed in only 5–9 % of all AS patients. Hematogenous metastatic spread is rather the exception and practically only occurs in AS patients with SO (19, 117).

The data pertaining to the frequency of disease recurrence are largely based on tumors that are primarily confined to the uterus. Despite substantial differences in terms of recurrence, 5-year OS among patients with AS with SO is not considerably shorter than that among patients without SO (60.7 vs. 69.3 %) (11). A different study (albeit with a smaller sample) revealed that the 2-year DFS and OS were both 20 % for patients with SO, and 100 % for patients without SO (106). A recent analysis (14) measured a median DFS and a median OS of 29.4 resp. 55.4 mo for AS with SO, compared to 105.9 resp. 112.4 mo for AS without SO. Among stage I disease patients, 77 % with SO and 22 % without SO showed recurrence. The difference was statistically significant.

In summary, the mesenchymal sarcomatous component dictates the immunohistochemical, clinical, and prognostic features and behavior of the AS. The role that the epithelium plays has long remained unresolved (91). More recent data (see pathogenesis) suggest that the epithelial elements are in fact "merely" glands that have been "trapped/captured" by the AS as it has developed in the endometrium (77). Thus, AS with SO and AS without SO differ significantly in terms of their prognosis. The former exhibits clinical features and prognostic behavior more reminiscent of HG-ESS and other high-grade sarcomas, while the latter more closely resembles LG-ESS from a clinical and prognostic perspective.

Adenosarcoma without sarcomatous overgrowth has a relatively favorable prognosis. Recurrences usually only arise late. The presence of sarcomatous overgrowth has a clear negative impact on prognosis and distant metastasis is more frequent in such tumors. Diagnosis is largely dictated by the sarcomatous component that is usually high-grade in adenosarcomas with sarcomatous overgrowth. Myometrial invasion, lymphovascular invasion, and the number of tumor cell necroses are further pivotal prognostic variables. Pelvic and para-aortic lymph nodes are only rarely positive, and the ovaries are only rarely primarily involved.

6.1.7 Primary surgery

Due to the rarity of AS, there are no therapeutic studies that specifically pertain to this type of neoplasm. Accordingly, there are no recommendations that satisfy the criteria for "evidence-based medicine". The NCCN Guidelines (69) give AS no consideration. The situation is even more unsatisfactory if one differentiates between AS with and without SO. Therapeutic decision-making is made somewhat easier, however, by the fact that AS and stromal sarcomas share certain clinical, microscopic, biochemical, and prognostic commonalities (97). AS without SO is more reminiscent of LG-ESS, while AS with SO more closely resembles HG-ESS or other high-grade sarcomas. Procedure should or can thus be guided by the procedure applied to the sarcomas to which the different AS variants bear close resemblance (35, 97, 113).

In accordance with the current NCCN Guidelines for LG-ESS and HG-ESS and the GCIG-Consensus (35, 69), THE without injuring the uterus with accompanying BSO is regarded as the adequate surgical approach to be applied, and thus as accepted standard practice. There is no indication for performing TVH when an AS has been diagnosed, due to the risk of injuring the uterus and the fact that this procedure does not allow for abdominal exploration. LAVH or TLH, when opted for, must be performed without causing injury to the uterus.

The SEER analyses and the lack of scientific evidence notwithstanding, there is nonetheless consensus among several studies that a BSO is more likely indicated when the tumor expresses HR positivity (5, 10, 36, 58). Reference should be had to the chapter on LG-ESS in this regard (cf. Vol. 1, Chapter 4). The data, when taken together, suggest that preserving the adnexa is at least a possibility, i.e. that a subsequent extirpation can be forgone. According to the NCCN Guidelines, in referring to LG-ESS, decisions for or against performing a BSO can be made on an individualized basis under consideration of patient's reproductive age or desire for fertility preservation (69). This statement is supported by the current GCIG Consensus (35). Patients with HR positive AS should, however, be informed of the potentially elevated risk of recurrence that is associated with ovarian preservation. Notwithstanding, when the data are all taken together, they do not truly suffice to reliably justify subjecting premenopausal women to a BSO. Patients must, however, be informed of the minor risk that remains (14). Said risk obviously only applies to uterus-preserving surgical procedures. A BSO is not necessary for AS with SO because the HR are usually negative in premenopausal women.

It is currently contested whether or not performing an LNE is necessary (49), not least because the share of cases with nodal involvement is low (see prognosis). Data stemming from smaller studies suggest that an LNE could potentially serve to reduce the number of pelvic recurrences (81, 108). These findings notwithstanding, the current SEER data do not serve to verify that performing an LNE has any benefits on OS (91), even in cases with nodal involvement. The biases that are inherent to the retrospective SEER studies do, however, need to be borne in mind. Further retrospective analyses, too, have been unable to verify that undergoing an LNE has a favorable impact on OS (11, 55). In the current NCCN Guidelines, LNE has been removed from the recommendations for all uterine sarcomas (69). Likewise, according to the current GCIG Consensus, the benefits of an LNE have yet to be scientifically proven. Routinely performing a systematic LNE is thus not recommended (35). However, the guidelines do indeed recommend the removal of all metastatic masses, which can be interpreted as a recommendation for performing selective LNE on enlarged LN on an individualized basis. It needs to be reiterated that the preceding statement is not supported by evidence-based data, and that it has yet to be scientifically proven to any degree that performing any form of LNE is beneficial for prognosis.

In summary, systematic LNE or LN sampling currently lack a sufficing and adequate scientific basis, and can thus not be defined as standard practice (14, 35, 36, 92). Moreover, it is not clear whether LN positivity is of any prognostic value in patients with AS confined to the uterus. Sampling enlarged LN is currently deemed a justifiable compromise. However, not performing an LNE cannot be regarded as erroneous practice. If an LNE is opted for, it must be borne in mind that no prognostic or therapeutic consequences can be deduced from the findings resulting from said course of action, even when the LN test positive. The patient must be unequivocally informed of this fact, as well as of the potential complications that can arise from undergoing an LNE.

Standalone TE, any form of morcellation, and any form of SHE all constitute inadequate surgical procedures for AS. As also applies for LG-ESS, HG-ESS, UUS and LMS, a negative impact on the prognosis has to be expected when such procedures are performed (12, 28, 76). Fifteen percent of patients who underwent completion surgery following inadequate primary surgical interventions were upstaged, though these higher stages were actually found in new tumor deposits, and were not necessarily evidence of an incorrectly staged primary lesion (28). A case has been reported in which the uterus was perforated during curettage, which allowed tumor material to enter the abdominal cavity and ultimately resulted in the development of a large recurrence of disease within a short period of time (67). The problems associated with inadequate modes of surgery including morcellation are discussed at length in Chapter 6 of Vol. 1, where a respective diagnostic flowchart is also provided.

Local resection appears to be an option in exceptional cases of young women who urgently desire fertility preservation and in whom the AS without SO is conveniently located within and confined to the uterus (19, 39, 63, 98). It is necessary that R0-esection margins are achieved beyond doubt in such cases. One study revealed that one patient who underwent curettage alone, and two patients who underwent SHE, had no recurrences (11). According to two further studies (13, 34), among 7 adolescents who underwent organ-sparing surgery for cervical AS, 5 developed recurrences. Conservative procedures are best suited for pedunculated tumors confined to the endometrium, under the condition that R0 resection is achieved (39). In general, patients must be thoroughly informed of the implications of such course of action, not least because preserving the ovaries when an HR positive AS has been subjected to inadequate surgery could potentially promote recurrence (as also applies to LG-ESS, Vol. 1, Chapter 4). A case has been reported in which adnexal preservation was not accompanied by recurrence in the follow-up period (63).

When TE or SHE have been opted for, the residual uterus should be resected without undue delay. For patients who wish to preserve their fertility, the THE should be performed no later than when that wish has expired. Adjuvant HT should be considered for patients who have undergone organ-sparing surgery or morcellation on HR positive AS (cf. LG-ESS and adjuvant and additive HT, Vol. 1, Chapter 4).

AS that have spread within the pelvis and the abdominal cavity should be subjected to maximal cytoreductive surgery. Retrospective studies, albeit referring to all uterine sarcomas, suggest that doing so is associated with improved OS (36). There is an account of a patient with an AS with SO that had spread to and within the pelvis, who underwent a total of three cytoreductive operations following THE with BSO plus cytoreduction plus hyperthermic intraperitoneal CHT with 50 mg/m^2 melphalan. The patient was still alive with disease after 55 mo (46). Notwithstanding the fact that experiences with sarcomas are limited in this regard, this method could nonetheless constitute a further therapeutic alternative in select applicable cases. However, it remains unclear in this case whether hyperthermic CHT actually had any effects. Drawing on findings relating to LG-ESS, it is fair to assume that performing maximal cytoreductive surgery will have favorable effects on survival (108). “Removal of all tumor” and “free resection margins” are deemed the most important prognostic factors for such tumors (70). For AS with SO, analogous to HG-ESS (cf. Vol. 1, Chapter 5), due to the absence of effective alternatives, maximal cytoreductive surgery should also be considered. According to the current NCCN 2A recommendations (that refer to all uterine sarcomas), the decision to surgically resect all tumor tissue can be made on an individualized i.e. case-specific basis, depending on symptoms, extent of disease, and resectability. LNE is deemed inadequate where there is extrauterine spread (69). There are currently no data available pertaining to the potential benefits of performing a selective LNE, even when the resection margins are tumor free.

More extensive surgical procedures, for example exenterations, are generally rejected on the grounds of the substantial complications that can arise and in light of the poorer prognosis with which especially AS with SO are generally associated. Pelvic exenteration should only be considered in exceptional cases, in which R0 resection (i.e. disease-free margins) can be achieved and the patient is young and in a good general state of health (50).

Total hysterectomy without injuring or damaging the uterus is regarded as the gold standard for surgically treating adenosarcoma. Clinically unsuspicious adnexa can be left in situ in premenopausal women. Especially in cases with inadequate surgery not removing the ovaries could increase the risk of recurrence when the primary tumor is hormone-receptor positive. Selective or systematic pelvic and para-aortic lymphadenectomy currently cannot be regarded or defined as standard practice. Not performing a lymphadenectomy can therefore not be deemed erroneous practice. Patients with clearly delineated tumors without sarcomatous overgrowth can undergo tumor extirpation if they wish to preserve their fertility. When opted for, the resection margins must be verifiably disease-free and patients must be subjected to rigorous follow-up. Hysterectomy should then be performed once the desire to preserve fertility has expired. In cases of advanced disease, subjecting all visible and palpable lesions to maximal cytoreductive surgery could improve survival. Said course of action should be considered for patients who are in a good general state of health. Subjecting such patients to systematic or selective lymphadenectomy has not yet been proven to be beneficial.

6.1.8 Adjuvant and additive radio-, chemo- and hormone therapy

It has yet to be scientifically substantiated beyond doubt that subjecting AS with/without SO that are confined to the uterus to postoperative RT has any effect on DFS and OS, so that this question currently remains unanswered (23). A randomized phase III trial (EORTC 55874) covering all types of uterine sarcomas (albeit without any AS in the sample) revealed that postoperative RT did not yield improvements in DFS and OS compared to the observation arm (80). However, since there were no AS in the EORTC study sample, no definitive conclusions can be drawn for this type of neoplasm specifically. This notwithstanding, the data gathered in the EORTC trial, the SEER analyses and a number of smaller retrospective studies can still be said to largely apply to AS. The aforementioned studies were unable to verify that postoperative RT offers any favorable prognostic effects (51, 93). A SEER analysis focusing solely on AS revealed that performing ERT had no influence on OS (7). Two larger retrospective analyses, covering either all types of uterine sarcoma (60) or only LG-ESS and HG-ESS (58), suggest that ERT effects only non-significant reductions in the rate of local recurrence, while having no impact on OS. Combining ERT with VBT is said to yield the most promising results in this regard (60). In one more recent retrospective analysis, no local recurrences occurred in patients with AS with SO who underwent pelvic ERT (11). However, the number of cases covered in said study was only relatively small, so that no definitive conclusions can be drawn from the results. There are, however, also reports (89) suggesting that RT is entirely ineffective. It would be conceivable to assume that subjection to standalone VBT could serve to lower rates of recurrence, however such a hypothesis has yet to be backed by respective scientific data. The favorable effects of RT on the rate of local recurrence and OS could not be confirmed in two further studies on AS (14, 86).

Summing up, in light of the presented data, there have been no valid studies or trials to date that are in favor of subjecting patients with AS to postoperative ERT. Accordingly, analogous to LG-ESS, the current NCCN 2A recommendations only recommend subjecting respective patients to observation (35, 69). According to a category 2B NCCN recommendation (69) for HG-ESS and UUS, administering ERT with or without VBT can be considered for AS with SO. However, said recommendation entirely lacks any scientific basis or supporting plausible data.

In general, there is no indication for subjecting patients with uterus-confined AS with/without SO to postoperative RT. Said course of action should be reserved to treating recurrent disease.

In a similar vein, there are no data which suggest that applying postoperative RT in advanced cases in which R0 and R1/2 resection has been achieved in primary surgery yields any favorable effects. Accordingly, there are no practice recommendations pertaining to AS in this regard. Drawing on what we know about the other types of uterine sarcoma, improved survival should not be reckoned with in such cases. However, targeted RT might serve to improve local control. Therefore, according to the current NCCN category 2A recommendation, subjecting the region in which the tumor is located to targeted ERT and/or BT can be considered an adequate option (69). Such course of action would be most likely conceivable for cases in which R1 resection margins have been achieved in primary surgery. Targeted RT can be combined with HT for AS with positive HR (69), though there are no valid data which suggest that doing so offers any benefits in terms of survival. Administering whole abdomen RT should be viewed critically due to the high frequency with which side effects are known to occur, which is likely the reason why said measure has been omitted from the NCCN recommendations. Patients who insist on whole abdomen RT must be unequivocally informed of the complications that can potentially arise as well as of the lack of scientifically proven benefits of doing so.

Administering adjuvant CHT to AS patients has yet to be proven to be associated with more beneficial outcomes. No positive impact on survival was recognizable in the few retrospective studies that have been published (56, 113). In a recent retrospective analysis, treating stage I to IV AS with SO with adjuvant CHT effected an (albeit statistically insignificant) improvement in both DFS and OS. The authors came to the conclusion that adjuvant CHT can be considered as a therapeutic option in such cases (14). Two further publications – one randomized study covering all types of uterine sarcoma except AS, and one meta-analysis on STS – failed to verify that adjuvant CHT has an influence on OS (74, 109). One publication reports a case in which disease progressed in a patient with cervical AS with SO under adjuvant CHT using ifosfamide plus doxorubicin. Changing CHT to gemcitabine plus docetaxel did not serve to halt progression, and the patient died 12 mo after diagnosis (89). AS are accorded no consideration in the current NCCN recommendations (69). Building on the assumption that stromal sarcomas and AS share numerous commonalities (91) and exhibit largely identical behavior, the criteria applied in the context of adjuvant CHT for stromal sarcomas must also be accepted for AS. The NCCN Guidelines make a category 2A recommendation to subject LG-ESS merely to observation (69). There are currently no arguments that go against applying this recommendation to AS without SO as well. Observation is also a recommended option for HG-ESS and UUS (2A recommendation). The NCCN Guidelines do also make a very weak 2B recommendation to consider adjuvant CHT as a possible course of action. However, this recommendation is based on a very small number of cases presented in retrospective studies and is thus already rather weak for HG-ESS (cf. Vol. 1, Chapter 5). The data situation pertaining to AS with SO is too poor to support administering adjuvant CHT as "evidence-based practice". A recent retrospective study (11) revealed no findings to suggest that CHT in this context offers any benefits.

In summary, there is wide consensus that subjecting patients with uterus-confined AS with/without SO to adjuvant CHT cannot be deemed standard practice, as there is currently no indication for doing so. If such treatment is nonetheless opted for on the basis of the aforementioned weak NCCN 2B recommendations, despite the lack of supporting data, then the patient must be unequivocally informed of the fact that adjuvant CHT in this context has yet to be scientifically proven to be beneficial.

No findings have yet been published that pertain to whether subjecting primarily R0/1/2 resected advanced AS (stages II and III) to postoperative CHT is prognostically beneficial. AS are not covered in the NCCN Guidelines (69). Since there are currently no recommendations concerning the subjection of patients with advanced AS with SO to postoperative CHT, general reference can be had to the respective data pertaining to HG-ESS and UUS, as they are closely morphologically, immunologically, clinically and prognostically related to AS with SO. Individual reports and so-called expert opinions support giving postoperative CHT to patients with advanced tumors (29, 36, 79). In the new NCCN Guidelines, administering standalone postoperative CHT to patients with LMS, HG-ESS and UUS has been degraded to a comparably weak category 2B recommendation (69). According to the stated recommendations, postoperative CHT can, however, be considered when there is spread in the abdominal cavity. There are isolated accounts of a highly toxic combination of dactinomycin, doxorubicin und cyclophosphamide being potentially effective in AS patients (113). In general, and according to the NCCN Guidelines, combining CHT with RT could be plausible in isolated cases (69). Both methods should be applied sequentially (for CHT regimens and dosages see palliative CHT).

The fact that AS without SO express HR almost without exception makes such tumors generally eligible for adjuvant HT, analogous to LG-ESS. Respective studies focusing specifically on AS in this context have yet to be published. Given the numerous commonalities, features and characteristics that uterine stromal sarcomas (97) and AS share, as well as their virtually identical behavior, the same criteria must be applied to the latter as to the former in regard to HT as well. Administering adjuvant HT to patients with LG-ESS primarily confined to the uterus, and whose tumors have been subjected to adequate primary surgery (R0 resection margins), has not yet been shown to be beneficial (cf. Vol. 1, Chapter 4). The current NCCN 2A recommendations concerning LG-ESS recommend subjecting such patients solely to observation (69). The guidelines do, however, make a very weak 2B recommendation that adjuvant HT can be considered, even though there is no evidence of beneficial outcomes to support such practice. Hence, there is no scientifically substantiated indication for adjuvant HT. When adjuvant HT is nonetheless opted for, the procedure should be designed analogous to that for LG-ESS (cf. Vol. 1, Chapter 4). Verified HR positivity is one precondition that must be fulfilled in order for HR to be permissible. Adjuvant HT is categorically ruled out if this is not the case. Patients with R0 primary resection margins who undergo adjuvant HT must be unequivocally and comprehensibly informed of the potential side effects, and of the fact that the procedure has not yet been scientifically proven beneficial.

Postoperative HT should be administered in RX situations (tumor injury, morcellation, TE), in cases of primarily advanced AS without SO and with positive HR (stages II and III), or in patients in whom primary surgery left R1/2 resection margins. Postoperative HT should also be given serious consideration for patients who have undergone forms of surgery (e.g. SLH, SAH) that are deemed inadequate. Reference can be made in this regard to the details pertaining to postoperative HT and LG-ESS (cf. Vol. 1 Chapter 4) (35, 97, 113). Within the current NCCN 2A guidelines (69), reviews and individual studies (22, 29, 36, 79, 113), there is overall agreement that HT should be given to patients whose primary resection margins are not free of disease and whose primary tumors were HR positive. Furthermore, postoperative HT should also be administered when tumors not confined entirely to the uterus have been resected, even when the resection margins are clear, i.e. R0 (89).

For premenopausal women, HT can consist of a BSO or progestin therapy. In the DKSM case materials, four consecutive patients with HR positive LG-ESS who were subjected to inadequate operations (TE and/or morcellation) relapsed within very short periods of time, despite having undergone a BSO. Against this backdrop, administering HT with progestins in addition to a BSO should be given serious consideration. Progestin therapy is regarded as the method of choice for postmenopausal women, and is recommended in the NCCN Guidelines (2A recommendation) (69). Long-lasting remissions of suboptimally resected AS have been observed under MPA therapy (40, 113). AI can be applied when the use of progestins is contraindicated, for instance when patients have type 2 diabetes or thromboses (further information is provided at length in the chapter on LG-ESS, Vol. 1, Chapter 4). The progestin DNG can be administered where contraindications prevent the use of the relatively highly dosed MPA or MGA. Whether or not GnRH analogues can actually serve to prevent recurrence in premenopausal patients who have not undergone a BSO remains insufficiently substantiated. GnRH analogues and AI are only administered “off-label” in Germany, and the former are only accepted in the USA in the form of a weak 2B recommendation (69). GnRH analogues can be a sensible therapeutic option for bridging the time period to a planned ex post BSO, not least because progestin therapy has to be discontinued in due time prior to surgical therapy, because of the risk of thromboses.

Patients in whom R1/2 resections have been achieved should continue therapy until they relapse, while 5 years of treatment might potentially suffice for patients whose advanced AS have been R0 resected and/or who have been subjected to inadequate modes of surgery. Overall, the duration of therapy should be designed in accordance with the approach adopted for other malignant, hormone-sensitive tumors. More details are provided in the subchapter on palliative HT.

In the current version of the NCCN Guidelines, subjecting patients with stage II or stage III disease, who have undergone maximal or submaximal cytoreductive surgery, to targeted postoperative RT, either as a standalone or as an additional therapeutic measure, has been downgraded to a weak 2B recommendation (69).

If a patient with an HR positive AS is under HRT or tamoxifen therapy at the time of initial diagnosis, then said therapies should be discontinued. Tamoxifen therapy that is being administered as treatment for breast cancer should urgently be switched over to an AI. Tamoxifen must be regarded as being contraindicated.

There is no evidence to suggest that subjecting adenosarcomas confined to the uterus with and without "sarcomatous overgrowth" to postoperative external irradiation prolongs survival. Overall, percutaneous irradiation is deemed not indicated. The few data available pertaining to achieving reductions in the rate of local recurrence are contradictory. Brachytherapy could possibly be beneficial in this regard and thus be taken into consideration as a possible option. Targeted external irradiation and/or brachytherapy can be considered for patients who have been subjected to R1/2 resections. Whole abdomen radiotherapy is not indicated due to the potential side effects and the fact that doing so has yet to be proven to promote favorable outcomes.

No valid, reliable data exist that suggest that adjuvant chemotherapy improves survival in patients with adenosarcoma confined to the uterus and who have undergone adequate surgery. Furthermore, there are no sufficiently tested and effective chemotherapeutic schedules or regimens. Consequently, there is currently no indication for adjuvant chemotherapy. The same largely applies to R0/1/2 resected advanced tumors.

Moreover, there is also no evidence that adjuvant hormone therapy or ovarectomy (as a form of adjuvant ablative hormone therapy) serve to improve survival in patients who have undergone adequate surgery on uterus-confined, hormone-receptor positive adenosarcomas.

Analogous to low-grade endometrial stromal sarcoma, subsequent hormone therapy is regarded as the treatment method of choice for cases in which hormone receptor positive adenosarcomas have been subjected to R1/R2 or RX resections or inadequate surgery. For premenopausal women, such hormone therapy can take the form of an ovarectomy or at least 5 years of progestin therapy. Some data suggest that supplementary progestin therapy is indicated despite ovarectomy. It has not yet been reliably proven that GnRH analogues achieve more favorable outcomes compared to those achievable via ovarectomy. Administering aromatase inhibitors is indicated if there is a contraindication for progestin therapy in postmenopausal women or women who have undergone ovarectomies. For R1/2 resections, hormone treatment should continue until disease progresses.

6.1.9 Primary radio-, chemo- and hormone therapy, approach in cases of general inoperability

Patients with primarily advanced AS with and without SO that are confined to the pelvis/the abdomen should undergo surgical therapy. Analogous to LG-ESS, HG-ESS, UUS and CS, pelvic ERT with or without BT can be considered if a patient with an AS confined to the uterus is generally inoperable. Evidence pertaining to the efficacy of said practice and to improved survival has yet to be published. If the tumor is localized outside of the uterus, but remains confined to the pelvis, targeted ERT can be administered with or without BT. Combining such therapy with CHT would also be a conceivable option. One publication recounts a case in which a CR was achieved in a generally inoperable patient under a combination of RT and carboplatin monotherapy (113). RT can also be considered, albeit without any curative aspirations, as a means of temporary symptom control when tumors are inoperable for technical reasons or when the patient refuses surgery (58, 60). Primary RT was found to be ineffective in one patient with AS with SO that had extended into the parametria (89). It is therefore urgently required that patients are unequivocally informed of the fact that subjecting operable tumors to RT offers no scientifically proven benefits. A combination of RT and CHT has served to effect a CR in isolated cases (see neoadjuvant CHT).

One publication reports two cases in which remission was achieved in AS under primary carboplatin CHT. The first case involved an AS without SO that was jointly treated with GnRH analogues, while the second patient had an AS with SO and also underwent RT (113). The reported remissions could thus also have been a consequence of the treatment with GnRH analogues and RT, respectively. Whether or not carboplatin is effective in this context therefore remains questionable. It should be noted, however, that therapy in these generally inoperable cases was not geared towards achieving operability.

Since achieving quick remission is the goal in the neoadjuvant context, poly-CHT regimens are the only option in practice. The few effective cytostatic agents that are available are described in the subchapter on palliative CHT. One study reports a case of an LG-ESS that had spread beyond the uterus, in which operability was successfully achieved (and surgery was subsequently performed) by administering neoadjuvant CHT using ifosfamide plus doxorubicin (42). Applying the highly tolerable combination of liposomal doxorubicin plus carboplatin (25) or doxorubicin plus trabectedin could also be a conceivable strategy for AS-SO in exceptional cases, especially when ifosfamide is contraindicated (cf. palliative therapy). However, it should not come as a surprise if there is no response. In one case of advanced cervical AS with SO, CHT with ifosfamide plus doxorubicin as well as subsequent gemcitabine plus docetaxel failed to achieve a response (89). Due to the bleak data situation, administering neoadjuvant CHT to achieve operability can currently only be regarded as a “therapy attempt” that cannot be assumed to be effective. All patients who are to undergo CHT must be unequivocally informed of the wide lack of previous clinical experience in this context.

For AS in which ER and PGR expression is strong throughout the entire tumor, HT can be attempted as a means for achieving tumor operability, either primarily or when CHT is contraindicated. Notwithstanding, there are no known reliable data which would support such an indication. Progestin therapy is the first option to be considered, and should be replaced with AI when progestins are contraindicated for postmenopausal patients. There are no usable data pertaining to the use (and benefits of the use) of GnRH analogues in premenopausal patients. Nor can any reliable statements currently be made as to whether HT achieves superior outcomes compared to neoadjuvant CHT. One collection of case histories describes how a good remission was achieved in a 79-year-old patient under a combination of carboplatin and GnRH analogues, though it remains unclear what the observed therapeutic effect was ultimately a consequence of. It should be noted that the purpose of therapy in the stated case was not to make the locally advanced tumor operable (113). It needs to be reckoned with that responses can be delayed under standalone HT. It is questionable whether or not this drawback can be compensated for by administering targeted RT to locally confined tumors. Overall, neoadjuvant HT must be regarded as unreliable, and applying it needs to be understood as a "therapy attempt" in which curative effects cannot be reliably assumed to follow, even when tumors are positive for HR. The hormone-therapeutic models correspond to those applied to recurrences and metastases.

There is currently no indication for subjecting generally operable patients with resectable adenosarcomas with and without "sarcomatous overgrowth" to primary radiation therapy. Irradiating only advanced tumors may serve to achieve temporary symptom control, however such practice has yet to be proven beneficial. Combining such targeted radiotherapy with chemotherapy might serve to improve the results.

No particular treatment method can be highlighted as constituting optimal therapy for generally inoperable patients. Percutaneous pelvic irradiation with or without brachytherapy can be performed on patients whose tumors are confined to the uterus and the pelvis. Such treatment can be combined with chemotherapy. Chemotherapy is indicated for all other instances, and can be combined with targeted radiotherapy when the tumor is localized in the abdominal cavity. Chemotherapy for generally inoperable patients should begin with a monotherapeutic regimen when symptoms are mild and the pressure to achieve a remission is not so great. Otherwise, a combination regimen should be opted for. Treatment can begin with hormone therapy if the hormone receptors are positive.

Neoadjuvant polychemotherapy with the option for surgery can be considered for inoperable adenosarcomas, though there is no evidence to support that doing so yields more favorable outcomes. No chemotherapeutic agents or regimens have yet been proven to be effective in AS for such an approach. In exceptional cases, reference can be made to the information pertaining to palliative therapy in this context.

Subjecting advanced adenosarcomas with positive hormone receptors to neoadjuvant hormone therapy will always merely constitute a therapy attempt with an uncertain outcome, and is essentially only an option for adenosarcomas without sarcomatous overgrowth. Neoadjuvant hormone therapy might possibly even be superior to chemotherapy in such cases. Whether better outcomes can be achieved in locally confined tumors by combining neoadjuvant hormone therapy with targeted radiation therapy remains unclear.

6.1.10 Aftercare, recurrences, metastases

Analogous to the other types and variants of uterine sarcoma, aftercare should be clinically guided by symptomatology via gynecological and general examination. Follow-ups should be conducted every 3 mo for 2 years, every 6 mo for the next 3 years, and every 12 mo thereafter. TVS and TAS can be among the applied modes of clinical examination (Fig. 6.1.11 (A)). Performing a CT of the thorax, abdomen and pelvis can be considered at the same intervals. Further measures should only be taken when follow-up reveals a need for them, or when patients present with symptoms. Complex laboratory chemical and technical examinations as well as a very early therapy have not yet been proven to reliably improve survival. Taking more intensive diagnostic steps is, therefore, only sensible if clinical and/or sonographic examination yields suspicious results, or when patients are symptomatic. No tumor markers are known that could serve as means for reliably monitoring the follow-up period. Determining the N/L ratio can be a helpful, easy and cheap means for detecting recurrences or for monitoring the progress of palliative treatment. It needs to be noted that the N/L ratio is not specific to AS, but rather also applies to the other uterine sarcomas, including CS. The cut-off value for uterine sarcomas is 2.12 (52). Tumors with values beyond 2.12 have a sensitivity, a specificity, a PPV, an NPV and an accuracy of 74.5, 70.3, 29.5, 94.3 and 60.6 %, respectively (cf. Vol. 1, Chapter 6). It is, however, entirely unclear which consequences can be deduced when the results from imaging diagnostic examinations are suspicious or when the N/L ratio is abnormal in asymptomatic patients. Consequently, such findings do not necessarily have any definitive therapeutic implications. Elevated LDH values have also been detected in advanced tumors in some cases (62, 111).

As a precaution, analogous to the other types of uterine sarcoma, patients who have been subjected to inadequate surgery or morcellation should undergo follow-up LSC within 3 to 6 mo, unless completion surgery via reresection is already planned.

It is strongly advised that HET not be given to patients who have undergone surgery on HR positive AS. Tamoxifen and toremifene therapy are both contraindicated due to their pathogenetic association with AS. AI or GnRH analogues (the latter for younger patients) can be administered in the usual dosages if adjuvant HT is indicated due to simultaneous or metachronic breast cancer.

In 70–100 % of cases, recurrences and metastases of AS are purely sarcomatous and are usually not as well differentiated as the primary tumor (Fig. 6.1.10 (B), (C)). Metastases from AS without SO can themselves exhibit SO (103). Furthermore, it is not uncommon for metastases to lack the HR that had previously been verifiable in the primary tumor. Due to the therapeutic consequences that could potentially result from not doing so, the metastases and recurrences should also be tested for HR. Assessing the presence of HR in recurrences and metastases is, however, superfluous when the primary tumor was HR negative. Local recurrences of AS without SO often arise up to 10 years after primary diagnosis, usually in the vagina, the lesser pelvis and in the abdominal cavity, and typically exhibit slow rates of growth. Distant metastasis is more frequently observed in patients with AS with SO, and usually involves the abdominal cavity and the lungs (11). Recurring AS with SO have a distinctly poorer prognosis, and are often only even identified as such upon detection of recurrent tumors and/or metastases. Patients in these cases have often already undergone HE for other reasons, during which the AS was overlooked. In certain circumstances, measuring the LDH value (62) and the L/N ratio can be drawn on as means for monitoring therapeutic progress and effects (for details, see LMS, Vol. 1, Chapter 2).

For adenosarcomas, aftercare and follow-up should be clinically guided by symptomatology via gynecological and general examination in combination with sonography. Follow-up should be conducted every 3 months for 2 years, every 6 months for the next 3 years, and every 12 months thereafter. Performing a CT on the thorax, the abdomen and the pelvis at these intervals can also be considered. Farther-reaching measures should only be initiated when examinations reveal suspicious findings or when patients present with symptoms. The increased risk of recurrence associated with inadequate operations requires particular attention and consideration. Subjecting patients who have undergone morcellation or whose tumors sustained injury during surgery to endoscopic follow-up might be sensible if completion surgery/reresection is not definitely planned. Hormone replacement therapy is contraindicated when hormone receptors are positive. Adjuvant tamoxifen therapy administered as treatment of mammary carcinoma should be replaced with aromatase inhibitors or GnRH analogues.

In general, recurrences and distant metastases should be histologically verified and examined for the presence of hormone receptors. Distant metastasis and recurrence are both more frequently observed in patients whose adenosarcomas exhibit sarcomatous overgrowth.

6.1.11 Surgical management and postoperative additive therapy for recurrences and metastatic disease

There is consensus that all of the measures described hereafter constitute adequate therapeutic measures, the adequacy of which is only based on clinical experience or "lower-level evidence".

Localized recurrences in the lesser pelvis and the abdominal cavity should, if technically possible, be subjected to surgical treatment analogous to stromal sarcomas. The key precondition is that R0 resection margins can be achieved according to the results from imaging diagnostic examination. Metastases in the abdominal cavity are usually well accessible, implying that surgery is relatively simple in many cases from a technical perspective (Fig. 6.1.11 (B)–(E)). The results from two retrospective studies suggest that cytoreductive surgery is superior or at the very least equally adequate to palliative CHT (11, 106). Women who underwent cytoreductive surgery showed a clearly (albeit not statistically significantly) longer PFI compared to those who did not (14, 106). Resection can also be considered in cases of solitary lung and liver metastases (57). A minimally invasive approach is also possible when more than one, but fewer than five metastases are present in the lungs and the liver. LITT, SIRT or chemoembolization are eligible options in this context, though no larger-scale studies or experiences have yet been published that refer specifically to AS. In principle, surgical management can correspond to that envisaged for the surgical treatment of recurrent and metastatic stromal sarcomas. Respective details for AS without SO can be found in the chapter on LG-ESS, while the relevant information for AS with SO is provided in the chapter on HG-ESS (cf. Vol. 1, Chapter 4 and 5). No valid data are

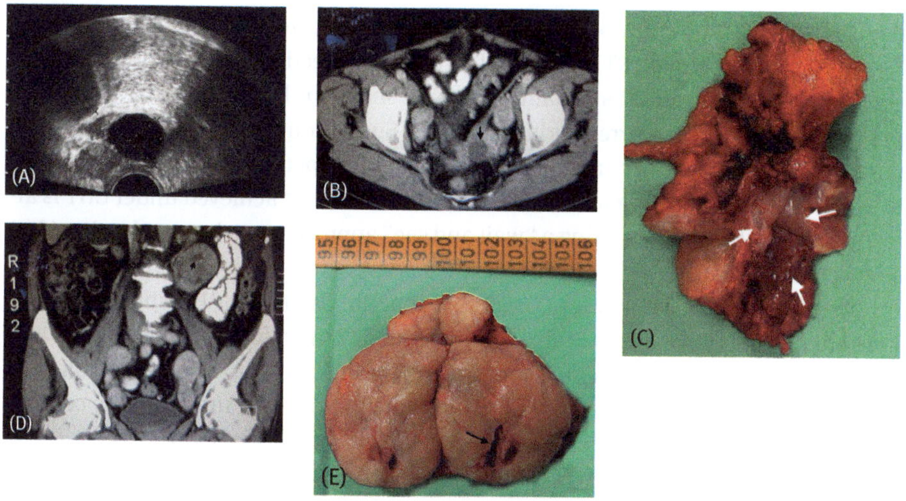

Fig. 6.1.11: Imaging of and surgery on pelvic recurrences and intraabdominal metastases. (A)–(C) vaginal sonography with solid and anechoic areas; axial CECT likewise reveals both a solid and a non-enhancing, cystic region (arrow); both structures are traceable in the macroscopic specimen (arrows indicate the margin of the opened "cyst"); (D) coronal CECT clearly reveals that the metastases in the upper abdomen and the pelvic recurrences are open to adequate resection, a finding that was intraoperatively confirmed; (E) The cystic sections (arrows) do not enhance in CECT and can be easily discerned in the presented metastatic lesion resected from the upper abdomen.

available pertaining to improved survival. Whether surgery is superior to systemic therapy cannot currently be confirmed definitively. The advantage of opting for the surgical route lies in the fact that the masses can usually be removed relatively easily and effectively, and that CHT (that is only barely effective, and when so only achieves short responses) can be kept in reserve.

The currently available evidence is insufficient to verify that subjecting patients whose recurrences and/or metastases have been R0/R1/R2 resected to postoperative RT or CHT offers any benefits in terms of OS. Against the backdrop of the fact that AS and stromal sarcomas exhibit largely identical behavior (91), the criteria applied in the context of additive therapy for uterine stromal sarcomas must also be accepted for AS. The approaches to additive therapy for AS with and without SO can thus largely mirror those adopted for LG-ESS and HG-ESS, respectively (cf. Vol. 1, Chapters 4 and 5). According to the current NCCN category 2A guidelines for these types of neoplasms, targeted postoperative ERT and/or BT are most likely justified in cases of localizable R1/R2 resected recurrences (69). CHT (for substances and dosages, see palliative CHT) can be considered when findings cannot be localized and the tumor is HR negative. It is vital that the potential side effects be borne in mind, given the fact that it is questionable whether or not postoperative CHT or RT will achieve a response, and that, when they are achieved, responses are short. Evidence has yet to be provided that postoperative CHT and/or RT offer any benefits when patients are postoperatively asymptomatic. The efficacy of performing RT and/or CHT after an R0 resection is thus highly questionable and lacks any scientific substantiation. CHT should be kept in reserve for renewed progression or further recurrences in such cases. Such a course of action is further supported by the fact that there are barely any chemotherapeutic agents that are known to achieve responses in AS patients, and the PFI that can be achieved under CHT is already very short as it is. Adopting a "wait and see" approach can thus not be classified as erroneous practice, not least because there are very few alternatives.

Based on what is known for LG-ESS, AS that are positive for HR should be subjected to postoperative HT, as is also recommended (2A recommendation) for LG-ESS in the current NCCN Guidelines (69). In general, an approach can be adopted that corresponds to that recommended for LG-ESS. Particularities pertaining to this context are discussed at length in the chapter on LG-ESS (cf. Vol. 1, Chapter 3).

Localized recurrent masses in the pelvis and the abdominal cavity should be subjected to surgery when technically feasible. Solitary lung and liver metastases can also be resected, under the condition that R0 resection margins will be achieved and that the patient is otherwise disease-free. The surgical strategic approach can correspond to the measures used for uterine stromal sarcomas. A minimally invasive approach can be opted for when there are more than one, but fewer than five metastatic lesions in the lungs and/or the liver. There is currently no evidence to suggest that the aforementioned measures are superior to systemic therapy with or without irradiation.

It has yet to be scientifically proven that subjecting patients who have undergone R0 resections to postoperative chemo- or radiation therapy yields prognostic benefits. Targeted external irradiation and/or brachytherapy can be considered as therapeutic options for localized (!) R1/R2 resected tumors. Postoperative chemotherapy can be considered if lung and liver metastases have been subjected to R1/R2 resection, or to targeted irradiation due to technical inoperability, though there are no data to verify that doing so yields more favorable outcomes. An observant approach can be adopted in place of chemotherapy if patients are asymptomatic. Doing so has not yet been associated with negative effects on overall survival. It is generally indicated that postoperative hormone therapy be subsequently administered whenever recurrences and metastases of hormone-receptor positive tumors are resected.

6.1.12 Palliative radio-, chemo- and hormone therapy, treatment with small molecules, supportive therapy

There have been only few experiences with palliative external RT and AS. Palliative external RT is indicated for localized (!) recurrences and distant metastases that are not surgically accessible/inoperable and that are ineligible for HT. Among the few cases that have been reported, there is one account in which local recurrences rapidly progressed under RT. In another case, subjecting a vaginal metastatic tumor to VBT achieved a CR (104). At the very least, applying targeted RT can achieve short-term palliative effects (11). Targeted RT, in the form of ERT or BT, provides an alternative to surgically treating local recurrences when surgery is not possible for whatever reason.

The few available data pertaining to the use of palliative CHT in AS patients are disappointing and come exclusively from retrospective studies. CHT is indicated when there is diffuse metastasis, for symptomatic patients, or when disease is located in threatening or risk-associated sites, and the operative, radiological and hormone-based options have been exhausted or are not applicable in the case at hand. In practice, this usually concerns AS with SO. As AS and uterine stromal sarcomas share various commonalities, the cytostatic agents should be those that are effective in achieving responses in uterine stromal sarcomas. Doxorubicin/epirubicin or a combination of ifosfamide and doxorubicin are the most noteworthy regimens in this regard (14, 104). These regimens are only rarely reported to have effected a CR (for 5 years in one case) (14), and PR are usually only for a short period. There are accounts in which both a CR and a PR were achieved under liposomal doxorubicin (24, 41, 62). Based on these data and several meta-analyses, liposomal doxorubicin monotherapy appears to be the most adequate regimen for the palliative context (41, 62). Ifosfamide could be administered as an alternative, especially when there are contraindications for liposomal doxorubicin. In one study, administering trabectedin effected a 13 mo PR in one patient, one case of SD for 3 mo, and no response in a third patient (87). Trabectedin monotherapy can thus also be considered, especially when no response can be achieved using doxorubicin or ifosfamide, or when these agents are contraindicated.

Experience has shown that the combinations carboplatin plus paclitaxel, ifosfamide plus paclitaxel, and ifosfamide plus carboplatin either only lead to short-term RR or SD that rarely last for longer than 3 mo, or they achieve no response at all (16, 110). In one study, a combination of ifosfamide, doxorubicin plus cisplatin only achieved a PFI of between 44 and 80 days (115). Similarly, gemcitabine plus docetaxel triggered no response except for one PR for 4.4 mo (87, 106). Positive responses were achieved in two cases using carboplatin in combination with HT and RT, respectively (113). In light of it having been administered simultaneous to HT or RT in these cases, the effectiveness of carboplatin must be deemed questionable.

Poly-CHT can achieve potentially better response rates than mono-CHT, and is thus indicated when achieving disease remission is urgently required or when patients present with severe symptoms. Analogous to LG-ESS, a combination of ifosfamide plus doxorubicin currently appears to be the regimen of choice. A combination of gemcitabine and docetaxel can also be considered for lack of alternatives (106), though it must be reckoned with that said regimen will fail to yield a response and that, when yielded, the PFI will be very short (89). Accounts of remissions that were achieved in AS by administering trabectedin and doxorubicin monotherapies (87, 106) render the combination of trabectedin and doxorubicin (a regimen that has been proven highly effective in LMS) a promising alternative for treating AS. For LMS, this combination has achieved an RR of 55 % and a CBR of 88 % with a PFI of 8.1 mo (75). In the DKSM materials database, in one advanced AS, PD under liposomal doxorubicin was followed by SD for 4 mo under trabectedin (end of follow-up). Administering the rather tolerable (in terms of toxicity and side effects) combination of liposomal doxorubicin plus carboplatin could be adequate in some isolated cases (25). However, the PFI under or following this CHT regimen is usually only a few months in duration. Poly-CHT is associated with toxicity-related detrimental effects on quality of life and usually only effects a very short PFI. It should, therefore, be regarded critically, and should only be administered when there is urgency to achieve remission. Combinations of three agents, for instance ifosfamide, epirubicin and cisplatin, should be the exception.

Therapy proposal: chemotherapy

Monochemotherapy	Ifosfamide or	1.5 g/m^2 i.v. 2 g/m^2 i.v.	(d 1–4) (d 1–3)	q 3–4 wk q 3–4 wk
	Peg-liposomal doxorubicin	40 mg/m^2 1 h i.v.	(d 1)	q 4 wk
	Trabectedin*	1.5 mg/m^2 i.v.	(d 1)	q 3 wk
Polychemotherapy	Ifosfamide 1.5 g/m^2 i.v. (d 1–4) + Doxorubicin 50 mg/m^2 i.v. (d 1) Ifosfamide 2 g/m^2 i.v. (d 1–3) + Epirubicin 40 mg/m^2 i.v. (d 1) + Cisplatin 60 mg/m^2 (d 1)			q 3 wk q 4 wk
	Doxorubicin 60 mg/m^2 i.v. D1+Trabectedin* 1.1 mg/m^2 3 h, d 1			q 3–4 wk
	Gemcitabine 900 mg/m^2 i.v. d 1 + Docetaxel 100 mg/m^2 i.v. d 8			q 3 wk
	Peg-liposomal doxorubicin 30–40 mg/m^2 1 h i.v. (d 1) + Carboplatin AUC 5–6 i.v. (d 1)			q 4 wk

* second line

Patients with HR positive AS can undergo palliative HT when all surgical options have been exhausted, when they are inoperable, or when there is diffuse metastatic disease. There is one report of a case in which a 10-year PR was achieved under MGA therapy (106). DNG is highly effective for treating endometriosis, and constitutes a more novel hormone-therapeutic option for AS (53). Due to its endocrinological characteristics (82), the virtual absence of influence on metabolism change, and its proliferation-inhibiting effects on endometrial stromal cells (73), DNG appears to be adequate for treating HR positive endometrial stromal sarcomas as well. There is one case report in which a marked PR with an SD of 21 mo and a parallel reduction of elevated CA-125 values was observed in an endometriosis-associated AS (107). In one of our own cases (54), a patient with recurrent and metastasized LG-ESS underwent intensive sequential hormonal pretreatment with BSO, MAG, AI and fulvestrant. After further recurrence, the patient was treated with DNG. She showed SD for more than 6 mo (end of follow-up). However, for lack of approved alternatives, DNG can be used as a therapy attempt when MPA and MGA are contraindicated (thrombosis) or fail. HR status should be re-evaluated prior to any HT, as their expression (as is also the case for other hormone-dependent tumors) can change for the worse. FES-PET-CT can be performed instead if HR expression cannot be assessed by other means, for whatever reasons (112, 118). FES-PET-CT has the advantage that it serves to determine the HR content of all filiae. An absence of receptors is regarded as a contraindication for HT. No further data are available that pertain to the effectiveness of HT in AS patients, as their incidence is so low. Given the fact that AS and stromal sarcomas both pathogenetically originate from the endometrial stroma (91) and that both of these neoplasms exhibit virtually congruent behavior, the same criteria can also be adhered to as are accepted for uterine stromal sarcomas in the context of palliative HT. Such a course of action is also supported by the literature (97, 113). Details pertaining to the agents and dosages applied are described at length in the chapter on ESS (cf. Vol. 1, Chapter 4) and can be transferred to AS. CHT is indicated if HT is ineffective or the options within that group of therapeutic measures have been exhausted.

Analogous to the other types of uterine sarcoma, in cases in which disease has spread, CHT can be replaced with the provision of best supportive care, an option that is also positively echoed in the current NCCN Guidelines (69).

While both AS types largely immunophenotypically correspond to the stromal uterine sarcomas, in contrast to the latter, only 5 % of AS express c-Kit (CD117) (97). Consequently, in contrast to stromal sarcomas (85), AS are not eligible or adequate for therapy with the c-Kit inhibitor and the TKI imatinib (97).

Palliative irradiation is most likely indicated for localized recurrences and distant metastases that are either inoperable or not eligible for hormone therapy.

Palliative chemotherapy is indicated when the surgical, radiological and hormone-based alternatives have been exhausted, when surgery is contraindicated, or when there is diffuse metastatic disease. Chemotherapy should first be administered as monotherapy when patients present with symptoms. Polychemotherapeutic regimens should only be opted for when remission must urgently be achieved and/or when patients present with severe symptoms and/or when disease is localized in threatening or risk-associated sites, or when disease progresses despite monotherapy.

Analogous to low-grade endometrial stromal sarcomas with positive hormone receptor expression, palliative hormone therapy is also regarded as the therapeutic option of choice for patients whose AS are hormone-receptor positive and who exhibit diffuse metastasis, or when all surgical alternatives have been exhausted. Ovarectomy should be performed first if the ovaries have not yet been removed. The first therapeutic step for patients who are under hormone replacement or tamoxifen therapy would be to discontinue such treatment. Progestins, aromatase inhibitors, and GnRH analogues (exceptionally for premenopausal patients) constitute the alternative therapeutic options in this regard. Palliative hormone treatment must be continuously rendered until there is renewed progression, upon which a switch to another hormone-based measure is possible. While no data are available pertaining to the use of fulvestrant in this context, off-label use as a “therapy attempt” could be feasible when progestins and aromatase inhibitors have failed.

Standalone best supportive care is an accepted therapeutic option for cases in which there is diffuse metastatic dissemination. Small molecule therapy has not yet been proven to be effective in adenosarcoma patients.

6.2 Extrauterine and extragenital adenosarcomas

Extrauterine AS have been reported to arise in the ovary, the fallopian tube, in the paraovarian tissue, the vagina, in the area of the ligamentum latum, and on the intestinal serosa (61). Clinical and pathologico-anatomical findings from numerous studies suggest that extrauterine AS with and without SO develop from or arise in extraovarian endometriosis in the majority of cases (6, 15, 27, 48, 59, 66, 68, 99). Women with extrauterine AS appear to be younger than women with uterine AS.

Extrauterine and extragenital adenosarcomas predominantly develop in or from an endometriosis.

6.2.1 Adenosarcomas of the ovary and the fallopian tube

The ovary appears to be the most common localization in which extrauterine AS arise. Notwithstanding, AS account for only 2.1 % (1 of 48) of all ovarian sarcomas in the DKSM material database (54). Among 40 reported cases, mean patient age was 54 years (30–84 years), which is lower than among patients with uterine AS. The same microscopic criteria apply as for uterine AS. Disease was unilateral in 39 of 40 cases, and tumor size ranged from 5.5 to 50 cm (27). Staging for OC is generally applied (95). The majority of such tumors are predominantly solid, while 10 % are predominantly cystic, and a further 10 % are entirely solid. Cyst diameters range from 0.2 to 12 cm (27) (Fig. 6.2.1).

The presence of SO is verified in 30 % of cases. Heterologous elements can be present in tumors both with and without SO, and usually consist of RMS or chondromatous, osteomatous or lipomatous sarcoma components. Analogous to uterine AS, sex cord-like elements can also occasionally be present (27).

Ovarian AS are characterized by features, findings and symptoms that are also typical of OC. Sixty percent of ovarian AS are recognized as malignancies at the time of primary diagnosis. Ovarian AF, cystadenofibroma and ovarian endometriosis are the most significant DD. Steps must be taken to rule out sex cord stromal tumors when sex cord-like components are present. From a differential diagnostic perspective, pure homologous and heterologous sarcomas can be difficult to discern from an AS with SO. Pure sarcomas must be extensively examined to determine whether or not they also contain epithelial structures, so as not to overlook an AS. CS must also be considered as an alternative diagnostic option when there are epithelial atypia.

Recurrences or metastases are observed in 62.5 % of ovarian AS within a mean time period of 2.6 years (median 2.2 years). Median survival is 7.3 years. Five, 10, and 15-year OS are 64, 46 and 30 %, respectively (27). Tumor ruptures and the presence of an SO with a high-grade (in part RMS) sarcomatous component are risk factors associated with an unfavorable impact on OS. Literature review reveals that prognosis is generally poorer than for the uterine types, likely caused by their free localization in

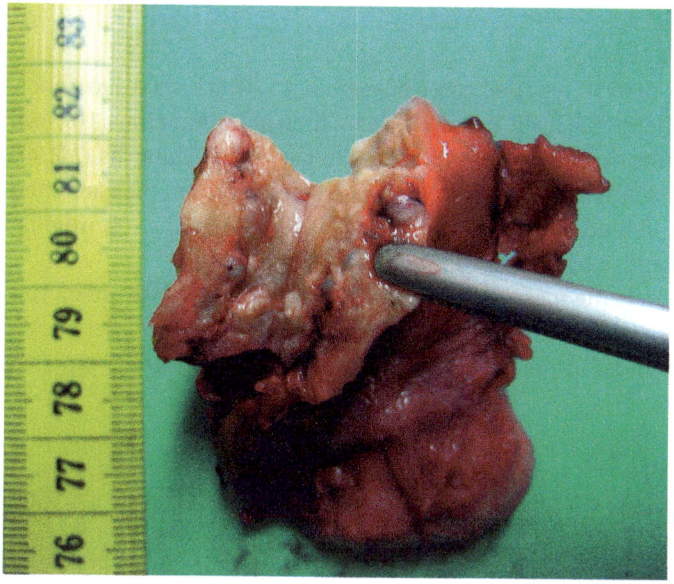

Fig. 6.2.1: Macroscopic features of an ovarian adenosarcoma. The epithelial cystic areas in the sarcomatous stroma are clearly visible.

the abdominal cavity, a higher proportion of tumors with SO, tumor perforations, and by the fact that tumors tend to be larger due to being detected and diagnosed comparably later. Patient age < 53 years is said to be an unfavorable prognostic factor (27).

Reliable R0 resection is the therapeutic method of choice. No data are available that could give insight as to whether an additional THE or an ovarectomy on the non-affected contralateral ovary would be beneficial. Uterine AS needs to have been ruled out via imaging diagnostics if the uterus is to be left in situ. However, uterine AS only exceptionally metastasize to the ovaries (see uterine AS). LNE or omentectomy are currently not indicated. Ovarian AS with extraovarian extension should also be subjected to R0 resection. Regarding the postoperative treatment of recurrences and metastases, the same criteria apply as described for uterine AS with and without SO.

AS of the fallopian tube is extremely rare and can barely be clinically discerned from ovarian AS. The same therapeutic criteria apply as to ovarian AS.

> The ovaries are the most common site of extrauterine adenosarcoma. Such tumors barely differ from ovarian carcinoma in terms of their clinical features and behavior. The more frequent presence of sarcomatous overgrowth in ovarian adenosarcomas, their free localization in the abdominal cavity and tumor perforations impact negatively on prognosis. Reliable R0 resection is the therapeutic method of choice. Performing further-reaching surgical and postoperative measures has not yet been proven to be beneficial in terms of prognosis. Recurrences and metastases are treated analogous to those of uterine adenosarcomas.

6.2.2 Adenosarcoma of the vagina

There have been fewer than 10 reported cases of vaginal AS, which serves to underline their rarity. AS of the vagina likely usually develop from an endometriosis (6, 48). There have been accounts of such neoplasms arising in patients as young as 17 (114). Since these sarcomas usually originate from the rectovaginal septum, they are often located retrocervically, behind or beside the uterus. AS arising from the rectovaginal pouch can breach into and subsequently fill the vagina (111).

Definite R0 resection is the therapeutic method of choice. Further treatment can be designed in accordance with the therapeutic strategies described for uterine AS. Locally confined recurrences in the vagina can be positively responsive to targeted irradiation (6).

Adenosarcomas of the vagina must be subjected to definite R0 resection. Apart from that, the approach corresponds to that followed for uterine adenosarcomas. Targeted irradiation is a further option for recurrences in the vagina.

6.2.3 Extragenital adenosarcomas

Accounts of AS arising from the pelvic and abdominal peritoneum have been described in the literature. According to a meta-analysis covering numerous individual publications, they can occur on the peritoneum of the entire abdomen including the mesentery and the greater omentum. Affected women have a median age of 45 years and are thus significantly younger than women with uterine AS. The development of the majority of extragenital AS is highly likely to be associated with endometriosis. Clinically speaking, extrauterine AS can usually be palpated at their respective site or they are incidental findings discovered during imaging diagnostic procedures. Endometriosis-associated AS are said to have a better prognosis than those with another genesis (41). Macroscopic and imaging diagnostic observations often reveal a cystic, lobulated soft mass. Due to the fact that they develop from an endometriosis, such tumors are frequently localized in the pouch of Douglas (Fig. 6.2.2). Malignant ovarian tumors are the most important differential diagnostic alternatives.

In one publication, median and mean survival were 24 resp. 30 mo in endometriosis-associated cases, while the figures were considerably worse in cases not associated to an endometriosis (12 resp. 15.8 mo) (41). Presence of SO does not appear to be an important prognostic factor in extragenital AS. AS of the mesentery as well as recurrences of such tumors can cause bowel obstruction (41). Maximal cytoreductive surgery leaving disease-free (i.e. R0) resection margins is among the most important prognostic factors. To date, as also applies to uterine and other genital AS, subjecting patients to postoperative therapeutic measures has yet to be scientifically proven as beneficial.

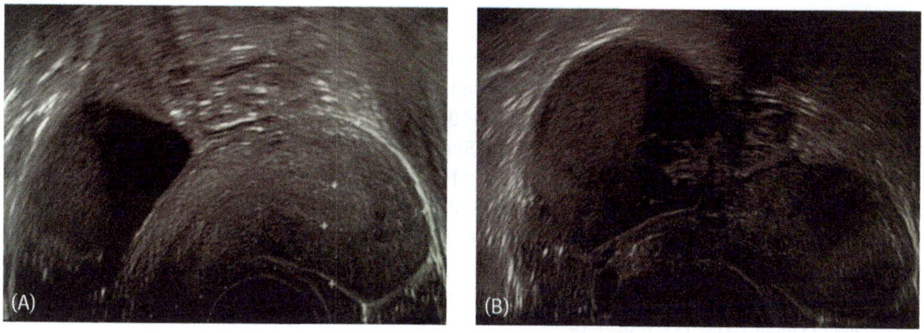

Fig. 6.2.2: Endometriosis-associated extrauterine peritoneal adenosarcoma. (A) sagittal vaginal sonography reveals a cystic tumor that is clearly localized in the Douglas pouch. The weak echoes in the cystic component of the tumor correspond to hemorrhages so identified intraoperatively. The small tumor in the uterus turned out to be leiomyoma; (B) transverse sonography shows that the tumor consists of solid and cystic or necrotic components. The hemorrhages are also clearly visible. A deep concretion with the serosa of the uterus was confirmed during surgery.

Regarding the treatment of recurrences and metastases, the same criteria apply as described for uterine AS.

Extragenital adenosarcomas arise in the entire abdomen. Reliable R0 resection is the therapeutic method of choice. Resorting to farther-reaching measures has yet to be proven beneficial. Recurrences und metastases are treated analogous to those of uterine adenosarcomas.

References

(1) Abeler VM, Røyne O, Thoresen S, Danielsen HE, Nesland JM, Kristensen GB. Uterine sarcomas in Norway. A histopathological and prognostic survey of a total population from 1970 to 2000 including 419 patients. Histopathology 2009; 54: 355–364

(2) Amant F, Steenkiste E, Schurmans K, Verbist L, Abeler VM, Tulunay G, Jonge E de, Massuger L, Moermann P, Vergote I. Immunhistochemical expression of CD10 antigen in uterine adenosarcoma. Internat J Gynecol Cancer 2004; 14: 1118–1121

(3) Amant F, Schurmans K, Steenkiste E, Verbist L, Abeler VM, Tulunay G, Jonge E de, Massuger L, Moermann P, Vergote I. Immunhistochemical determination of estrogen and progesterone receptor positivity in uterine adenosarcoma. Gynecol Oncol 2004; 93: 680–685

(4) Amant F, Vloeberghs V, Woestenborghs H, Debiec-Rychter M, Verbist L, Moerman P, Vergote I. ERBB-2 gene overexpression and amplification in uterine sarcomas. Gynecol Oncol 2004; 95: 583–587

(5) Amant F, De Knijf A, Van Calster B, Leunen K, Neven P, Berteloot P, Vergote I, Van Huffel S, Moerman P. Clinical study investigating the role of lymphadenectomy, surgical castration, and adjuvant hormonal treatment in endometrial stromal sarcoma. Br J Cancer 2007; 97: 1194–1199

(6) Anderson J, Behbakht K, De Geest K, Bitterman P. Adenosarcoma in a patient with vaginal endometriosis. Obstet Gynecol 2001; 98: 964–966

(7) Arend R, Bagaria M, Lewin SN, Sun X, Deutsch I, Burke WM, Herzog TJ, Wright JD. Long-term outcome and natural history of uterine adenosarcomas. Gynecol Oncol 2010; 119: 305–308
(8) Arici DS, Aker H, Yildiz E, Tasyurt A. Mullerian adenosarcoma of the uterus associated with tamoxifen therapy. Arch Gynecol Obstet 2000; 164: 105–107
(9) Bansal S, Lewin SN, Burke WM, Deutsch I, Sun X, Herzog TJ, Wright JD. Sarcoma of the cervix: natural history and outcomes. Gynecol Oncol 2010; 118: 134–138
(10) Berchuk A, Rubin SC, Hoskins WJ, Saigo PE, Pierce VK, Lewis JL jr. Treatment of endometrial stromal tumors. Gynecol Oncol 1990; 71: 60–65
(11) Bernard B, Clarke BA, Malowany JI, McAlpine J, Lee CH, Atenafu EG, Ferguson S, Mackay H. Uterine adenosarcomas: A dual-institution update on staging, prognosis and survival. Gynecol Oncol 2013; 131: 634–639
(12) Bonvalot S, Rivoire M, Castaing M, Stoeckle E, Le Cesne A, Blay JY, Laplanche A. Primary retroperitoneal sarcomas: A multivariate analysis of surgical factors associated with local control. J Clin Oncol 2009; 27: 31–37
(13) Buyukkurt S, Guzel AB, Gumurdulu D, Vardar MA, Zeren H, Sucu M. Mullerian adenosarcoma of the uterine cervix in an adolescent girl. J Pediatr Adolesc Gynecol. 2010; 23: e13–15
(14) Carroll A, Ramirez PT, Westin SN, Soliman PT, Munsell MF, Nick AM, Schmeler KM, Klopp AH, Fleming ND. Uterine adenosarcoma: An analysis on management, outcomes, and risk factors for recurrence. Gynecol Oncol 2014; 135: 455–461
(15) Chang HY, Changchien CC, Chen HH, Lin H, Huang CC. Extrauterine müllerian adenosarcoma associated with endometriosis and rectal villotubular adenoma: report of a case and review of the literature. Int J Gynecol Cancer 2005; 15: 361–365
(16) Choi YJ, Jung MH, Park YK, Lee BY, Huh CY. Uterine müllerian adenosarcoma with sarcomatous overgrowth and lung metastasis in a 25-year-old woman. Eur J Gynaecol Oncol 2011; 32: 91–94
(17) Chourmouzi D, Boulogianni G, Zarampoukas T, Drevelengas A. Sonography and MRI of tamoxifen-associated müllerian adenosarcoma of the uterus. AJR Am J Roentgenol 2003; 181: 1673–1675
(18) Chung YW, Bae HS, Han SI, Song JY, Kim IS, Kang JS. Endometrial mullerian adenosarcoma after toremifene treatment in breast cancer patients: A case report. J Gynecol Oncol 2010; 21: 269–272
(19) Clement P, Scully R. Mullerian adenosarcoma of the uterus: A clinico-pathologic analysis of 100 cases with a review of the literature. Hum Pathol 1990; 21: 363–381
(20) Clement PB, Oliva E, Young RH. Mullerian adenosarcoma of the uterine corpus associated with tamoxifen therapy: A report of six cases and a review of tamoxifen-associated endometrial lesions. Int J Gynecol Pathol 1996; 15: 222–229
(21) Clement PB, Young RH. Atlas of Gynaecologic Surgical Pathology. Saunders Elsevier 2014
(22) Dahhan T, Fons G, Buist MR, ten Kate FJW, van der Velden J. The efficacy of hormonal treatment for residual or recurrent low grade endometrial stromal sarcoma. A retrospective study. Eur J Obstet Gynecol Reprod Biol 2009; 144: 80–84
(23) D'Angelo E, Prat J. Pathology of mixed Müllerian tumours. Best Pract Res Clin Obstet Gynaecol 2011; 25: 705–718
(24) Del Carmen MG, Lovett D, Goodman A. A case of Müllerian adenosarcoma of the uterus treated with liposomal doxorubicin. Gynecol Oncol 2003; 88: 456–458
(25) Du Bois A, Pfisterer J, Burchardi N, Loibl S, Huober J, Wimberger P, Burges A, Stähle A, Jackisch C, Kölbl H. Arbeitsgemeinschaft Gynäekologische Onkologie Studiengruppe Ovarialkarzinom; Kommission Uterus. Combination therapy with pegylated liposomal doxorubicin and carboplatin in gynecologic malignancies: A prospective phase II study of the Arbeits-

gemeinschaft Gynäekologische Onkologie Studiengruppe Ovarialkarzinom (AGO-OVAR) and Kommission Uterus (AGO-K-Ut). Gynecol Oncol 2007; 107: 518–525

(26) Duggal R, Nijhawan R, Aggarwal N, Sikka P. Mullerian adenosarcoma (heterologous) of the cervix with sarcomatous overgrowth: A case report with review of literature. J Gynecol Oncol 2010; 21: 125–128

(27) Eichhorn JH, Young RH, Clement PB, Scully RE. Mesodermal (müllerian) adenosarcoma of the ovary: A clinicopathologic analysis of 40 cases and a review of the literature. Am J Surg Pathol 2002; 26: 1243–1258

(28) Einstein MH, Barakat RR, Chi DS, Sonoda Y, Alektiar KM, Hensley ML, Abu-Rustum NR. Management of uterine malignancy found incidentally after supracervical hysterectomy or uterine morcellation for presumed benign disease. Int J Gynecol Cancer 2008; 10: 1065–1070

(29) El Maalouf G, Duvillard P, Rey A, Morice P, Haie-Meder Ch, Lhommé C, Pautier P. Clinical features, recurrence patterns and treatment in endometrial stromal sarcomas: A thirty-year single-institution experience. J Clin Oncol 2008; 26: Abstr. 10574

(30) Fait T, Zivny J, Freitag P, Kuzel D. Adenosarcoma of the uterine body in a 19-year-old woman—three year survival: case report. Eur J Gynaecol Oncol 2001; 22: 61–63

(31) Farhat MH, Hobeika EM, Moumneh G, Nassar AH. Uterine mullerian adenosarcoma with sarcomatous overgrowth fatal recurrence within two weeks of diagnosis: A case report. Med Case Reports 2007; 25: 103

(32) Farhat F, Fakhruddine NA. A case of synchronous relapse of breast cancer and uterine müllerian adenosarcoma post tamoxifen in a premenopausal woman. Eur J Gynaecol Oncol 2008; 29: 95–97

(33) FIGO Committee on Gynecologic Oncology: FIGO staging for uterine sarcomas. Int J Gynecol Obstet 2009; 104: 179

(34) Fleming NA, Hopkins L, de Nanassy J, Senterman M, Black AY. Mullerian adenosarcoma of the cervix in a 10-year-old girl: case report and review of the literature. J Pediatr Adolesc Gynecol 2009; 22: 45–51

(35) Friedlander ML1, Covens A, Glasspool RM, Hilpert F, Kristensen G, Kwon S, Selle F, Small W, Witteveen E, Russell P. Gynecologic Cancer InterGroup (GCIG) consensus review for mullerian adenosarcoma of the female genital tract. Int J Gynecol Cancer 2014; 24(9 Suppl 3): 78–82

(36) Gadducci A, Cosio S, Romanini A, Genazzani AR. The management of patients with uterine sarcoma: A debated clinical challenge. Crit Rev Oncol Hematol 2008; 65: 129–142

(37) Gallardo A, Prat J. Mullerian adenosarcoma: A clinicopathologic and immunohistochemical study of 55 cases challenging the existence of adenofibroma. Am J Sur Pathol 2009; 33: 278–288

(38) Gollard R, Kosty M, Bordin G, Wax A, Lacey C. Two unusual presentations of müllerian adenosarcoma: case reports, literature review, and treatment considerations. Gynecol Oncol 1995; 59: 412–422

(39) Han XY, Xiang Y, Guo LN, Shen K, Wan XR, Huang HF, Pan LY. Clinicopathological analysis of mullerian adenosarcoma of the uterus. Chin Med J (Engl) 2010; 123: 756–759

(40) Hines BJ, Porges RF, Mittal K, Muggia FM, Curtin JP. Use of medroxyprogesterone acetate in the treatment of Müllerian adenosarcoma: A case report. Gynecol Oncol 2002; 85: 192–195

(41) Huang GS, Arend RC, Sakaris A, Hebert TM, Goldberg GL. Extragenital adenosarcoma: A case report, review of the literature, and management discussion. Gynecol Oncol 2009; 115: 472–475

(42) Ihnen M, Mahner S, Jänicke F, Schwarz J. Current treatment options in uterine stromal sarcoma: report of a case and review of the literature. Int J Gynecol Cancer 2007; 17: 957–963

(43) Inoue M, Fukuda H, Tanizawa O. Adenosarcomas originating from sites other than uterine endometrium. Int J Gynaecol Obstet 1995; 48: 299–306

(44) Ioffe YJ, Li A J, Walsh CS, Karlan BY, Leuchter R, Forscher C, Cass I. Hormone receptor expression in uterine sarcomas: prognostic and therapeutic roles. Gynecol Oncol 2009; 115: 466–471
(45) Jessop FA, Roberts PF. Müllerian adenosarcoma of the uterus in association with tamoxifen therapy Histopathology 2000; 36: 91–92
(46) Jimenez WA, Sardi A, Nieroda C, Gushchin V. Cytoreductive surgery and hyperthermic intraperitoneal chemotherapy in the management of recurrent high-grade uterine sarcoma with peritoneal dissemination. Am J Obstet Gynecol 2014; 210: 259.e1-8. DOI: 10.1016/j.ajog.2013.11.002
(47) Jones S, Stransky N, McCord CL, Cerami E, Lagowski J, Kelly D, Angiuoli SV, Sausen M, Kann L, Shukla M, Makar R, Wood LD, Diaz LA Jr, Lengauer C, Velculescu VE. Genomic analyses of gynaecologic carcinosarcomas reveal frequent mutations in chromatin remodelling genes. Nat Commun 2014; 5:5006. DOI: 10.1038/ncomms6006
(48) Judson PL, Temple AM, Fowler WC Jr, Novotny DB, Funkhouser WK Jr. Vaginal adenosarcoma arising from endometriosis. Gynecol Oncol 2000; 76: 123–125
(49) Kaku T, Silverberg SG, Major FJ, Miller A, Fetter B, Brady MF. Adenosarcoma of the uterus: A Gynecologic Oncology Group clinicopathologic study of 31 cases. Int J Gynecol Pathol 1992; 11: 75–88
(50) Khoury-Collado F, Einstein MH, Bochner BH, Alektiar KM, Sonoda Y, Abu-Rustum NR, Brown CL, Gardner GJ, Barakat RR, Chi DS. Pelvic exenteration with curative intent for recurrent uterine malignancies. Gynecol Oncol 2012; 124: 42–47
(51) Kim WY, Lee JW, Choi CH, Kang H, Kim TJ, Kim GB, Lee JH, Bae DS. Low grade endometrial stromal sarcoma: A single center's experience with 22 cases. Int J Gynecol Cancer 2008; 18: 1084–1089
(52) Kim HS, Han KH, Chung HH, Kim JW, Park NH, Song YS, Kang SB. Neutrophil to lymphocyte ratio for preoperative diagnosis of uterine sarcomas: A case-matched comparison. Eur J Surg Oncol 2010; 36: 691–698
(53) Köhler G, Faustmann TA, Gerlinger C, Seitz C, Mueck AO. A dose-ranging study to determine the efficacy and safety of 1, 2, and 4 mg of dienogest daily for endometriosis. Int J Gynaecol Obstet 2010; 108: 21–25
(54) Köhler G, Belau, A, Dennis K, Evert K, Evert M, Hesse J, Hegenscheid K, Köller M, Krichbaum J, Kühnast M, Lehnhoff H, Lehr A, Linke L, Marcinek A, Müller S, Riechmann C, Schalitz S, Simon J, Spring P, Schädler, J, Ständer C, Trojnarska D, Wilcke S, Witte N, Zygmunt M.; Deutsches klinisches Kompetenzzentrum für genitale Sarkome und Mischtumoren an der Universitätsmedizin Greifswald (DKSM) und Kooperationspartner VAAO Deutschland und FK Frankfurt/Sachsenhausen. Datenbank und Promotions- und Forschungsgruppe genitale Sarkome, Greifswald 2016, http://www.medizin.uni-greifswald.de/gyn/dksm/
(55) Koivisto-Korander R, Butzow R, Koivisto AM, Leminen A. Clinical outcome and prognostic factors in 100 cases of uterine sarcoma: Experience in Helsinki University Central Hospital 1990–2001. Gynecol Oncol 2008; 111: 74 – 81
(56) Krivak TC, Seidman JD, McBroom JW, MacKoul PJ, Aye LM, Rose GS. Uterine adenosarcoma with sarcomatous overgrowth versus uterine carcinosarcoma: comparison of treatment and survival. Gynecol Oncol 2001; 83: 89–94
(57) Levenback C, Rubin SC, McCormack PM, Hoskins WJ, Atkinson EN, Lewis JL. Resection of pulmonary metastases from uterine sarcomas. Gynecol Oncol 1992; 45: 202–205
(58) Li N, Wu LY, Zhang HT, An JS, Li XG, Ma SK. Treatment options in stage I endometrial stromal sarcoma: A retrospective analysis of 53 cases. Gynecol Oncol 2008; 108: 306–311
(59) Liu L, Davidson S, Singh M. Müllerian adenosarcoma of vagina arising in persistent endometriosis: report of a case and review of the literature. Gynecol Oncol 90 2003; 90: 486–490

(60) Livi L, Paiar F, Shah N, Blake P, Villanucci A, Amunni G, Barca R, Judson I, Lodge N, Meldolesi E, Simontacchi G, Piperno G, Galardi A, Scoccianti S, Biti GP, Harmer C. Uterine sarcoma: twenty-seven years of experience. Int J Radiat Oncol Biol Phys 2003; 57: 1366–1373

(61) Löning T. Funktionelle Morphologie und Pathologie des Myometriums. In: Löning T, Riethdorf L (eds.). Pathologie der weiblichen Genitalorgane III – Pathologie des Uterus der Vagina und Vulva. Springer, Berlin – Heidelberg – New York 2001; pp. 652–704

(62) Maeda M, Mabuchi S, Matsumoto Y, Hisamatsu T, Ohashi H, Kimura T. Activity of pegylated liposomal doxorubicin for extragenital mullerian adenosarcoma with sarcomatous overgrowth: A case report and a review of the literature. Eur J Gynaecol Oncol 2011; 32: 542–546

(63) Manoharan M, Azmi MA, Soosay G, Mould T, Weekes AR. Mullerian adenosarcoma of uterine cervix: report of three cases and review of literature. Gynecol Oncol 2007; 105: 256–260

(64) McCluggage WG, Ganesan R, Herrington CS. Endometrial stromal sarcomas with extensive endometrioid glandular differentiation: report of a series with emphasis on the potential for misdiagnosis and discussion of the differential diagnosis. Histopathology 2009; 54: 365–373

(65) Mikami Y, Hata S, Kiyokawa T, Manabe T. Expression of CD10 in malignant müllerian mixed tumors and adenosarcomas: An immunohistochemical study. Mod Pathol 2002; 15: 923–930

(66) Milam MR, Atkinson JB, Currie JL. Adenosarcoma arising in inguinal endometriosis. Obstet Gynecol 2006; 108: 753–755

(67) Mills SE, Sugg NK, Mahnesmith RC. Endometrial adenosarcoma with pelvic involvement following uterine perforation. Diagn Gynecol Obstet 1981; 3: 149–154.

(68) Murugasu A, Miller J, Proietto A, Millar E. Extragenital mullerian adenosarcoma with sarcomatous overgrowth arising in an endometriotic cyst in the pouch of Douglas. Int J Gynecol Cancer 2003; 13: 371–375

(69) National Comprehensive Cancer Network: NCCN Practice Guidelines in Oncology – V.2.2016, Uterine neoplasms. www.nccn.org

(70) Nordal R, Kristensen GB, Kaern J, Stenwig A, Pettersen EO, Tropé CG. The prognostic significance of surgery, tumor size, malignancy grade, menopausal status, and DNA ploidy in endometrial stromal sarcoma. Gynecol Oncol 1996; 62: 254–259

(71) Oda Y, Nakanishi I, Tateiwa T. Intramural müllerian adenosarcoma of the uterus with adenomyosis. Arch Pathol Lab Med 1984; 108: 798–801

(72) Özcan J, Dülger Ö, Küpelioğlu L, Gönenç Aİ, Erşahin A. Uterine sarcoma in a 14 year-old girl presenting with uterine rupture. Gynecol Oncol Rep 2014; 10: 4–46

(73) Okada H, Nakajima T, Yoshimura T, Yasuda K, Kanzaki H. The inhibitory effect of dienogest, a synthetic steroid, on the growth of human endometrial stromal cells in vitro. Mol Hum Reprod 2001; 7: 341–347

(74) Omura GA, Blessing JA, Major F, Lifshitz S, Ehrlich CE, Mangan C, Beecham J, Park R, Silverberg S. A randomized clinical trial of adjuvant adriamycin in uterine sarcomas: A Gynecologic Oncology Group Study. J Clin Oncol 1985; 3: 1240–1245

(75) Pautier P, Floquet A, Cupissol D, Lacas B, Bompas E, Chevreau C, Selle F, Weber BE, Guillemet C, Penel N, Duffaud F. A phase II single-arm multicenter study of doxorubicin in combination with trabectedin as a first-line treatment of advanced uterine leiomyosarcoma (u-LMS) and soft tissue LMS (ST-LMS): First results in patients with u-LMS. J Clin Oncol 2013; 31: abstr 10505

(76) Perri T, Korach J, Sadetzki S, Oberman B, Fridman E, Ben-Baruch G. Uterine leiomyosarcoma: does the primary surgical procedure matter? Int J Gynecol Cancer 2009; 19: 257–260

(77) Piscuoglio S, Burke KA, Ng CK, Papanastasiou AD, Geyer FC, Macedo GS, Martelotto LG, de Bruijn I, De Filippo MR, Schultheis AM, Ioris RA, Levine DA, Soslow RA, Rubin BP, Reis-Filho JS, Weigelt B. Uterine adenosarcomas are mesenchymal neoplasms. J Pathol. 2016; 238: 381–388

(78) Prat J. FIGO staging for uterine sarcomas. Int J Gynecol Obstet 2009; 104: 177–178
(79) Reed NS. The management of uterine sarcomas. Clin Oncol 2008; 20: 470–478
(80) Reed NS, Mangioni C, Malmström H, Scarfone G, Poveda A, Pecorelli S, Tateo S, Franchi M, Jobsen JJ, Coens C, Teodorovic I, Vergote I, Vermorken JB. Phase III randomised study to evaluate the role of adjuvant pelvic radiotherapy in the treatment of uterine sarcomas stages I and II: A European organisation for research and treatment of cancer gynaecological cancer group study (protocol 55874). Eur J Cancer 2008; 44: 808–818
(81) Riopel J, Plante M, Renaud MC, Roy M, Têtu B. Lymph node metastases in low-grade endometrial stromal sarcoma. Gynecol Oncol 2005; 96: 402–406
(82) Ruan X, Seeger H, Mueck AO. The pharmacology of dienogest. Maturitas. 2012; 71: 337–344
(83) Sadeghi R, Zakavi SR, Hasanzadeh M, Treglia G, Giovanella L, Kadkhodayan S. Diagnostic performance of fluorine-18-fluorodeoxyglucose positron emission tomography imaging in uterine sarcomas: systematic review and meta-analysis of the literature. Int J Gynecol Cancer 2013; 23: 1349–1356
(84) Sale E. Adenosarcoma. In: Hricak HH, Akin O, Sala E, Ascher SM, Levine D, Reinhold C (eds.). Diagnostic Imaging Gynecology. Amyrsis 2007; 2/166–2/171
(85) Salvatierra A, Tarrats A, Gomez C, Sastre JM, Balaña CA. A case of c-kit positive high-grade stromal endometrial sarcoma responding to Imatinib Mesylate. Gynecol Oncol 2006; 101: 545–547
(86) Sampath S, Schultheiss TE, Ryu JK, Wong JY. The role of adjuvant radiation in uterine sarcomas. Int J Radiat Oncol Biol Phys 2010; 76: 728–734
(87) Schroeder BA, Rodler ET, Loggers ET, Pollack SM, Jones RL. Clinical benefit of trabectedin in uterine adenosarcoma. Med Oncol 2013; 30: 501
(88) Scott McMeekin, D. Sarcoma of the uterus. In: DiSaia PJ, Creasman WT (eds.). Clinical Gynecologic Oncology. 7th edn. Mosby Elsevier 2007; pp. 185–199
(89) Seagle BL, Falter KJ, Lee S, Frimer M, Samuelson R, Shahabi S. Mullerian adenosarcoma of the cervix: Report of two large tumors with sarcomatous overgrowth or heterologous elements. Gynecol Oncol Case Rep 2014; 9: 7–10
(90) Seidman JD, Wasserman CS, Aye LM, MacKoul PJ, O'Leary TJ. Cluster of uterine mullerian adenosarcoma in the Washington, DC metropolitan area with high incidence of sarcomatous overgrowth. Am J Surg Pathol 1999; 23: 809–814
(91) Seidman JD, Chauhan S. Evaluation of the relationship between adenosarcoma and carcinosarcoma and a hypothesis of the histogenesis of uterine sarcomas. Int J Gynecol Pathol 2003; 22: 75–82
(92) Shah JP, Bryant CS, Kumar S, Ali-Fehmi R, Malone JM, Morris RT. Lymphadenectomy and ovarian preservation in low grade endometrial stromal sarcoma. Obstet Gynecol 2008; 112: 1102–1108
(93) Sharma P, Kumar R, Singh H, Jeph S, Sharma JB, Jain SK, Sharma DN, Bal C, Malhotra A. Role of FDG PET-CT in detecting recurrence in patients with uterine sarcoma: comparison with conventional imaging. Nucl Med Commun 2012; 33: 185–190
(94) Shi Y, Liu Z, Peng Z, Liu H, Yang K, Yao X. The diagnosis and treatment of Mullerian adenosarcoma of the uterus. Aust N Z J Obstet Gynaecol 2008; 48: 596–600
(95) Sobin LH, Gospadarowicz MK, Wittekind CH (eds.). TMN Classification of Malignant Tumours, 7th edn. John Wiley and Sons; 2009
(96) Sölder E, Huter O, Müller-Holzner E, Brezinka C. Adenofibroma and adenosarcoma of the uterus in young women. Geburtshilfe Frauenheilkd 1995; 55: 118–120
(97) Soslow RA, Ali A, Oliva E. Mullerian adenosarcomas: An immunophenotypic analysis of 35 cases. Am J Surg Pathol 2008; 32: 1013–1021

(98) Stadsvold JL, Molpus KL, Baker JJ, Michael K, Remmenga SW. Conservative management of a myxoid endometrial stromal sarcoma in a 16-year old nulliparous woman. Gynecol Oncol 2005; 99: 243–245

(99) Stern RC, Dash R, Bentley RC, Snyder MJ, Haney AF, Robboy SJ. Malignancy in endometriosis: frequency and comparison of ovarian and extraovarian types. Int J Gynecol Pathol 2001; 20: 133–399

(100) Stolnicu S, Balachandran K, Aleykutty MA, Loghin A, Preda O, Goez E, Nogales FF. Uterine adenosarcomas overgrown by sex-cord-like tumour: report of two cases. J Clin Pathol 2009; 62: 942–4. DOI: 10.1136/jcp.2008.063727

(101) Swisher EM, Gown AM, Skelly M, Ek M, Tamimi HK, Cain JM, Greer BE, Muntz HG, Goff BA. The expression of epidermal growth factor receptor, HER-2/Neu, p53, and Ki-67 antigen in uterine malignant mixed mesodermal tumors and adenosarcoma. Gynecol Oncol 1996; 60: 81–88

(102) Szklaruk J, Tamm EP, Choi H, Varavithya V. MR imaging of common and uncommon large pelvic masses. Radiographics 2003; 23: 403–424

(103) Taçkin S, Bozaci EA, Sönmezer M, Ekinci C, Ortaç F. Late recurrence of uterine Mullerian adenosarcoma as heterologous sarcoma: Three recurrences in 8 months increasing in number and grade of sarcomatous components. Gynecol Oncol 2006; 101: 179–182

(104) Taga S, Sawada M, Nagai A, Yamamoto D, Hayase R. A case of adenosarcoma of the uterus. Case Rep Obstet Gynecol 2014; Article ID 342187, 4 pages. DOI: 10.1155/2014/J42187

(105) Takeuchi M, Matsuzaki K, Yoshida S, Kudo E, Bando Y, Hasebe H, Kamada M, Nishitani H. Adenosarcoma of the uterus: magnetic resonance imaging characteristics. Clin Imaging 2009; 33: 244–247

(106) Tanner EJ, Toussaint T, Leitao MM Jr, Hensley ML, Soslow RA, Gardner GJ, Jewell EL. Management of uterine adenosarcomas with and without sarcomatous overgrowth. Gynecol Oncol 2013; 129: 140–144

(107) Tasaka N, Matsumoto K, Satoh T, Minaguchi T, Onuki M, Ochi H, Tanaka YO, Sakata A, Noguchi M, Yoshikawa H. Therapeutic effect of dienogest on adenosarcoma arising from endometriosis: A case report. Springerplus 2013; 2: 618

(108) Thomas MB, Keeney GL, Podratz KC, Dowdy SC. Endometrial stromal sarcoma: treatment and patterns of recurrence. Int J Gynecol Cancer 2009; 19: 253–256

(109) Tierney JF, Mosseri V, Steward LA, Souhami R, Parmar MK. Adjuvant chemotherapy of soft-tissue sarcoma: review and meta-analysis of the published results of randomised clinical trials. Br J Cancer 1995; 72: 469–475

(110) Tirumani SH, Ojili V, Shanbhogue AK, Fasih N, Ryan JG, Reinhold C. Current concepts in the imaging of uterine sarcoma. Abdom Imaging 2013; 38: 397–411

(111) Toyoshima M, Akahira J, Moriya T, Hayakawa S, Yaegashi N. Primary vaginal adenosarcoma with sarcomatous overgrowth. Gynecol Oncol 2004; 95: 759–761

(112) van Kruchten M, Hospers GA, Glaudemans AW, Hollema H, Arts HJ, Reyners AK. Positron emission tomography imaging of oestrogen receptor-expression in endometrial stromal sarcoma supports oestrogen receptor-targeted therapy: case report and review of the literature. Eur J Cancer 2013; 49: 3850–3855

(113) Verschraegen CF, Vasuratna A, Edwards C, Freedman R, Kudelka AP, Tornos C, Kavanagh JJ. Clinicopathologic analysis of mullerian adenosarcoma: the M.D. Anderson Cancer Center experience. Oncol Rep 1998; 5: 939–944

(114) Wang Y, Huang YW, Li YF. Primary vaginal sarcoma: Experience of a regional cancer center in China. J Obstet Gynaecol Res 2015; 41:1463–14688

(115) Yamagami W, Susumu N, Ninomiya T, Kuwahata M, Takigawa A, Nomura H, Kataoka F, Tominaga E, Banno K, Tsuda H, Aoki D. A retrospective study on combination therapy with

ifosfamide, adriamycin and cisplatin for progressive or recurrent uterine sarcoma. Mol Clin Oncol 2014; 2: 591–595.
(116) Yoshizako T, Wada A, Kitagaki H, Ishikawa N, Miyazaki K. MR imaging of uterine adenosarcoma: case report and literature review. Magn Reson Med Sci 2011; 10: 251–254
(117) Zaloudek CJ, Norris HJ. Adenofibroma and adenosarcoma of the uterus: A clinicopathologic study of 35 cases. Cancer 1981; 15: 354–366
(118) Zhao Z, Yoshida Y, Kurokawa T, Kiyono Y, Mori T, Okazawa H. 18F-FES and 18F-FDG PET for differential diagnosis and quantitative evaluation of mesenchymal uterine tumors: correlation with immunohistochemical analysis. J Nucl Med 2013; 54: 499–506

Image references

Batka M, Lederer A. Gynäkologie, Barmherzige Brüder Krankenhaus Salzburg, Salzburg (Österreich). Fig. 6.1.8 (A), (B)

Beyer P, Schwärzler P. Asklepios-Klinik Barmbeck, Gynäkologie und gynäkologische Onkologie, Hamburg. Fig. 6.1.8 (I)

Brüning R. Asklepios-Klinik Barmbeck, Abteilung für Radiologie und Neuroradiologie, Hamburg. Fig. 6.1.8 (G), (H)

Evert M, Evert K. Universitätsmedizin Greifswald, Institut für Pathologie, Greifswald. Figs. 6.1.1 (A), (B); 6.1.2 (A)–(C); 6.1.3 (A)–(F); 6.1.4 (A)–(D); 6.1.5; 6.1.9; 6.1.10 (A); 6.1.10 (C)

Hessler PA, Kuhfus S, Dennis K. Krankenhaus Sachsenhausen, operative Gynäkologie, Frankfurt/Main. Fig. 6.1.6 (B)

Hosten N, Hegenscheid K. Universitätsmedizin Greifswald, Institut für Diagnostische Radiologie und Neuroradiologie, Greifswald. Figs. 6.1.10 (B); 6.1.11 (B), (D)

Kaufmann L, Job H. Theresienkrankenhaus und St. Hedwigs-Klinik GmbH, Gynäkologie und Geburtshilfe, Mannheim. Fig. 6.2.2 (A), (B)

Köhler G, Zygmunt A. Universitätsmedizin Greifswald, Klinik Frauenheilkunde und Geburtshilfe, Greifswald. Figs. 6.1.11 (A), (C), (E); 6.2.1

Krentel H. St. Anna Hospital Herne, Klinik für Frauenheilkunde und Geburtshilfe, Herne. Fig. 6.1.6 (D)

Lederer A, Bakta M. Barmherzige Brüder Krankenhaus Salzburg, Abteilung Gynäkologie, Salzburg (Österreich). Fig. 6.1.8 (A), (B)

Münch M, Weiss E. Klinikverbund Südwest, Krankenhaus Böblingen Frauenklinik, Böblingen. Fig. 6.1.7 (A)

Owidh A, Konieczny M, Brum K. Mathilden Hospital Herford, Klinik für Frauenheilkunde u. Geburtshilfe, Herford. Fig. 6.1.7 (C), (D)

Ruhwedel W. St. Vinzenz-Hospital Köln, Klinik für Gynäkologie und Geburtshilfe, Köln. Fig. 6.1.6 (A)

Schaffler D. Abteilung Radiologie und Nuklearmedizin, Barmherzige Brüder Krankenhaus Salzburg, Salzburg (Österreich). Fig. 6.1.8 (C)–(F)

Stibora M. Marienhospital Gelsenkirchen, Klinik für Gynäkologie und Geburtshilfe, Gelsenkirchen. Figs. 6.1.6 (C); 6.1.7 (B)

Zeidler B. Pastor S. Asklepios Südpfalzklinik. Abt. Frauenheilkunde u. Geburtshilfe, Germersheim. Fig. 6.1.1 (C)

Günter Köhler, Katja Evert, Marek Zygmunt and Matthias Evert

7 Carcinosarcoma

Carcinosarcoma (CS) consists of a malignant epithelial (carcinomatous) and a malignant mesenchymal (sarcomatous) component and is thus classified as a malignant mixed tumor. CS are most commonly localized in the uterine corpus. Fewer than 3 % of uterine CS originate in the cervix (43). The ovaries are the most common extrauterine genital site. CS can occasionally also arise in the fallopian tube, and can sometimes occur in the region of the peritoneum of the pelvis or the abdominal cavity. Primary CS of the vagina virtually do not arise. On closer observation, the few CS that are found there are likely to be metastatic lesions (219).

Carcinosarcoma consists of a malignant epithelial (carcinomatous) and a malignant mesenchymal (sarcomatous) component and predominantly occurs in the uterus.

7.1 Uterine carcinosarcoma

7.1.1 General, epidemiology, etiology, pathogenesis, staging

Recent findings suggest that uterine CS (UCS) originating in the endometrium are largely highly malignant EC with sarcomatous dedifferentiation. From a clinical and prognostic perspective, the attributes of UCS, however, more closely correspond to those of sarcoma. Accordingly, the majority of publications and studies cover UCS in the context of sarcoma, and occasionally also in the context of high-risk EC. High-risk EC and UCS share numerous epidemiologic, prognostic, clinical and therapeutic commonalities. Due to its particular characteristics, however, UCS should be investigated in separate studies.

UCS account for fewer than 5 % of all uterine malignancies (224). Black women are said to be affected to a significantly greater degree than white women (142). More recent data from the USA, however, suggest that 71 % of patients are white women (201). The majority of UCS occur in postmenopausal women – 66 % of women are older than 60 and 58.7 % are older than 65. In 10 % of cases, UCS presents before the patient has reached 40 years of age. The age of the women in 329 DKSM consultation cases (128) ranged from 34–92 years (median 65, mean 63.3 years). Other studies have revealed median ages of 67 (201) and 72 years (206), respectively. Etiologically, analogous to EC, previous or ongoing tamoxifen exposure plays a non-negligible role (12, 68, 63, 236, 255). The same applies to LG-ESS, HG-ESS, UUS and LMS (cf. Vol. 1, Chapters 2, 4 and 5). Accordingly, following tamoxifen exposure, EC and uterine sarcomas can coincide (35), which can theoretically form the basis for UCS to develop through collision (see below). The median time interval between the onset of tamoxifen therapy and UCS is 120 (32–140) mo (127). In the etiologic context, a tamoxifen-induced modification of the p53 protein likely plays a role. UCS are sometimes associated with the risk factors pertaining to endometrioid adenocarcinoma, for example hypertension, adiposity and nulliparity (107). Other data suggest an association with prior nativities (68). Anamnesis occasionally reveals a history of prior pelvic RT (260). Endocrinic and radiogenic etiologies have, however, not yet been definitively substantiated.

In terms of formal pathogenesis, there are several theories. On the one hand, there is the less frequently observed "multifocal tumorigenesis" (8–15 % of cases) (215, 224, 264), which implies that CS develops biclonally from a separate carcinoma and a separate sarcoma, thus constituting a collision tumor (collision theory) (Fig. 7.1.1).

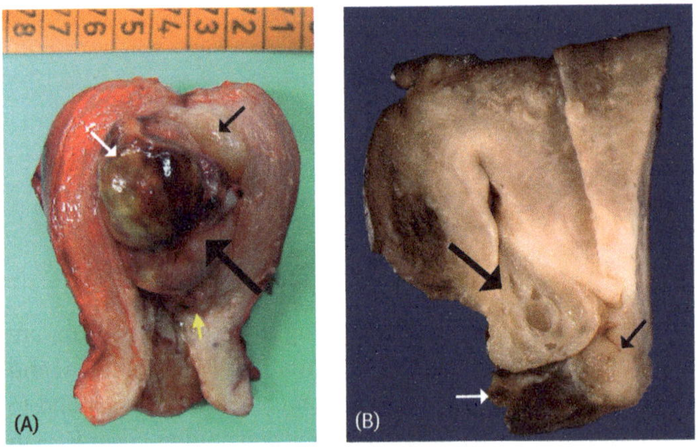

Fig. 7.1.1: Carcinosarcoma – identical case of a collision tumor. (A) carcinomatous (short yellow arrow) and sarcomatous (small white arrow) components forming a collision tumor (large black arrow), with an additional fibroglandular-cystic polyp of the corporal mucous membrane (small black arrow); (B) fixed specimen cut in another plane, fibroglandular-cystic polyp (large black arrow), carcinomatous (short black) and sarcomatous component (short white arrow).

Conversion theory, by contrast, implies that both tumor components originate monoclonally and unifocally from an EC (92). Both monoclonal and biclonal genesis theories have been verified via genetic testing (90, 112, 264). Monoclonal formation hypothesizes metaplastic transformation or transdifferentiation of the epithelial carcinoma cells into malignant mesenchymal cells. This process of "epithelial-mesenchymal transition" constitutes an important source for the genesis of mesenchymal cells in the context of embryologic development that later also occurs in malignant cells (114). This is supported by the fact that the metaplastically formed sarcomatous component expresses both epithelial (cytokeratins) and mesenchymal markers (vimentin). Interestingly, EC is among the few types of carcinoma that continuously express the intermediate filament protein vimentin, even when the tumor is well differentiated. In contrast, vimentin is barely present in the epithelial cells of most other carcinomas, and can thus be regarded as a factor suggestive of the presence of mesenchymal cells. Therefore, the joint expression of cytokeratin and vimentin in the epithelial cells can at least be regarded as an indirect indication of their metaplastic potential for sarcomatous transdifferentiation. The fact that both the sarcomatous and the carcinomatous component express identical genetic changes (e.g. p53 and KRAS mutations) serves to further substantiate conversion theory and the common origin that this theory implies (90, 92, 131, 120, 238). Loss of expression or functionality of epithelial cell marker and cell adhesion molecule E cadherin can be regarded as further signs for transdifferentiation (279). Furthermore, analogous to EC, the tumor suppressor gene PTEN (phosphatase and tensin homolog) is frequently mutated in UCS. In contrast, PTEN is rather rarely mutated in pure uterine sarcoma (6). Prognosis primarily depends on the epithelial factors (grading, histologic type). Moreover, both locoregional and distant metastases are purely carcinomatous or carcinosarcomatous in 94 % of cases, and are only rarely purely sarcomatous (231).

VEGF can be found in the epithelial tissue in up to 100 %, and in the mesenchymal tissue in up to 93 % of cases. In contrast to high-risk EC, VGEF-A-m-RNA expression has been shown to be significantly more frequent in UCS (67), with expression being particularly elevated in the epithelial component of the tumor. From a molecular-biological perspective, this distinguishes UCS from EC, their identical clonal origins notwithstanding. Recent genetic and molecular-biological studies have in fact associated UCS more closely with uterine sarcoma than with EC (38), which would also serve to better account for its clinical behavior and overall/general chemoresistance.

A combination of an AS and an EC is also possible (215). Recent data (195) pertaining to the pathogenesis of AS (see Chapter AS) serve to clarify that the development of a UCS from an AS is rather unlikely, but that such neoplasms can nonetheless coincide. However, it cannot be ruled out that a UCS can develop in or from an AS as a consequence of malignant transformation of its benign epithelial component. AS components have been found in 15 % of UCS (215, 224). Metastases and recurrences of AS occasionally present as CS (42, 128). The DKSM materials database also included cases in which a UCS developed from adenomyosis or adenomyoma.

A large SEER analysis covered a total of 128 cases of cervical UCS. Fewer than 65 cases of primary cervical UCS have been published (1, 20, 143, 158). Patients have a median age of 64 years (25–93) (20, 271). Only 8 % of cervical UCS are said to actually originate in the cervix (22). Cervical UCS normally stem from cervical adenocarcinoma, sometimes from squamous cell cervical carcinoma, in such cases. Pathogenetically, prior infection with the human papilloma virus (HPV) is often said to play a role (20, 218). The carcinomatous component is of mesonephric origin in 16 % of cases (143, 158). Mesonephric CS are considered not to be HPV induced (122).

New binding FIGO staging was introduced for UCS in 2009 (Tab. 7.1.1). This new staging is identical to that for endometrial carcinoma and takes the origination of UCS from EC into consideration (70, 227). In contrast to pure sarcoma, stage II UCS is limited to the uterus. Instances in which only the cervical glands (intraluminal growth into the cervix without invasion of the cervical stroma) are affected by the UCS are classified as stage I. The intraperitoneal cytological findings (see also prognosis) are not taken into consideration in staging, but should nonetheless be recorded separately. Likewise, since 2010, the UICC TNM staging system for UCS (Tab. 7.1.2) has corresponded to the classification for EC (227). Analogous to EC, staging is performed surgically and cannot be replaced by imaging.

Tab. 7.1.1: FIGO staging for uterine carcinosarcoma.

I	Involvement of corpus uteri and/or cervical glands
IA	Involvement of endometrium with no or less than half (< 50 %) myometrial invasion
IB	Invasion equal to or more than half (> 50 %) of the myometrium
II	Cervical stromal involvement
III	Local and/or regional pelvic spread (positive cytology to be assessed separately)
IIIA	Invasion of the serosa and/or the adnexa
IIIB	Vaginal and/or parametrial involvement
IIIC	Pelvic and/or para-aortic lymphadenopathy
$IIIC_1$	Positive pelvic lymph nodes
$IIIC_2$	Positive para-aortic lymph nodes with/without positive pelvic lymph nodes
IV	Involvement of organs and/or distant metastasis
IVA	Bladder and/or rectal mucosal involvement
IVB	Distant metastases incl. intraabdominal involvement and/or involvement of inguinal lymph nodes or intraabdominal lymph nodes other than pelvic/para-aortic nodes

Tab. 7.1.2: TNM classification for uterine carcinosarcoma according to the UICC.

T1	Involvement of corpus uteri and/or cervical glands
T1a	Involvement of endometrium with no or less than half (< 50 %) myometrial invasion
T1b	Invasion equal to or more than half (> 50 %) of the myometrium
T2	Cervical stromal involvement, no extrauterine involvement
T3	Local pelvic spread (positive cytology to be assessed separately)
T3a	Invasion of the serosa and/or the adnexa (direct spread or metastases)
T3b	Vaginal and/or parametrial involvement (direct spread or metastases)
N1	Metastases in pelvic and/or para-aortic lymph nodes
T4	Bladder and/or rectal mucosal involvement
M1	Distant metastases incl. intraabdominal involvement and/or involvement of inguinal lymph nodes or intraabdominal lymph nodes other than pelvic/para-aortic nodes

Uterine carcinosarcoma predominantly arises in postmenopausal women. Anamnesis often reveals previous exposure to tamoxifen. In terms of pathogenesis, dedifferentiation from an endometrial carcinoma predominates over collisions of pure sarcoma with endometrial carcinoma. Staging for carcinosarcoma corresponds to that for endometrial carcinoma.

7.1.2 Macroscopic and microscopic features

UCS have a polypoid, fleshy and usually very soft macroscopic appearance. Such tumors are noticeably sludgy decomposed, gray to reddish-gray exophytic masses with hemorrhages, necroses and cystic areas that are also clearly visible in sonography. In addition, hyaline tumor material as well as tumor tissue that appears to be relatively solid/hard can also be observed. The different sarcomatous and epithelial components can result in a particularly polymorphous appearance that bears great resemblance to G3-EC. On occasion, a UCS can also develop within an endometrial or cervical polyp. In terms of macroscopic and imaging features, UCS is predominantly observed as a tumor in the endometrial cavity. It exhibits a conspicuously fast rate of polypoid growth, often completely filling the cavity. From there, it visibly proceeds to infiltrate the entire myometrium. In collision tumors, the different sarcomatous and carcinomatous components can be recognizable to the naked eye (Fig. 7.1.1 (A), (B)). Once UCS have reached a certain size, they can protrude from the cervix into the vagina and be subsequently mistaken for (necrotic) endometrial or cervical polyps. Rapid growth all the way up to the vulva can occasionally result in an inversion of the uterus (97, 225) (Fig. 7.1.2 (A)–(F)).

The pressure emitted by the tumor's rapid growth is often so great that it can ooze or quickly protrude from the incision when the uterus is cut open. The tumor can also visibly penetrate/rupture through the myometrium (Fig. 7.1.3 (A), (B)).

Though a rather less common growth pattern, the tumor can sometimes completely invade the myometrium and rupture the serosa (Fig. 7.1.4 (A), (B)).

As with other uterine malignancies, tumor bleeding can result in hematometra.

Cervical CS has the same polypoid, hemorrhagic and necrotic macroscopic appearance as CS originating in the corpus uteri (137).

A UCS is classified as homologous when its sarcomatous component derives from uterine tissue. The mesenchymal component consists of HG-ESS or UUS in the majority of cases, followed by LG-ESS and (rarely) LMS. If the mesenchymal component consists of non-uterine tissue, the UCS is deemed heterologous. The heterologous component usually consists of chondrosarcoma (Fig. 7.1.5 (B), (C)), RMS (Figs. 7.1.2 (E), 7.1.5 (A)), or (very rarely) osteosarcoma.

LS and FS can also be found in rare cases. In the DKSM materials database, the heterologous component consists of chondrosarcoma, RMS and osteosarcomas in 51 %, 30 % and 7 % of cases, respectively. It can also occur that multiple sarcomatous components can be found within one tumor. Homologous UCS can also contain heterol-

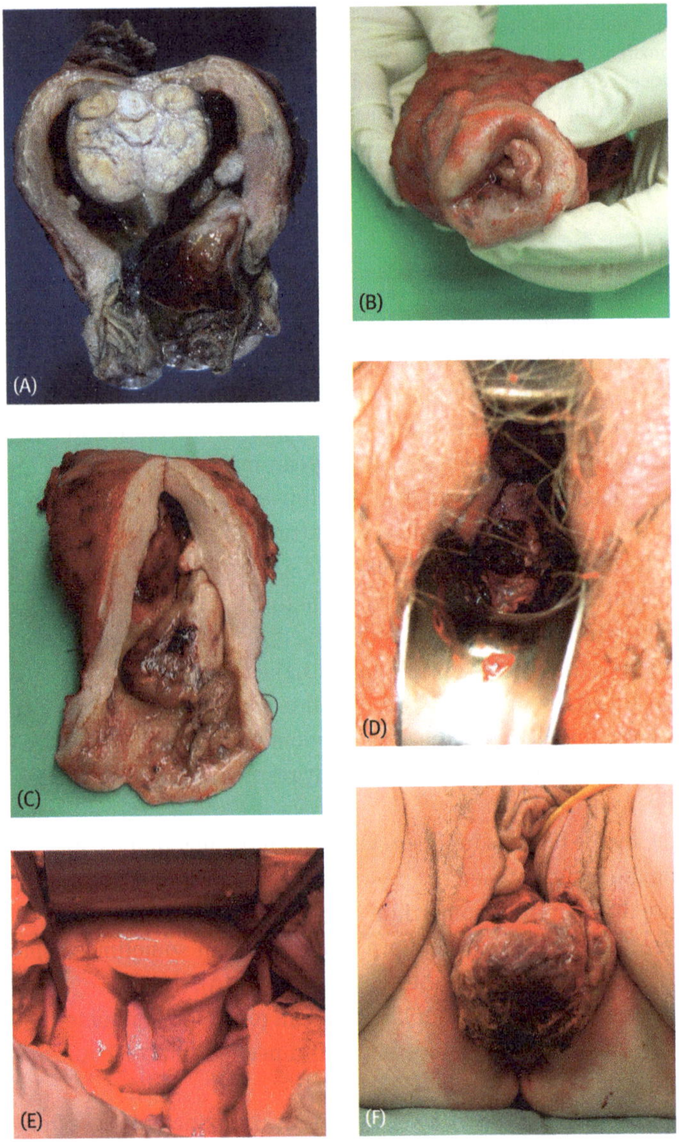

Fig. 7.1.2: Carcinosarcoma – macroscopic aspect. (A) polypoid carcinosarcoma in lower left segment of the uterus, along with common (despite suspicious gross appearance) leiomyoma in the fundus; (B), (C) identical intact and opened uterus with broad-based pedunculated carcinosarcoma; (D) carcinosarcoma with a macroscopic appearance resembling a necrotic cervical polyp; (E), (F) uterine inversion in a 79-year-old patient with a huge heterologous (in this case rhabdomyosarcoma) carcinosarcoma, (E) laparotomy findings showing the inverted uterine fundus; (F) corresponding tumor that has prolapsed from the vagina outside of the vulva.

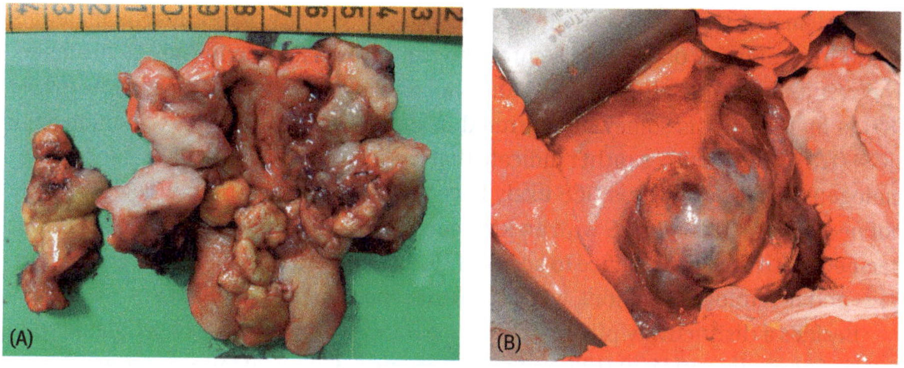

Fig. 7.1.3: Carcinosarcoma – macroscopic aspect. (A) the cut-open uterus stands agape, suggestive of substantial growth-induced mechanical pressure; distended cervix visible in lower part of the image; (B) penetration of the uterine wall with tumor extension into the Douglas.

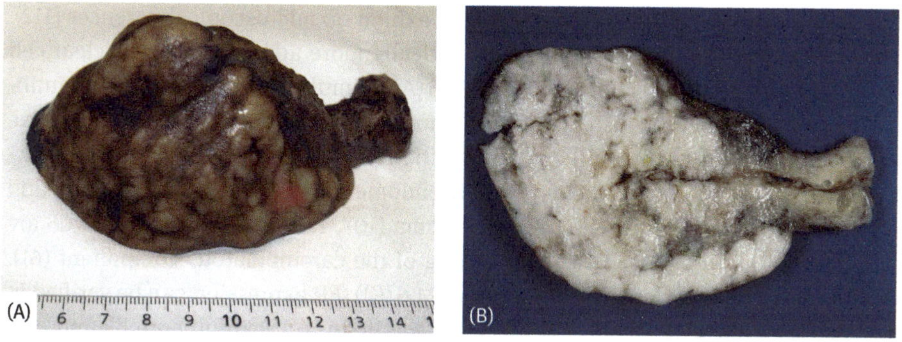

Fig. 7.1.4: Carcinosarcoma – macroscopic aspect. (A), (B) unopened and opened uterus, the tumor has invaded the entire myometrium; the uterine wall including the serosa has been ruptured.

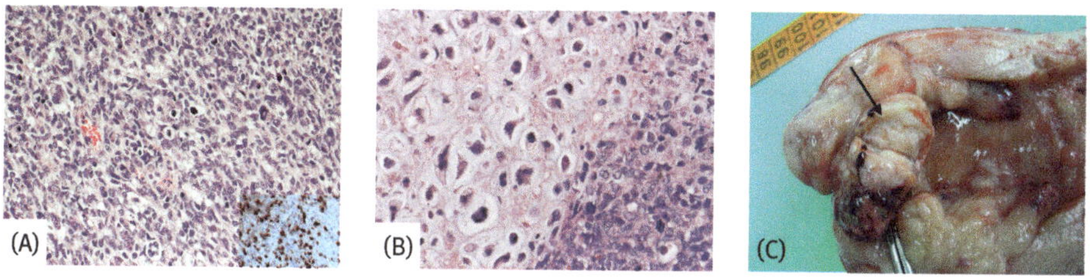

Fig. 7.1.5: Heterologous carcinosarcomas, microscopic and macroscopic aspects. (A) heterologous sarcoma component corresponding to pleomorphic rhabdomyosarcoma, inset at the lower right shows immunohistochemical staining with myogenin which is specific for rhabdomyosarcoma (identical with the case depicted in Fig. 7.1.2 (E)); (B) heterologous chondrosarcomatous component, a small residual of an undifferentiated stromal sarcoma component remains in the bottom right of the image; (C) identical case, the whitish-gray color (arrow) and the more solid cut surface are already grossly suggestive of a chondrosarcoma component.

ogous elements that can be easily overlooked. Accordingly, heterologous materials found in specimens obtained via curettage can be untraceable in the HE specimen. The results from one study suggest that homologous UCS is more common (69 %) (89), a finding that is somewhat mirrored in the DKSM materials (65 % homologous UCS) (128). Other sources rather indicate that the distribution is largely balanced. Homologous and heterologous UCS likely have an identical prognosis, though this may not necessarily apply to UCS with an RMS component (see prognosis). From a clinical perspective, it may thus suffice to speak of UCS and to differentiate between homologous and heterologous tumors, without further specification (182, 224).

Besides a distinctively pleomorphic appearance, a high degree of cellular atypia, an MI of normally > 10 M/10 HPF, and the occurrence of atypical mitoses are key microscopic characteristics for all CS. Myometrial invasion, LVI and VI can be observed in most cases. The epithelial component of UCS can be either endometrioid carcinoma of different grading and squamous partial differentiation, or mucinous, adenosquamous, papillary-serous, parvocellular, clear cell, squamous cell and undifferentiated carcinoma. Monoclonal and biclonal tumors exhibit no microscopic differences (112). G3 endometrioid EC as well as the prognostically more adverse serous or clear cell carcinomas are frequently observed (Fig. 7.1.6 (A)). Simultaneous occurrence of multiple epithelial elements is also possible and not uncommon. Further aberrations have also been observed in the epithelial differentiation (e.g. embryonal glandular structures). The carcinoma component is purely endometrioid in up to 50 % of cases, and occasionally takes the form of G1/G2 carcinoma (107, 120). Nonetheless, all UCS are classified as G3, independent of the grading of the carcinomatous component (61). UCS can also express steroid receptors (Fig. 7.1.6 (C)). ER expression can be verified in up to 44 % of cases, up to 19 % express PGR, and up to 24 % exhibit both ER and PGR expression (108, 265). Hardly any usable and reliable data are available that pertain to receptor distribution in and among both tumor components. Menopausal status and whether the sarcoma is heterologous or homologous apparently have no influence on receptor expression (265).

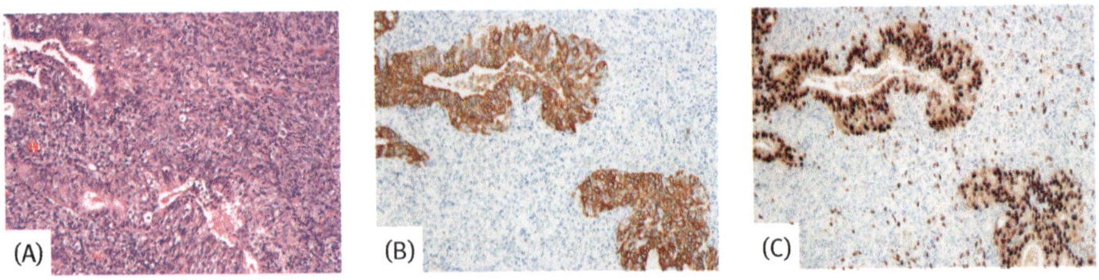

Fig. 7.1.6: Carcinosarcoma – microscopic aspect. (A) "standard" histology with malignant endometrial glands and malignant stroma in the style of an undifferentiated (homologous) uterine sarcoma; (B) cytokeratin immunohistochemistry serves to nicely visualize the glands; (C) only the carcinoma cells and benign stromal cells are estrogen receptor positive, while the sarcomatous cells are not.

Both the carcinomatous and the sarcomatous component can be predominant with UCS (188), with a ratio of 59 % to 41 % (120). The carcinomatous component can account for less than 1 % of total tumor volume. Accordingly, the presence of carcinomatous cells in specimens obtained via curettage or HE can result in a misdiagnosis as pure uterine sarcoma (see DD). Whether sarcomatous overgrowth is prognostically relevant (analogous to AS, see Chapter 6) remains unclear. It could, however, imply poorer responsivity to CHT (188). The morphologic and immunohistochemical transformation of the carcinoma glands into sarcoma cells (see conversion theory) can sometimes be nicely visible under the microscope.

IHC findings have shown that the sarcomatous component is strongly positive for vimentin in 100 % of cases, and focally positive for CK7 in 36 %. The epithelial component has expressed a strong reaction to CK7 in 100 % of cases, and a weak reaction to CK20, vimentin and CA-125 (Figs. 7.1.6 (B), 7.1.7 (B), (C)) (131). Some pure sarcomas can contain a rudimentary degree of cytokeratin expression, which serves as a possible indicator for an epithelial origin. CD10, by contrast, is only expressed in the stromal component (Fig. 7.1.7 (D)).

EGFR expression in the epithelial and mesenchymal components has been measured at 13–30 % and 45–67 %, respectively (24, 41), and at up to 71 % in whole tumors without discernment between the two components (23). Available data on Her-2/neu

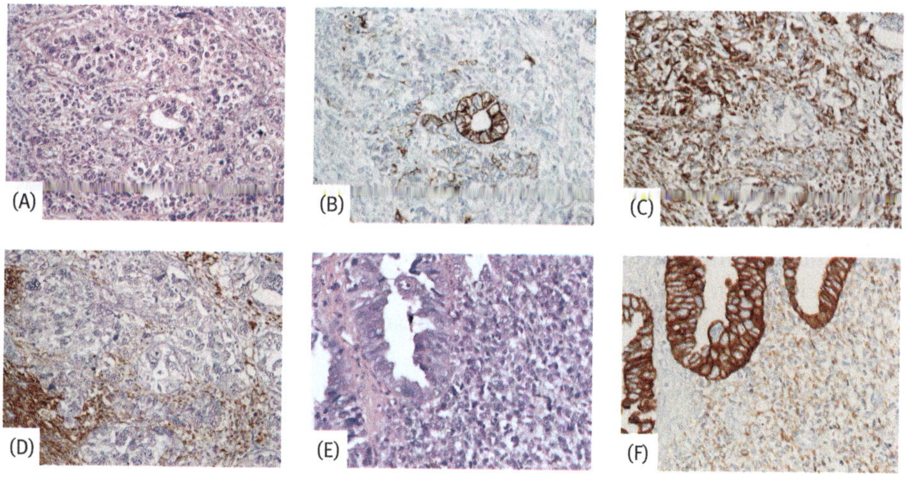

Fig. 7.1.7: In collision tumors, intermingling of the two components can often be observed, as can the morphologic and immunohistochemical transformation of carcinoma glands into sarcoma cells in some instances; (A) well-differentiated and poorly differentiated carcinoma glands that gradually pass over into the sarcomatous components, a picture strongly mirrored in immunohistochemistry, (B) cytokeratins: epithelium > stroma; (C) vimentin: epithelium < stroma; (D) CD10: only stroma; (E) rudimentary, usually only focal cytokeratin expression often remains in the sarcomatous components (carcinoma left, sarcoma right); (F) serial section of (E) with corresponding cytokeratin expression [antibody clone MNF116].

▸ Fig. 7.1.8: Carcinosarcoma – collision tumor. (A) digital specimen scan of the collision tumor presented in Fig. 7.1.1 (A), (B) that, besides the corporal polyp revealed in macroscopy, in fact consisted of three histologically different malignant components. The right part (double arrow) corresponded to the sarcoma (high-grade endometrial stromal sarcoma) that had already been partly removed via curettage, while the left part (arrow) was grade 1 endometrioid adenosarcoma. In the middle (arrow head), a very rare uterine small cell (neuroendocrine) carcinoma that is clearly delineated from the other two components; (B) adenocarcinomatous component under strong magnification; (C) sarcomatous component; (D)–(F) the small cell carcinoma from (A); (E) as is typical for such neoplasms, cytokeratins [antibody clone AE1/3] visualize as dots, which serves to reflect the epithelial origin of the tumor; (F) neuroendocrine differentiation [synaptophysin]). Despite the similarities in the results from (H) and (E) staining for the sarcoma (C) and the small cell carcinoma (D), histologic analysis revealed that these two components were clearly topographically delineated from each other, which in turn makes it seem possible that the two components each had an independent pathogenesis (collision tumor). (G) and (H) show the sharp, clear borders without fluent or gradual transitions between the sarcomatous component (top right) and the synaptophysin positive, neuroendocrine carcinomatous component (bottom left).

overexpression are rather contradictory. Studies have reported rates of Her-2/neu overexpression ranging from 0 to 56 to 100 % in the epithelial component, and from 6 to 83 % in the sarcomatous component. Generally, overexpression is greater in the epithelial component (8, 172, 213, 278).

Tissue specimens obtained via curettage can contain both carcinomatous and sarcomatous elements, while individual tissue samples collected via biopsies can contain only sarcomatous or only carcinomatous materials. Such findings are to be deemed suggestive of a collision tumor if more or less independent or separate carcinomatous and sarcomatous components can be found in the specimen yielded from HE as well. The surface of the area in which the two components of collision tumors are intermingled or mixed with each other need only be very small (231). It is not uncommon for only carcinoma or only sarcoma to be traceable in the surgical tissue specimen. Regardless, the diagnosis of UCS reached on the basis of curettage must be maintained (Figs. 7.1.1 (A), (B), 7.1.8 (A)–(H)).

Since the majority of UCS are dedifferentiated highly malignant EC, and thus constitute conversion-type tumors, up to 94 % of the corresponding metastases are either carcinomatous or a mix of carcinomatous and carcinosarcomatous, though purely carcinomatous metastases prevail (70 %). In the majority of cases, the pattern of metastasization corresponds to the characteristics and features of the respective tumor components. Analogous to EC, the carcinoma component lymphogenically metastasizes to the LN, the ovaries and the vagina. Accordingly, LN metastases are almost exclusively of epithelial origin (231). Analogous to serous EC, metastatic involvement of the omentum and the abdominal cavity are very common when the carcinomatous component is serous. Purely sarcomatous metastases develop hematogeneously and are thus predominantly found in the lungs and occasionally in the abdominal cavity.

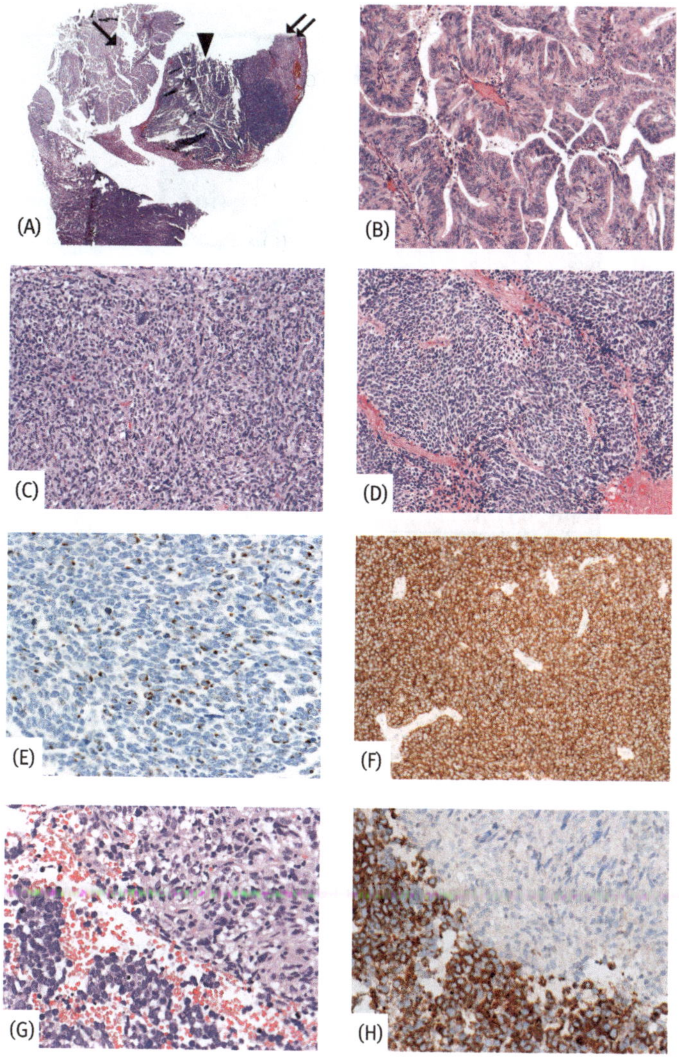

With the rarer collision tumors, both tumor components can invade the myometrium independently of each other and thus generate histologically different metastases. Generally, therefore, findings from microscopic examination of the metastases do not necessarily allow for the primary tumor to be definitively deduced (cf. DD) (Fig. 7.1.9 (A)–(I)).

Microscopically, the carcinomatous element of cervical UCS can be poorly differentiated squamous epithelial carcinoma, adenocarcinoma or undifferentiated carcinoma (158). In some instances elements of both squamous epithelial carcinoma and adenocarcinoma can be present simultaneously (143). In 16 % of cases, adenocarcinomas originate from mesonephric rests. Cervical UCS can equally occur as homolo-

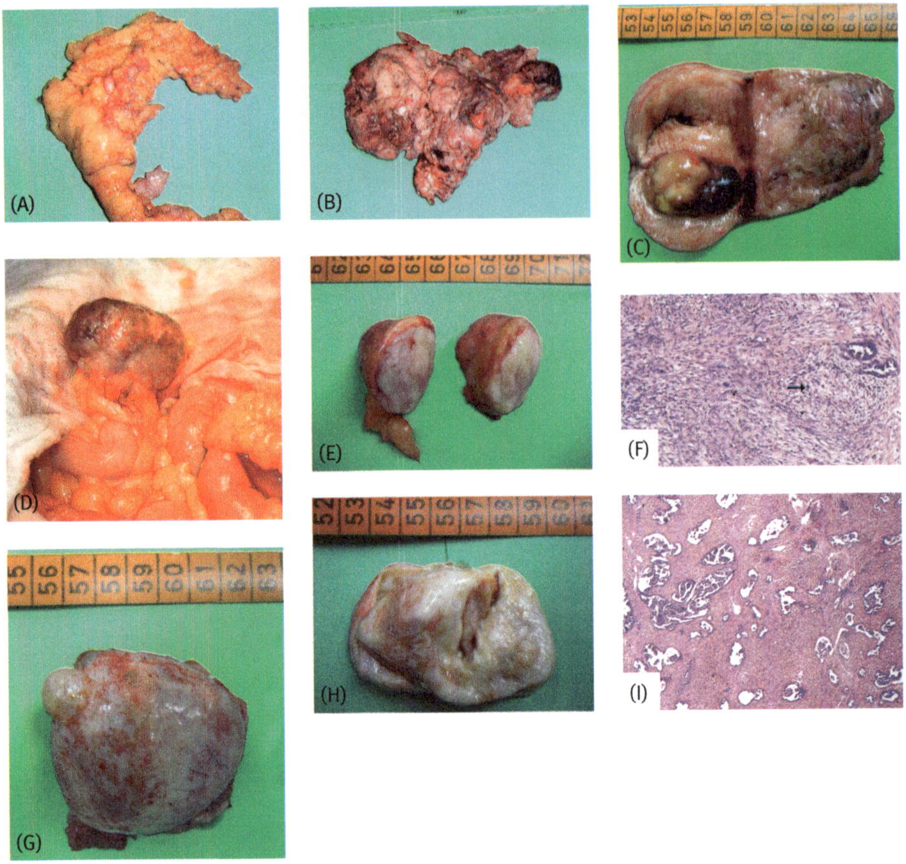

Fig. 7.1.9: (A), (B) in this case of carcinosarcoma (primary tumor see Fig. 7.1.2 (B)), the omental (A) und adnexal (B) metastases were purely carcinomatous; (C) primary collision tumor consisting of a high-grade papillary-serous carcinoma and a high-grade endometrial stromal sarcoma with distinct separate metastasization. Draining the hematocervix has left the cervix considerably dilated; (D)–(F) intact and opened mesenteric metastatic lesion that is predominantly sarcomatous, the arrow points to a mitosis of a sarcoma cell; (G)–(I) intact and opened ovarian metastatic mass that was revealed to be pure carcinoma via histologic analysis.

gous and heterologous tumors. Spindle cell sarcoma, chondrosarcoma, osteosarcoma and RMS have all been encountered as sarcomatous elements of CS originating in the cervix and the mesonephron (271).

Carcinosarcoma can generally not be discerned from G3 endometrial carcinoma on the basis of gross appearance alone. Carcinosarcomas are characterized as decomposing necrotic tumors exhibiting very rapid growth with a primarily central localization in the uterine cavity.

The epithelial component of carcinosarcoma usually consists of G3 type I or type II endometrial carcinoma. The sarcomatous component can be either homologous or heterologous (non-uterine tissue) sarcoma. Carcinosarcomas are characterized by a distinct degree of pleomorphism, a mitotic index of usually >10 mitoses/10 HPF and the presence of atypical mitoses. Myometrial, lymphatic and vascular invasions are usually present. Locoregional metastatic disease usually takes the form of carcinoma, while distant metastases are usually sarcomatous. Epithelial mesenchymal markers can always be immunohistochemically verified. Hormone receptors are positive only in rare cases.

7.1.3 Clinical presentation, diagnostics, screening

Postmenopausal bleeding or premenopausal AUB are the cardinal symptoms of UCS, sometimes in connection with lower abdominal pains. The uterus is often enlarged or dilated due to the rapid growth of the CS or due to hematometra/hematocervix (Fig. 7.1.9 (C)). An enlarged, relatively soft uterus can be the only finding. Overall, any uterus exhibiting postmenopausal growth should be considered suspicious for a malignant mesenchymal tumor. Like for pure uterine sarcomas, polypoid tumor masses protruding from the cervix, and occasionally from the vulva, are also characteristically suggestive of UCS. Very large UCS and LMS can even effect an inversion of the uterus (47, 97) (Fig. 7.1.2 (E), (F)). The urinary bladder is often unable to adapt to the rapid growth of the uterus, so that an otherwise unexplainable mictional urge can be among the symptoms. The dilatation of the cervix is a constitutive cause for the lower abdominal pains (Fig. 7.1.10)

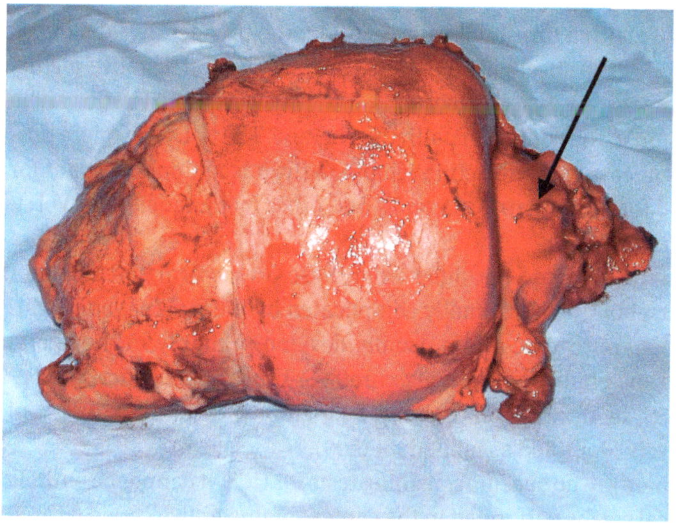

Fig. 7.1.10: Carcinosarcoma with maximally enlarged cervix, corpus (arrow), and both adnexa. The corpus has been massively suppressed by, and is consequently considerably smaller than the cervix, and generates the impression that it is merely superimposed.

Cervical UCS usually present as tumors in the cervical wall (271), with symptomatology that corresponds to that of cervical carcinoma. The principal symptom is AUB.

Speculum examination, rectovaginal palpation and TVS or TAS are followed by HSC with biopsy or fractional curettage. Where sonographic findings suggest a high probability for a UCS, it appears to be safer to dispense with the HSC (see prognosis). The dissemination of tumor cells that occurs in the course of said procedure may well be more relevant for UCS than it is for EC. In cases of tumors protruding from the cervix, a sufficiently large amount of tissue should be taken via biopsy. If not, it can occur that only the epithelial or the stromal component of the tumor can be microscopically detected. Due to the exceptionally high rate at which UCS grow, it is not rare that only necroses can be found in the samples gathered via biopsy or curettage. Due to the rapid rate of hematogeneous metastasization, up to 50 % of cases already present with distant metastasis at the time of initial diagnosis (4, 64). Consequently, the diagnosis is not seldom formed primarily on the basis of the distant metastases, predominantly those observed in the lungs.

Due to the advanced stage at which UCS are often initially diagnosed, contrary to common EC, imaging-based staging of pelvis, abdomen and thorax using CT and/or MRI are indicated in order to plan reasonable and adequate treatment strategies.

CA-125 levels are elevated in many UCS, and continue to rise as tumor growth progresses (103, 105). Elevated CA-125 levels can frequently be observed at the time of initial diagnosis and are for the most part an expression for an advanced stage of disease (105). The preoperative CA-125 levels have a sensitivity of 52.3 % and a specificity of 50.5 % at a cut-off value of ≥ 27.5 U/ml. UCS and pure uterine sarcoma can also exhibit elevated N/L ratios. With a threshold value of ≥ 2.12, the preoperative diagnosis has a sensitivity of 74.5 % and a specificity of 70.3 %. The positive and negative predictive values are 29.5 % and 94.3 %, respectively (125). CA-125 levels and N/L ratio can be used to monitor remission in the context of palliative therapy. The N/L ratio might possibly be an appropriate measure for detecting relapse early. It is not only relevant for CS specifically, but also for pure uterine sarcomas and other malignancies (cf. Vol. 1, Chapter 6).

Diagnostics for cervical UCS do not differ from those for cervical carcinoma or CS of the uterine corpus, but are occasionally complicated by the fact that adenocarcinoma and CS of mesonephrogenic origin usually develop primarily in the lateral cervical wall and can thus elude detection via curettage-based diagnostics. In contrast to LMS and LG-ESS, by drawing on cytology, sonography, CT and MRI, 94 % of UCS can be preoperatively identified as malignant (209).

Analogous to EC, there are no specific screening tests for UCS. It cannot be entirely ruled out that cytological swabs performed in the context of preventive cervical carcinoma screenings might yield endometrial or mesenchymal tumor cells, the presence of which will require further clarification. UCS show positive cytological results from swabs of the endometrial cavity in about 65 % of cases (209). Sarcomatous cells have been found in about 50 % of cases (109). The pertinence of performing transvaginal sonography on high-risk patients, for example those with prior or ongoing tamoxifen therapy, is disputed. For asymptomatic women with a fitting medical history and conspicuous sonographic findings, it could be expedient to perform an endometrial biopsy using the Pipelle device. The positive likelihood ratio for endometrial carcinoma, however, lies at roughly 65 % (257).

The sensitivities and specificities for CA-125 and the N/L ratio (see symptoms and findings) apply to all sarcomas and EC and are thus inadequate for use in targeted/specific UCS screenings.

Cytological screening can incidentally reveal cervical UCS. However, such findings are most likely to be understood as signs of adenocarcinoma or squamous cell carcinoma, if they are not simultaneously accompanied by malignant mesenchymal cells. In one study, cytological swabs taken from patients with sarcomatoid carcinoma only contained carcinoma cells (29).

Postmenopausal bleeding or additional/irregular bleeding in premenopausal women are the cardinal symptoms of carcinosarcoma. The uterus is usually significantly enlarged, and the tumor often protrudes from the cervix. Speculum examination, rectovaginal palpation, and sonography followed by hysteroscopy with biopsy or fractional curettage represent the most important diagnostic measures. CA-125 values and the neutrophil-lymphocyte ratio are often elevated. The fact that carcinosarcomas have frequently already spread beyond the uterus at primary diagnosis makes comprehensive imaging-based diagnostics imperative. Analogous to EC, there is no particular screening for UCS.

7.1.4 Imaging

An important factor that helps to distinguish UCS from pure sarcoma is that the former develops centrally in the region of the endometrium, and not within the myometrium. For all imaging methods, the presence of a large, broad-based lesion within the uterus, accompanied by (usually) visible myometrial invasion, is regarded as the most significant feature suggestive of UCS, but also of AS (cf. Chapter 6).

Analogous to the clinical presentation of UCS, an unusually enlarged uterus is also at the center of attention in the majority of cases from a sonographic perspective. Because UCS originate in the endometrium, a central localization in the endometrium in close proximity to the cavum is typical in sonography in the early stages of disease. Early tumor growth is often only represented by a homogeneous echogenic thickening of the endometrium. In correspondence to its genesis from an EC, young UCS is predominantly hyperechoic. In most cases, within a short period of time, the cavity is filled by a tumor that is at first primarily hyperechoic to the myometrium, and that has a recognizably papillary surface. Unlike polyps, the connection to the myometrium is almost always broad-based. The mean largest dimension of the intracavitary tumors has been measured at between 5.4 and 8.5 cm (246). UCS can also exhibit rapid infiltrative growth into the myometrium and ultimately fill the entire uterus, thus exhausting the whole myometrium. Accordingly, most tumors cannot be easily or reliably demarcated from the myometrium (135). In such cases the architecture of the uterus is lost both clinically and in imaging, so that neither the endometrium nor the myometrium can be clearly discerned.

As tumor growth progresses, the echotexture becomes increasingly heterogeneous, as the presence of hyperechoic and hypoechoic to anechoic areas increases. Examination of surgical tissue specimens generally reveals the poorly circumscribed hypoechoic to anechoic areas with irregular margins to be necroses and/or hemorrhages (135). Ultimately, what results is a bizarre heterogeneous sonographic texture with irregularly distributed hyperechoic and anechoic areas. According to a larger study, these tumors are predominantly isoechoic or hypoechoic compared to the endometrium (135). However, this difference can no longer be discerned when the CS has infiltrated or exhausted the endometrium entirely. Microscopic examinations suggest that the hypoechoic areas are attributable to the sarcomatous component, while the hyperechoic areas are attributable to the glandular epithelial elements (Fig. 7.1.11) (135). The anechoic clefts and fissures or small cysts represent dilated glands (135), but also vessels in some cases. Doppler sonography can provide easy clarification in this regard. In polypoid tumors protruding into the cavum, Doppler sonography clearly shows a larger nutritive vessel.

In most cases, the tumor exhibits expansive irregular vascularity in the solid components. RI ranges from 0.25–0.57 (65, 135, 242) with a mean of 0.41 (17, 135). It is the hypoechoic sarcomatous elements in particular that express a prominent degree of vascularity. Generally, whether anechoic clefts/fissures or small cysts are in fact vessels or dilated glands can usually be accurately verified in Doppler sonography. They usually have a narrow hyperechoic margin in gray-scale sonography. Overall, CS has a strikingly ostentatious appearance in sonography (31, 65, 135, 242, 246) (Tab. 7.1.3) and thus results in the correct diagnosis in 73 % of cases (Fig. 7.1.12 (A)–(D)).

The sonographic appearance is similar to that of high-risk EC and of AS originating in the endometrium. Endometrioid EC only rarely reach the metric dimensions of UCS and exhibit a central, predominantly hyperechoic structure compared to the latter.

Without exception, the dilatation of the endocervical canal by the tumor masses can be successfully visualized via imaging technologies. However, at the same time, such dilatation is also typical for pure uterine sarcomas and AS. Combining sonography with CA-125 analysis, particularly in more advanced stages of disease, can help to distinguish CS from pure sarcoma, but does not allow a reliable differentiation from advanced EC in particular.

CT is not an adequate measure for diagnosing particular neoplastic entities, and is instead used in the context of extrapelvic staging in particular.

Almost without exception, CT reveals an intracavitary, occasionally ill-defined mass (246). Analogous to the findings from sonography, CT reveals a dilatation of the cavum uteri caused by a usually broad-based lesion. The myometrium is often

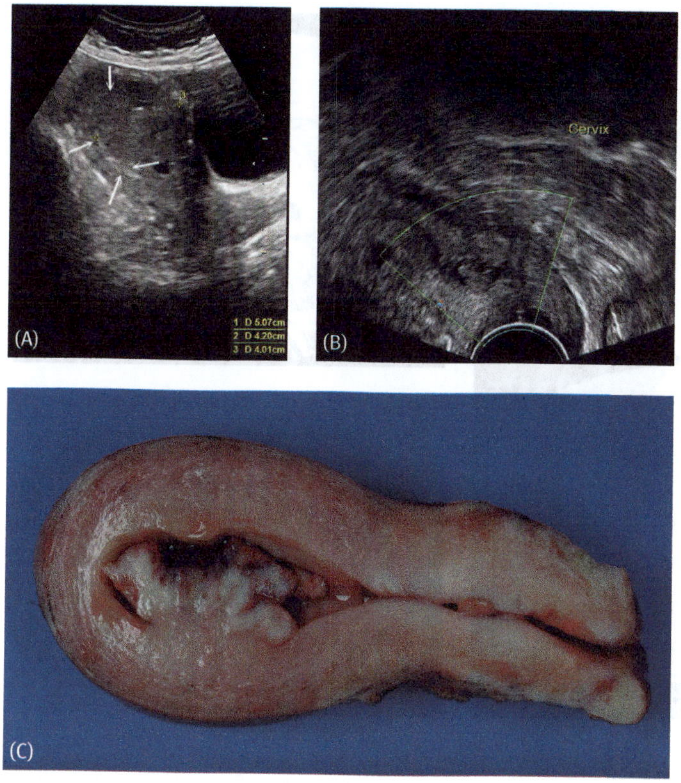

Fig. 7.1.11: Sonographic appearance of carcinosarcoma; (A) this carcinosarcoma is almost entirely confined to the cavum. Its posterior, lateral and anterior walls (transabdominal sonography) are surrounded by a margin that is clearly hyperechoic compared to the tumor and that corresponds to the endometrium (arrows). Endometrial hyperplasia already described in corresponding histologic analysis can be seen on the posterior wall (face to face arrows). The tumor transitions into the myometrium immediately beside said hyperplasia. The tumor itself is characterized by an unobtrusive heterogeneous echogenicity that is hypoechoic to the myometrium, a finding that serves to differentiate carcinosarcoma from endometrioid carcinoma, which itself is usually hyperechoic. The visible hypoechoicity is said to stem from the sarcomatous component and to be suggestive of a more advanced tumor; (B) the heterogeneous echogenicity of the tumor with bizarre, interrupted margins between the areas of differing echoicity are even easier to recognize in color Doppler sonography. Perfusion appears to be low and did not constitute a particularly significant factor in this case. The anechoic voids most likely correspond to necroses, that in fact rendered the tumor at hand a very soft specimen; (C) the specimen depicted here clearly mirrors the features described under (A). The tumor is located and has spread in the cavum. The cavum is visibly lined with the endometrium, which also appears to be thickened at the point at which it clearly infiltrates the myometrium.

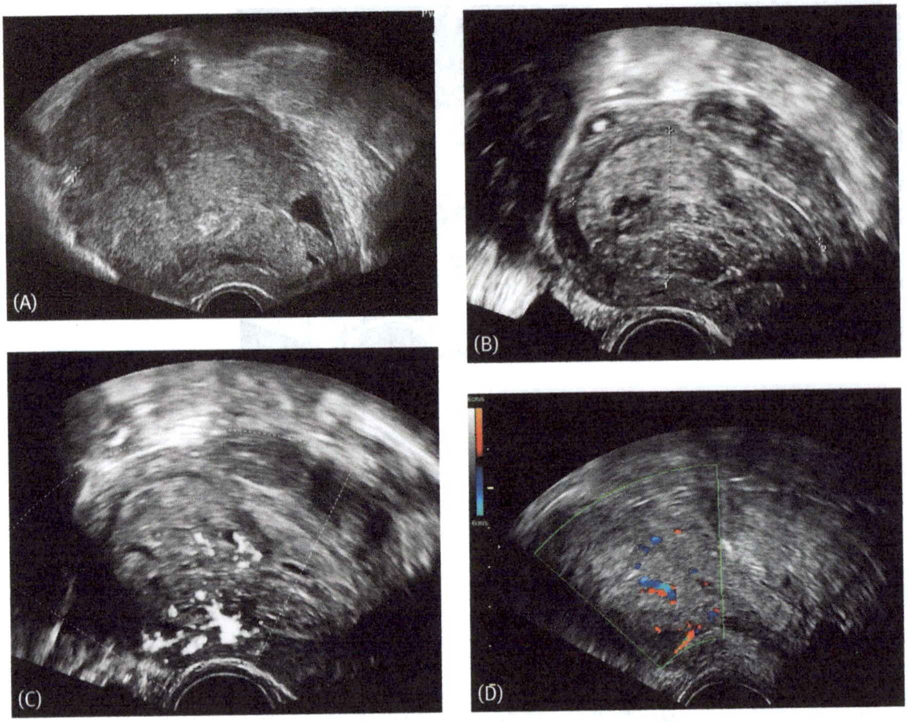

Fig. 7.1.12: Carcinosarcoma in sonography; (A) carcinosarcoma that has already metastasized into the abdominal cavity and the lungs, the endometrium has been entirely infiltrated/exhausted, observing the surgical specimen revealed that the tumor had widely ruptured the serosa in numerous locations; (B) a different tumor that completely fills the cavum and which infiltrates the myometrium at the lower anterior wall of the uterus; the carcinosarcoma is predominantly hyperechoic to normal myometrium, the anechoic clefts/voids correspond to vessels or necroses; (C) the aforementioned well-vascularized infiltration into the myometrium can be easily discerned in Doppler sonography, the anechoic voids correspond to numerous vascular lumina; (D) in a further case, the predominantly hyperechoic tumor exhibits irregular central vascularization, the infiltrative/pushing margins to the myometrium are ill-defined.

Tab. 7.1.3: Sonographic features of uterine carcinosarcoma.

Early stages	Centrally localized tumor with unclear margins that is hypoechoic to endometrium and hyperechoic to myometrium
Advanced stages	Heterogeneous echogenic centrifugally spread tumor with expansive hyperechoic sections, hypo- and anechoic areas and clefts with in part unclear margins, margins to myometrium often irregular or unclear
Doppler sonography	Irregularly distributed vascularity within the tumor, RI mostly < 0.4

compressed to a narrow band or strip. UCS appear hypodense to myometrium. Some few UCS have been shown to contain areas of hyperdensity that did not, however, constitute 50 % of the respective mass. With the exception of smaller lesions, the majority of UCS appears heterogeneous (246). CECT usually shows a heterogeneous enhancement that is, however, weaker than the enhancement of the myometrium (Fig. 7.1.13).

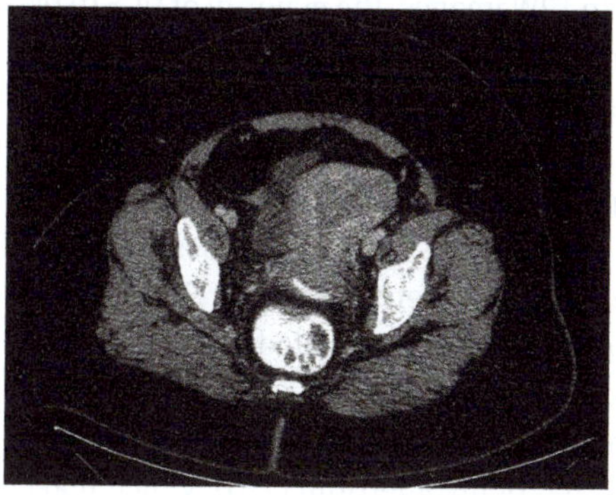

Fig. 7.1.13: Carcinosarcoma in axial CECT exhibiting heterogeneous enhancement that is significantly weaker than that of normal myometrium, and which reveals an infiltration in the left anterior wall that almost reaches up to the serosa.

The hypodense necroses that are so frequently observed show no enhancement in CECT (184).

Overall, the CT features of UCS are very unspecific – LMS can generate a largely identical image. However, the latter is primarily localized within the myometrium. In one analysis pertaining to diagnostics and UCS, CT yielded ambiguous or suspicious findings in 72 % of cases, however further specification was not possible (209).

MRI is the imaging method of choice for precisely diagnosing local disease spread, and should always be applied instead of CT in cases in which sonography yields suspicious results. In MR images, too, the primarily central localization of UCS in the region of the endometrium or the uterine cavity is an important criterion for distinguishing UCS from pure uterine sarcomas, from LMS and LG-ESS in particular (cf. Vol. 1, Chapters 2 and 4). Tumors that appear to be cervical in CT or MR imaging should be closely examined as to the presence of a pedunculated, stem-like connection to the cavum (broccoli-sign). A positive finding in this regard would corroborate the suspected diagnosis of a prolapsed UCS (111). Regarding metric tumor size or the degree of cavitary dilatation caused by the UCS, the statements made in the context of sonography and CT also apply to MRI. In fact, in one study, dilatation of the endometrial cavity, defined as a dilatation of more than 5 mm in the sagittal plane (151), was observed in 98 % of cases and was thus the most consistent finding (22). One factor that strongly alludes to UCS is when the diameter of the tumor within the cavity of the uterus is distinctly larger. The ratio of tumor thickness to maximum anteroposterior diameter of the uterus can be decisive for discerning between EC and CS. Where the ratio is higher than 0.63, forming a diagnosis of UCS should be considered (84). Tumors that fill the entire cavum uteri typically have a broad-based connection to the myometrium. The tumor epicenter is in the endometrium in 88 % of cases, in the myometrium in 4 % of cases and in the cervix in the remaining 8 % (22).

On T1W images, UCS appear isointense to both myometrium and endometrium in approx. 75 % of cases. SI is heterogeneous in one third of cases, sometimes with hyperintense areas or foci. The latter are usually hemorrhages. There have also been accounts in which a homogeneously low SI has been described (220). Hemorrhages appear as pouches or regions with strong SI. In T2W images, the majority of UCS (92 %) appear heterogeneous and hyperintense compared to normal myometrium (Fig. 7.1.14). Fifty-five percent of UCS are hypointense to endometrium, and 43 % appear isointense (22). The share with low SI can sometimes predominate (240). As tumor size increases, so too does heterogeneity in T2W images, in particular due to the increased presence of areas with higher SI that usually constitute hemorrhages and/or necroses. Generally, hemorrhages, necroses and cystic structures are characterized by high SI in T2W images. It is not uncommon for larger tumors to exhibit large fluid-filled or cystic sections with high SI (220). Necroses are the exception in early UCS.

While sometimes homogeneous, SI is heterogeneous in T1WC images in the majority of cases, and is generally weaker than that of myometrium (220), which makes myometrial invasion easier to recognize. Hemorrhages, necroses or cystic regions usually show no enhancement and remain hypointense. To date, there is no evidence to suggest that heterologous and homologous UCS differ in terms of their MRI characteristics.

In diffusion weighted MR images, the complex tissue structure of UCS, with its necroses and different histologic components, is demonstrated by strongly heterogeneous SI. Accordingly, it has been recommended that diffusion weighted imaging methods be incorporated into routine MRI diagnostics for uterine neoplasms (118). However, such methods are only rarely applied in clinical practice pertaining to gynecologic malignancies due to a lack of standardization, substantial overlap between benign and malignant tumors, and poor image quality (251).

In 88 % of cases, UCS exhibit the same MRI characteristics as EC (220). Consequently, the latter constitute the most important imaging-based differential diagnosis. Virtually all UCS exhibit early focal or diffuse sustained/delayed enhancement that is stronger or identical to that of the myometrium (Fig. 7.1.14). Endometrioid EC does not exhibit these characteristics. This is regarded as a clear sign of UCS and should set alarm bells ringing (22). MR imaging of EC only rarely reveals necroses.

UCS, AS and EC generally differ from pure uterine sarcomas in that they are usually primarily centrally localized in the uterus. Unlike LG-ESS, both UCS and EC almost always invade the LM (which are clearly discernable due to their hypointensity), a finding that can serve to distinguish UCS and EC from LG-ESS. The MR image that LMS generates is similar to that of UCS, though the former is usually primarily localized in the myometrium and generally exhibits more necroses than the latter. However, it is often not possible to reliably differentiate between these two entities on the basis of imaging alone (22, 45, 184, 217, 237, 240, 246, 251). While early-stage UCS still bear a

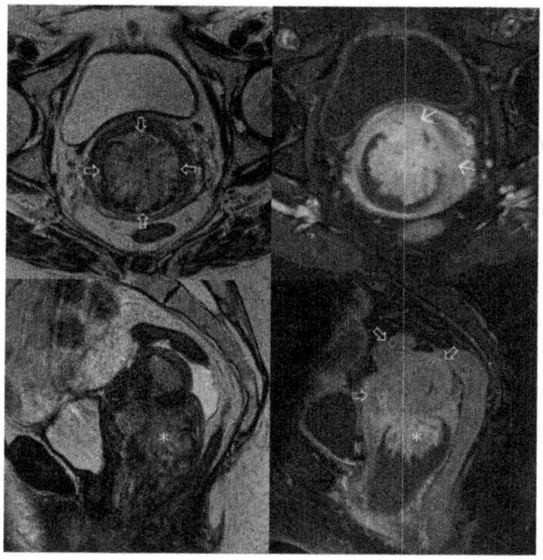

Fig. 7.1.14: MRI of the patient from Fig. 7.1.2 (E), (F); as described, the tumor prolapsed from the vulva causing uterine inversion two days after this MRI was taken; axial and sagittal T2 weighted images (upper and lower left) show a tumor that is heterogeneously hyperintense to the smooth musculature. Upon i.v. administration of contrast agent and fat suppression, the axial and sagittal T1 weighted images (upper and lower right) reveal a tumor with a diameter of no more than 5 cm. The tumor presents with an actiniform growth pattern in all images (large arrows) and protrudes from the uterus into in vagina (stars). The tumor causes the vagina to expand. In addition, the left side of the vagina has been infiltrated by the tumor (thin arrows). Urinary bladder and rectum are not involved.

close resemblance to EC, in more advanced stages of disease, the MRI characteristics associated with LMS, like necroses and hemorrhages, become increasingly manifest (240). LM can be easily distinguished from UCS in the majority of cases due to their well-defined margins, intramural localization and low homogeneous SI. Degenerated submucosal myoma can be problematic, as they are often characterized by heterogeneous SI.

There are currently no sufficiently validated data and thus no justifications for the routine use of PET-CT in staging (203, 208). CS are characterized by a high SUV in FDG-PET-CT. In individual cases, opting for PET-CT can be sensible as a means for diagnosing recurrence or for monitoring adjuvant or palliative CHT. False negative findings must be reckoned with when very small lesions are involved, as must false positive findings when inflammatory processes are involved (113).

In sonography, carcinosarcomas present as centrally localized tumors with a centrifugal growth pattern. They are usually predominantly hyperechoic, but also heterogeneously echogenic with anechoic areas (necroses, cysts).

In CT, uterine carcinosarcomas are usually hypodense to the myometrium with occasional hyperdense sections. They generally exhibit inhomogeneous enhancement in CECT that is weaker than that of the myometrium. CT is not suitable for diagnosing specific neoplastic entities. Instead, it is predominantly used in the context of extrapelvic staging and spread diagnostics.

In T1W-MRI, carcinosarcomas are usually isointense to both myometrium and endometrium. One third of cases exhibit noticeable heterogeneous signal intensity with in part hyperintense foci that constitute hemorrhages. In T2W-MRI, the majority of carcinosarcomas are hyperintense to the myometrium, while equal shares of such tumors are hypointense or isointense to endometrium. As tumor size increases, so too does heterogeneity in T2W images. In contrast MRI, most carcinosarcomas have heterogeneous SI (though SI can be homogeneous in less common cases) that is lower than that of normal myometrium. Hemorrhages, necroses or cystic components generally do not enhance and remain hypointense.

There is currently no justification for routinely using PET-CT as a means of staging. In isolated cases, PET-CT can be a useful tool for diagnosing recurrences or for monitoring neoadjuvant or palliative therapy.

7.1.5 Differential diagnostics

Early findings resulting from clinical sonographic examination and HSC can be mistakenly interpreted as evidence for EC, endometrial polyps or cervical polyps (see imaging). For polypoid tumors protruding from the cervix, the differential diagnostic options are: all other uterine sarcomas, AF, necrotic polyps and fibroids in statu nascendi. UCS can still be confused with (necrotic) endometrioid or cervical polyps, pedunculated fibroids or other uterine sarcomas on the basis of observation/assessment of the cut-open surgical specimen (Fig. 7.1.2 (B)–(D) and Fig. 7.1.15).

UCS can be barely discernible from G3-EC (9), HG-ESS, UUS, and (occasionally) LMS (cf. Vol. 1, Chapters 2, 4 and 5) on gross observation of the surgical specimen alone. G1/2 EC usually have a consistent macroscopic appearance without considerable invasion, which serves to differentiate them from UCS, which by contrast have a predominantly polymorphous appearance (Fig. 7.1.16 (A)–(C)).

In general, a UCS should always be considered in cases in which the entire cavum uteri is dilated by what appears to be a large endometrial carcinoma, especially in light of the fact that diagnoses formed on the basis of curettage are susceptible to being erroneous in such cases (see microscopic findings and below). It is often the case that the tissue obtained from fast-growing, voluminous tumors via curettage only contains evidence of necrosis. Widespread necrosis is always suggestive of UCS or a particularly aggressive form of sarcoma.

Where HT is planned as treatment for EC, the tumor tissue should be removed as completely and fully as possible via curettage and subsequently subjected to particularly thorough analysis, so as to avoid overlooking an early UCS. An unsuspected or overlooked UCS can grow relatively quickly when exposed to conservative progestin therapy (74).

When the tumor has invaded the abdominal cavity, OCS is also a possible differential diagnosis in terms of clinical presentation. Synchronous occurrence of CS in both the uterus and the ovaries could point to actual tumor synchronicity, but could also

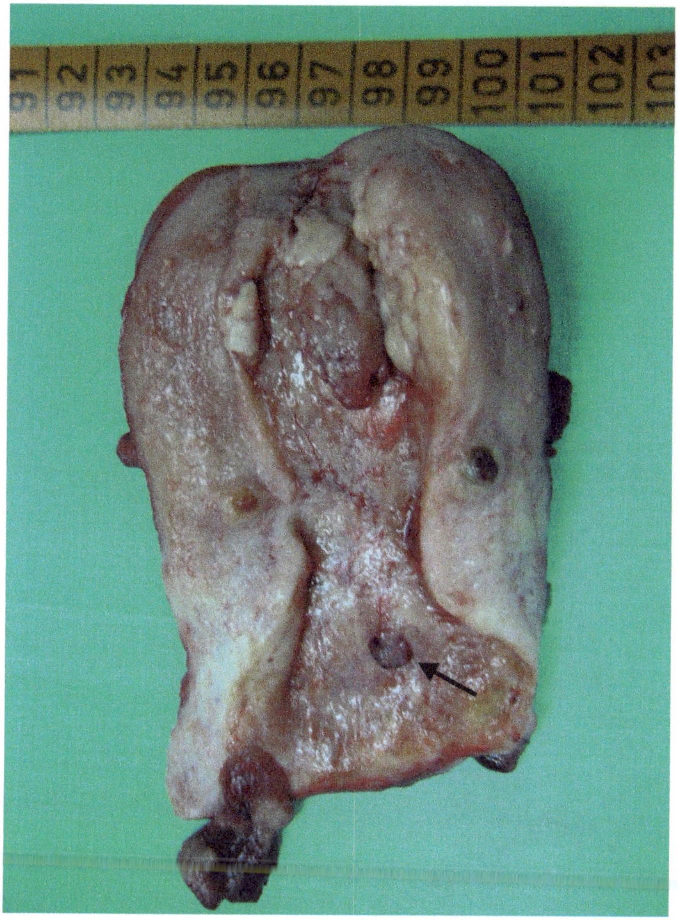

Fig. 7.1.15: Unusual case of an endometrioid adenocarcinoma of the corpus with synchronous presence of a tiny, almost purely sarcomatous carcinosarcoma (arrow) (with a gross appearance closely resembling a tiny cervical polyp) that later recurred and took a fatal course. Extensive analysis failed to detect any sarcomatous tissue within the endometrioid carcinoma. This served to rule out the possibility of canalicular metastasis and instead verified that the lesion was in fact a synchronous double tumor.

be due to metastatic spread of CS from the uterus to the ovaries or vice versa (cf. OCS). Tumors occurring simultaneously in both the uterus and the ovaries/the pelvis should be regarded as separate entities when also accompanied by endometriosis (268).

Cervical squamous cell carcinoma and adenocarcinoma of the cervix are key clinical differential diagnoses. Whether a CS is primarily cervical or corporal depends on the site in which the majority of the tumor volume is located, on the findings from palpation and imaging, and ultimately on the pathologico-anatomical diagnosis reached following analysis of the hysterectomy specimen. Tumors in the lateral cervical wall

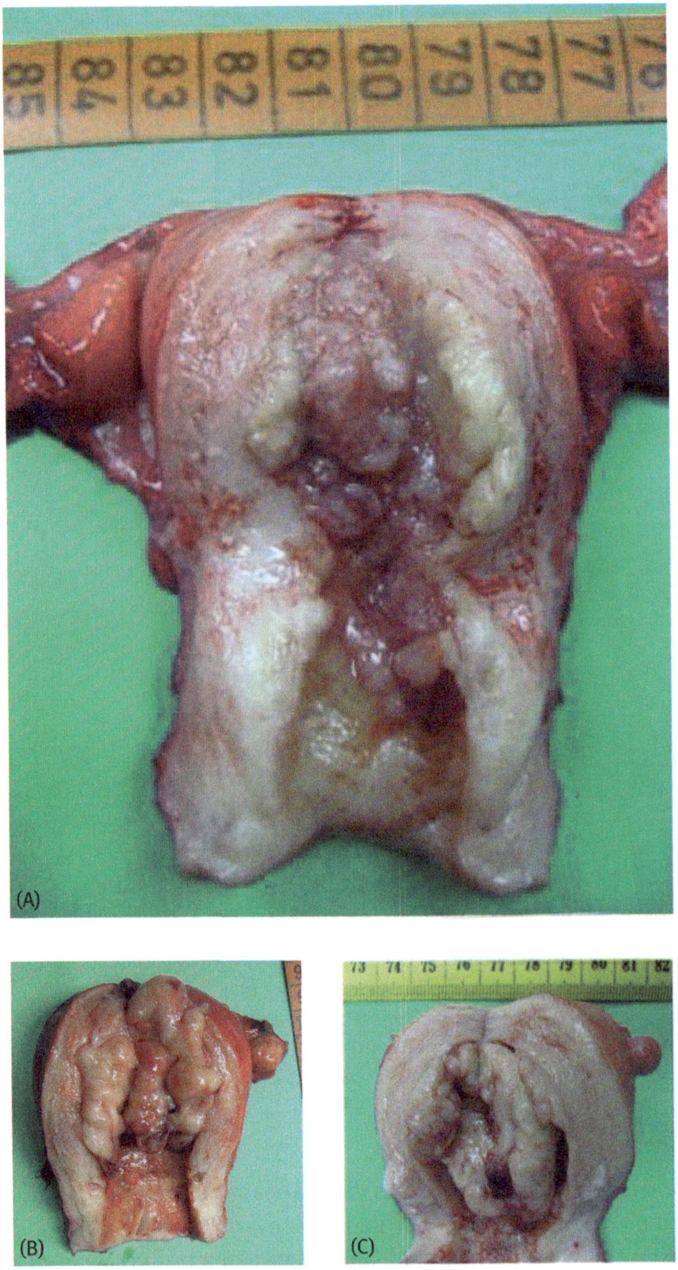

Fig. 7.1.16: Grossly differentiating carcinosarcoma from G3 endometrioid carcinoma is barely possible; (A) carcinosarcoma; (B), (C) G3 and G1 endometrioid carcinoma.

suggest a mesonephric origin. Very large lesions in the cervical walls are more likely to be CS than carcinoma.

DD can be very difficult at the microscopic level. Where the epithelial component has only developed focally or when there is "sarcomatous overgrowth", the curettage specimen, the surgical specimen or a recurrent tumor can be mistakenly interpreted as pointing to a pure homologous or heterologous uterine sarcoma. The true diagnosis then usually only becomes evident when the disease takes a suspicious clinical course, or because recurrent tumors or metastases exhibit epithelial structures. The literature and the DKSM material database recount multiple cases in which heterologous UCS with a rhabdomyomatous sarcoma component were primarily classified as RMS (57). Since RMS of the corpus uteri are very rare in adults, such tumors should be subjected to thorough examination, not least because the therapeutic consequences for RMS and UCS differ substantially. Primary tumors in which the epithelial component is predominant can be misdiagnosed as EC, especially when the diagnosis is based on findings from curettage. In cases of collision tumors, only the endometrial or only the sarcomatous component might be traceable in the available tissue specimens, which in turn could result in a primary misdiagnosis. Since UCS can focally contain normal glandular tissue, they can be wrongly diagnosed as AS (see Chapter 6) or as LG-ESS (cf. Vol. 1, Chapter 4) with extensive glandular differentiation. Such cases are not rare, and constitute examples for well-known pitfalls in the context of DD.

In the DKSM database, of the UCS that were definitively diagnosed as such following surgery, only 72 % had been diagnosed as UCS on the basis of the tissue specimens obtained via curettage. Among the remainder, 18 % had been diagnosed as EC, 5 % as pure sarcoma (LG-ESS, UUS), 1 % as AS and 4 % as benign or other neoplasms (128). Endometrioid EC sometimes contain heterologous chondroid and osteoid elements that, when regarded on their own, are insufficient grounds on which to base a diagnosis of UCS (63). Also, UCS can be confused with endometrioid EC when spindled epithelial cells are present in the latter (166). Such cases normally involve low-grade endometrial (G1/G2) and low-grade spindle cell components that, while exhibiting mitotic activity and high cellularity, are not strikingly atypical. Moreover, the clinical presentation of this entity does not correspond to that of UCS (63).

Occasionally, it can occur that an atypical polypoid adenomyoma is mistaken for UCS, especially when the cell-rich stroma is interpreted as a sarcomatous component, and the numerous atypia and mitoses in the epithelium are mistakenly interpreted as implying a carcinomatous component. Distinguishing cervical UCS from sarcomatoid carcinoma of the cervix can be challenging, not least because these two entities have a very similar macroscopic appearance. The spindle cells of the latter express unlike to all other mesenchymal tumors keratin, and also vimentin in some cases (29). They lack the glandular or basaloid morphology and exhibit direct transition of the squamous cell into a spindle cell component. Heterologous elements are not visible. Cervical UCS are occasionally also confused with cervical AS. Likewise, the possibility of a primary tumor in the corpus or the ovary that has subsequently metastasized must be borne in mind (181).

Endometrioid carcinoma is the cardinal clinical differential diagnostic alternative for uterine carcinosarcoma. Ovarian carcinosarcoma must also be considered as an option when tumors have spread within the abdominal cavity. A misdiagnosis as endometrioid carcinoma or as homologous or heterologous sarcoma is possible when diagnosis is based on tissue specimens gathered via curettage. Whenever a rare heterologous uterine sarcoma is diagnosed (rhabdomyosarcoma, liposarcoma, fibrosarcoma), effort must be devoted to reliably assessing whether or not epithelial components are present, because heterologous carcinosarcomas occur much more frequently than heterologous uterine sarcomas do, and these two neoplasms require different treatment approaches.

7.1.6 Course, prognosis

As is also the case for sarcoma, disease stage is the most important primary independent prognostic factor for UCS patients (4, 107, 201, 206). Achieving R0 resection margins, regardless of the stage of disease, appears to be equally, if not even more pivotal (3, 107). Advanced patient age is associated with a negative impact on prognosis (4, 165), while parity – when adjusted for age and clinical stage – appears to have no prognostic influence (4). A previous medical history of breast cancer and/or tamoxifen therapy has been shown to constitute a significant independent prognostic factor (68, 255). Whether the UCS has developed through collision or through conversion is of no clinical or prognostic significance. From a morphologic perspective, the carcinomatous component constitutes the driving force for prognosis, not least because proliferative activity is higher in the carcinomatous component than in the sarcomatous component (89, 216). Accordingly, analogous to EC, serous, clear cell or G3 EC components, myometrial invasion, LVI, VI, stromal involvement of the cervix and extrauterine dissemination are associated with a poor prognosis (52, 89, 148, 179, 224, 231, 274). Serous and clear cell carcinomatous components are regarded as the most significant prognostic factors (179, 224).

While some studies suggest that ER positive UCS could be associated with a slightly more favorable prognosis (108), other studies have not been able to confirm this effect (129, 277).

Irrespective of the considerable impact that the epithelial component has on prognosis, tumors with a well-differentiated sarcomatous component (e.g. LG-ESS) are associated with significantly longer PFS than tumors in which the sarcomatous component is poorly differentiated (e.g. HG-ESS and UUS). This applies to both homologous and heterologous UCS (148). Homologous UCS are said to be associated with significantly superior OS compared to their heterologous counterparts (69), though this may only apply to heterologous UCS with an RMS component. The experience of the DKSM (128), too, has shown that this entity tends to exhibit particularly rapid clinical growth (Fig. 7.1.2 (E)). According to a recent study, UCS with an RMS component have a median DFS of 13 mo and a median OS of 23 mo (150). The respective values for a control group were 15 and 67 mo (149, 150). According to other sources, the extent of the sarcomatous component, and whether the tumor is homologous or heterologous, are of no prognostic significance (55, 179, 224, 274). The question if prognosis is affected by whether a component is homologous or heterologous therefore remains unresolved. Research suggests that patients with a predominating sarcomatous component show poorer responses to CHT (188). MI apparently has no prognostic impact (148, 179). HR status (123, 265), Ki-67 and p53 expression (123) and Her-2 overexpression (199) apparently have no influence on prognosis. WT-1 overexpression is regarded as an independent prognostic marker for both DFS and OS (46).

Elevated CA-125 values prior to surgery are suggestive of primary extrauterine involvement and/or a serous epithelial component. Persistently high postoperative CA-125 values are deemed a predictor for a particularly poor prognosis (103, 105).

Overall, UCS is a highly aggressive neoplasm. Complete staging reveals myometrial invasion in 22–37 % and adnexal involvement in 5–23 % of stage I UCS patients. In 15–45 % of cases, disease has already spread to the pelvic LN, while para-aortic LN are involved in 8–27 % of patients (9, 148, 170, 273, 274). In the DKSM database, 29 % of cases had nodal involvement (128). Forty-one to forty-six percent of patients present with stage III or stage IV disease at the time of initial diagnosis, and the tumor has transgressed the boundaries of the uterus at least microscopically in up to 61 % of cases. Distant metastasis is already present in 24–45 % of patients at the time of primary diagnosis (4, 25, 107, 165, 274). According to most recent data from the National Cancer Database, covering 10,609 UCS, 28.2 % of patients presented with stage I disease at initial diagnosis, 6.1 % were stage II, 19.2 % had stage III disease and 12.4 % were in stage IV. No stage could be specified in 34.1 % of cases (201). Therefore, stages I and II occur with roughly the same frequency as stages III and IV. Sixty-one percent of first recurrences occur outside of the lesser pelvis or as distant metastasis (32, 148). The pelvis is affected alone or in combination with distant metastasization in only 30 % of cases. Autopsy reveals local metastasis in 55.6 % and distant metastasis in 62.9 % of cases (4). Analogous to EC, the vagina is the most frequently involved pelvic organ. The high frequency of pulmonary and hepatic metastasization is also noteworthy (Fig. 7.1.17 (A)–(G)).

In UCS patients, the LN are involved much more frequently compared to women with pure uterine sarcomas. The number of positive LN is at its highest when the epithelial component consists of serous carcinoma or clear cell carcinoma. Furthermore, LN involvement significantly correlates with involvement of the adnexa, the cervix and the isthmus as well as with myometrial invasion of over 50 %, but not with tumor size or MI (148). LN positivity is associated with a significantly poorer 5-year OS. However, whether it is the pelvic or the para-aortic LN that are affected appears to have no bearing on the prognosis (81). Prognosis is superior when only the LN are affected than when there is intraperitoneal disease spread (27). Please refer to the subsection on “primary surgery” for the prognostic relevance of an LNE. Positive peritoneal cytology is associated with a significantly poorer 5-year OS, and with a worsening of the prognosis that is identical to that caused by involvement of

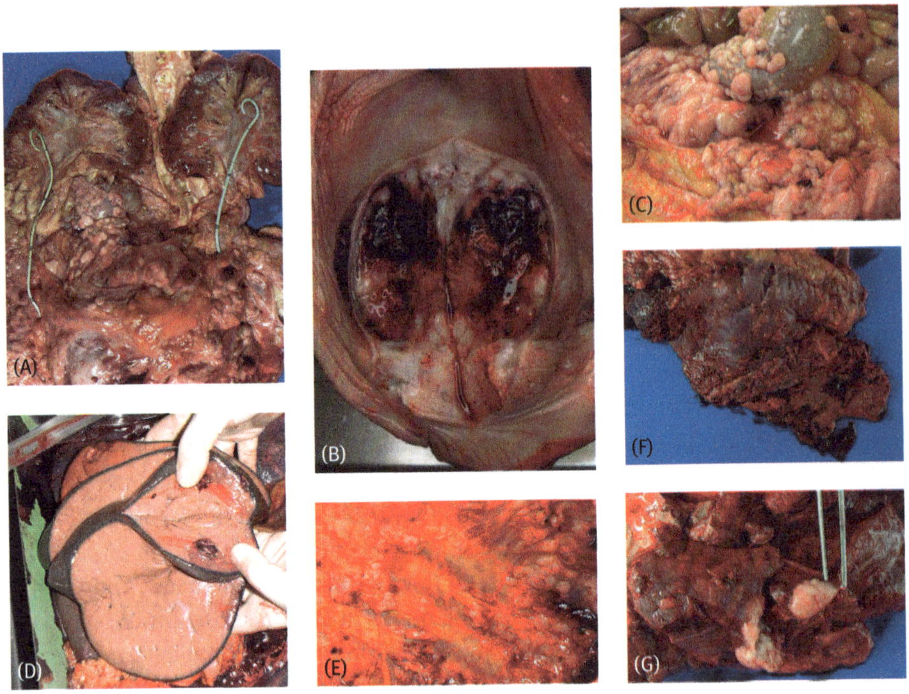

Fig. 7.1.17: Autopsy findings pertaining to the primary tumor in Fig. 7.1.15; (A), (B) Tumor dissemination in the lesser pelvis including retroperitoneum and vagina; (C), (D) spread over the entire upper abdomen (peritoneal carcinosis or sarcomatosis) and to the liver; (E)–(G) metastatic disease on the parietal and visceral pleurae and in the lung.

the uterine serosa or the adnexa (81). The clinical consequences of LN involvement and positive cytology, however, remain entirely unclear, and currently do not allow appropriate therapeutic measures to be deduced. In fact, only 13.3 % of recurrences and metastases are limited to the LN, while metastasis/recurrence is (also) distant in 73.3 % of cases, with pulmonary involvement being particularly frequent (206). In advanced (!) UCS, neoadjuvant CHT, deep myometrial invasion, VI, LVI, cervical, adnexal or parametrial involvement, positive intraperitoneal cytology, enlarged affected LN, the epithelial cell component and the presence of a heterologous sarcomatous component no longer have any prognostic consequences (206, 241).

Recurrences and metastases occur within the first 2 years in 53.3 % of cases, and within the first year in 43.3 % (206). According to other sources, 61 % of UCS recur within 10 mo of surgery. Forty percent of patients with stage I UCS relapse with 3 years. There have been numerous accounts of UCS recurring within only a few weeks of surgery (55). Median OS is 26 mo in stages I and II, and only 18–25 mo in stages I–IV (80, 256). Another study measured a median OS of 40 mo among patients with stage I–III disease (177). According to further research (197), median OS was 1,066 days for stage I, 648 for stage II and 641 for stage III patients. Five-year OS for all stages has been found to range from 25 up to 55 %. According to SEER data, disease-specific OS is 59 % for stage IA, 54 % for stage IB, 38 % for stage IC, 35 % for stage II, 22 % for stage III and 10 % for stage IV (FIGO before 2009) (19). One publication suggests that race negatively impacts on prognosis. Black women in the study had a median DFS of 13.6 mo and median OS of 25.4 mo, compared to 77.4 mo and 94.7 mo, respectively, for white women (66). The risk of recurrence and mortality in stages I and II is significantly greater for black than for white women. This difference does not carry over into higher stages of disease (66).

Based on the available literature, the prognosis for UCS patients is apparently identical to that for patients with serous EC (228), but significantly worse than for patients with high-grade endometrioid EC, which itself is already characterized by a poor prognosis (24, 69, 280). More recent studies suggest that UCS has significantly poorer DFS and OS compared to serous (55, 280) and clear cell EC (280). G3 endometrioid EC has a median OS of 78 % for stage IA disease, 83 % for stage IB, 68 % for stage IC, 60 % for stage II, 45 % for stage III and 17 % for stage IV (FIGO before 2009) (19). Other reports suggest that there is no discernible difference between UCS and G3 endometrioid EC in terms of OS (3). In general, there is wide consensus that UCS constitutes a highly aggressive variant of EC that should be regarded as an independent entity in the context of prognosis as well (9, 85, 256, 280). Overall, the survival data for UCS more or less correspond to those associated with LMS and UUS (cf. Vol. 1, Chapters 2 and 5), and are dramatically worse than for LG-ESS patients (cf. Vol. 1, Chapter 4). According to the current GCIG Consensus, the prognosis for UCS has not improved over the past two years (21).

Compared to UCS of the corpus uteri, primary cervical UCS are less frequently initially diagnosed in advanced stages of disease – 31 % are initially diagnosed in stages III and IV. This is apparently because the latter are easier to recognize clinically, and patients with cervical UCS show symptoms earlier. Research suggests, however, that cervical UCS originating in the mesonephron are associated with a poorer prognosis than their adenocarcinoma equivalents (10, 18). Nineteen percent of patients with primary cervical UCS have nodal metastases (20). However, what this implies for therapy is unclear. Upon critical review of the literature, which in total covers only a small number of cases, it appears as though the prognosis for cervical UCS is no worse than for UCS of the corpus uteri.

Carcinosarcoma is a highly malignant neoplasm. Five-year overall survival across all stages of disease is between 25 % and 55 %. Stage of disease and disease-free resection margins are the cardinal prognostic factors. Prognosis is primarily driven and determined by the epithelial component of the tumor. Serous, clear cell, or poorly differentiated carcinomatous components are associated with a poorer prognosis. Prognosis is better for tumors with less aggressive sarcomatous components (e.g. low-grade endometrial stromal sarcoma) than for tumors with more aggressive histologic types (e.g. undifferentiated uterine sarcoma, leiomyosarcoma, rhabdomyosarcoma). Nodal involvement is commonplace in carcinosarcoma, though the clinical consequences of this feature remain entirely unclear. High CA-125 levels are suggestive of extrauterine involvement. Recurrences and metastases involve distant metastasization in the majority of cases. It currently cannot be reliably discerned whether performing lymphadenectomy has any prognostic impact.

7.1.7 Primary surgery

For UCS that are confined to the uterus (stages I and II), performing THE with BSO is the smallest common denominator in terms of surgery. The current NCCN Recommendations Uterine Neoplasms Version recommend (2A recommendation) complete staging analogous to OC, consisting of THE, BSO, pelvic and para-aortic LNE, omentectomy as well as peritoneal biopsies and peritoneal cytology (175). This recommendation, however, is based solely on retrospective data that are subject to numerous biases, and lacks a clear scientific foundation. TAH with BSO is accorded a relatively high degree of recommendation in the Japanese Guidelines. Regarding LNE, the Japanese guidelines state that, though it has yet to be proven to have a positive therapeutic impact, LNE can be considered for use in the context of staging (169). The lack of evidence that measures beyond THE with BSO have any positive effect on DFS and OS is well exemplified by the classification as a 2A Recommendation ("based upon lower-level evidence, there is uniform NCCN consensus that the intervention is appropriate") (175). Like the NCCN Guidelines, the current GCIG Consensus (21) recommends complete staging be performed analogous to staging for OC. The recommendation is not backed by sufficient data, an insecurity that is underlined by the careful wording used: "adequate lymphadenectomy seems needed for both staging and therapeutic reasons". The German guidelines (54) are noncommittal in this regard, merely stating that retrospective studies suggest that LNE might have an impact on OS. There have in fact been no randomized studies to date that have proven that the recommended staging would be beneficial in terms of OS. There is also no evidence to suggest that systematic pelvic and para-aortic LNE prolongs survival. A retrospective survey with a small sample found that median/mean DFS and OS were only significantly improved when more than 11 LN were removed (245). Univariate analyses conducted in the context of a comparative retrospective evaluation of all (!) uterine sarcomas in 17 Japanese institutions revealed a significantly prolonged OS following LNE, though the results fail to take (in part substantial) biases into consideration (3). The data cannot, however, be said to apply to UCS without further ado. According to a SEER analysis, LNE was associated with a statistically significant improvement in 5-year OS and median OS (177). Beyond the fact that the study was retrospective and thus tied to different forms of bias, the data are also flawed with inconsistencies. No differentiation was made between pelvic and para-aortic LNE, and on average only 12 (1–90) LN were removed. Neither the number of removed LN, nor whether they were positive or negative, showed any recognizable significant effect on OS. Accordingly, the authors make no (!) recommendation on the basis of the data to perform LNE as routine practice, and warn that these results should be interpreted with caution (177). In a more recent SEER analysis, risk of mortality was 33 times lower for women who underwent LNE than for patients who did not. However, due to insecurities in the context of data collection, the authors refrained from definitively clarifying whether or not this had in fact been a therapeutic effect (80). Further retrospective research suggests that performing LNE in stages IIIC1/2 (81) and stage II (not stage I) (82) is associated with a statistically significant improvement in OS. Multivariate analysis conducted in the context of another study also revealed improved survival (95). However, a larger share (20 %) of the patients who underwent LNE had also received CHT-RT compared to the observation arm or the patients who underwent standalone CHT or RT. The extent of the LNE, the number of LN, and the proportion of cases with positive LN are not mentioned in the publication (95). Improvements in OS following LNE were also observed in a recent analysis (201) by the National Cancer Database, covering a total of 10,609 UCS. Since the study was marred by numerous biases, the authors refrained from drawing any definitive conclusions as to whether or not an LNE should be performed. Taken together, the presented retrospective studies do not allow any definitive statements to be made in terms of the prognostic impact of LNE. The benefits of performing pelvic and para-aortic LNE can be questioned, not least because, in many cases, occult distant metastatic disease has already developed at the time of surgery, and in 50 % of cases, distant metastatic dissemination can already be clinically verified (4). Distant metastasization is already present at the time of primary diagnosis in 27 % of corresponding cases in the DKSM database (128). Metastases in the abdominal cavity or distant metastasization are present in 70 % of cases in which the LN test positive (231). Tumor cell dissemination still occurs relatively swiftly after complete staging has been performed, even despite an absence of nodal involvement. In a further retrospective study, undergoing LNE appeared to have no positive effects on OS, while at the same time, early distant metastases could be found despite negative results from LNE (107, 130). Combining LNE with VBT does not appear to impact favorably on the rates of local and distant relapse (30). While 10–12 % of relapses occur as recurrences in the pelvic region, in around 90 % of cases, relapse involves metastases in the upper abdomen or distant metastases with and without pelvic recurrences. Sixty-one percent of women already exhibit extrauterine tumor dissemination at the time of primary diagnosis (274). According to other sources, 83 % of first recurrences are distant metastases with/without pelvic involvement (273) and recurrences are confined exclusively to the pelvis, including the vagina, in max. 25 % (148) resp. 11.3 % (55) of cases. OS is thus essentially determined by extrapelvic dissemination. The fact that an association between performing LNE in UCS patients per se and improved survival has yet to be scientifically proven is largely congruent with the results from two randomized studies on intermediate and high-risk EC (16, 190). LNE did not result in improvements in DFS or OS in either of the two studies. It should not be overlooked that these studies, too, have their flaws, and have repeatedly been the subject of critical enquiry (154, 176). The findings are remarkable nonetheless, because compared to UCS, EC much less frequently develop distant metastases or spread beyond the uterus. Accordingly, it would have been fully plausible to expect LNE to be beneficial for patients with EC. Despite a lack of reliable and/or valid data, for high-risk EC there is nonetheless the general recommendation not to go beyond LNE until need for another course of action has been proven beyond doubt (48).

Whether or not LNE offers any benefits in the context of staging or as a therapeutic measure remains contested (148). According to the available literature and clinical practice, LNE is nonetheless performed in 35 % to 100 % of cases (77, 81, 189, 201, 206, 263), with most sources stating frequencies ranging from 35 % to 57 % (189, 263). Sixty-seven percent of corresponding patients covered in the DKSM database (122) were subjected to LNE. Two recent studies report rates of 68.7 % and 80 %, respectively (95, 201).

Taken together, the available data do not suffice to prove that performing systematic pelvic and para-aortic LNE on UCS patients yields any benefits. For UCS, whether the LN are positive or negative currently has no therapeutic consequences or implications (see adjuvant and postoperative therapy). LNE thus currently serves only as a prognostic tool and for precisely determining the stage of disease. This purpose can also be achieved (albeit with limitations) using MR imaging or by removing enlarged LN via selective LNE. As long as no therapeutic consequences can be generally deduced from LN status, there is currently also no clear indication for sentinel LN biopsy. The guidelines only consider sentinel LN biopsy worthy of a category 3 recommendation (175). Whether reducing overall tumor burden by removing enlarged LN serves to improve OS is unclear. At the same time, it is rather unlikely, given the biology of UCS.

To recapitulate, there are currently no valid and reliable data that suggest performing systematic or selective pelvic and para-aortic LNE as standard practice. Nonetheless, taken together, the literature shows a certain consensus in that LNE should be considered in suitable fit patients (203). In such cases, the patient must be comprehensively and unequivocally informed of the possible complications that can arise, and that the benefits of the procedure have not been scientifically proven.

The only condition that the NCCN Guidelines state regarding THE is that the procedure is performed without causing injury to the uterus. (175). TLH is thus not categorically excluded. However, this contradicts the NCCN recommendation to subject the whole abdomen to detailed palpatory examination, which includes the retroperitoneal spaces. Furthermore, "port site" metastases should be reckoned with when endoscopic procedures are opted for (51). Laparotomy is recommended for patients with metastatic UCS, with large uteri, those who are morbidly obese, and/or elderly patients (175).

Though still practiced in many parts of the world, RAH is not recommended or considered in the NCCN Guidelines (175). In fact, there are no valid data that suggest that performing this measure would be beneficial in cases in which disease is confined to the uterus. Notwithstanding, in a retrospective Japanese study, both extended and RAH were associated with significantly improved OS (130). However, the study involved an analysis of all uterine sarcomas in stages I–IV that does not allow the share of stage I and II UCS to be deduced.

The available data pertaining to omentectomy are contradictory. Omental involvement is found in 9–13 % of cases at the time of initial diagnosis (79, 100). The omentum can be removed when there is a clear cell or serous epithelial component (139). In a recent retrospective study (88), multivariate analysis revealed that, in addition to stage of disease, undergoing complete staging with pelvic and para-aortic LNE as well as omentectomy was associated with longer OS. However, numerous biases and a relatively small sample size prevent us from drawing any definitive conclusions from the results. The NCCN Guidelines also suggest performing an omentectomy (category 2A recommendation). The German guidelines (54) at least question the sense behind such practice. According to the DKSM database (128), omentectomies are performed in 49 % of cases in Germany. In the USA, the figure is 42 % (95). Overall, due to the lack of reliable data and sound scientific substantiation, performing omentectomy cannot be deemed standard practice. At the same time, it is not subject to any definitive contraindications either.

The results from the recommended intraperitoneal cytological examinations currently have no therapeutic implications or consequences.

Where a UCS is only diagnosed as such after surgery, subsequent systematic LNE or omentectomy need not necessarily be performed due to a lack of respective benefits having been scientifically proven to that end. However, they should be performed if the patient so requests after having been comprehensively and clearly informed of that lack of proven benefits. It should generally be reckoned with that even patients with stage I disease who undergo extensive surgery including systematic pelvic and para-aortic LNE, omentectomy and parametrial resection are likely to relapse very early (Fig. 7.1.18 (A)–(D)).

Analogous to EC, the adnexa should also be excised, as they are often affected by metastatic infestation and/or synchronous CS (see prognosis).

The data situation pertaining to surgical therapy for cervical UCS is particularly poor. As is also the case for all other types and forms of sarcoma, it is key that cervical UCS are resected leaving no residual disease (i.e. R0 resection margins). Upon critical review of the literature, it appears that performing RAH with concurrent removal of the parametria is only advisable when there is extracervical dissemination. The benefits of performing LNE are also questionable and far from having been scientifically substantiated (20, 271).

Analogous to advanced OC and EC, at least maximal tumor debulking is recommended for UCS that have spread in the pelvis and the abdominal cavity (139, 149, 269, 273). The current NCCN Guidelines (2A recommendation), the GCIG Consensus and the German guidelines all recommend maximal cytoreduction for advanced tumors (21, 54, 175). These recommendations are primarily based on retrospective studies with no focus on extensive surgery, and/or that included all uterine sarcomas (130). In a retrospective review of 44 patients with UCS in stages IIIC–IVB, the median PFI following cytoreductive surgery was 8.6 mo in the total sample (241). Complete gross cytoreduction was associated with a median PFI of 14.3 mo, compared to 7.1 mo among patients with gross residual disease. The respective OS were 52.3 versus 8.6 mo. Maximal cytoreduction was achieved in 40 % of cases, while optimal tumor debulking was possible in 30 %. As expected, the further course also depended on the volume of residual disease. The results were better for patients in whom metastasis is limited to enlarged, bulky LN (stage IIIC), versus patients with peritoneal dissemination. Optimal cytoreduction and (independent of the extent of surgery) the subsequent administration of CHT or CHT-RT were the only independent factors to be associated with positive effects on OS. Interestingly, the precise forms of adjuvant therapy administered – CHT or CHT-RT – did not produce differing results. Therefore, and due to selection biases, the authors expressly advise not to overvalue the positive data yielded for postoperative adjuvant therapy.

Neoadjuvant CHT, deep myometrial invasion, cervical, vaginal or parametrial invasion, positive intraperitoneal cytology, LN involvement, a heterologous sarcomatous element, and the epithelial component all had no prognostic impact on the further course following cytoreduction in advanced UCS. In the authors' opinion, the overall results suggest that surgical resection should be considered when there is a strong likelihood of achieving complete gross resection (241). Since prognosis is not determined or guided by nodal involvement (81), whether or not it makes sense to resect enlarged LN is indeed a disputed issue. In practice, LN are in fact resected in only about 50 % of cases. Postoperative complications arise following cytoreductive surgery in about 36 % of cases (241).

Opting for a primarily surgical approach for treating advanced UCS can be justified by the fact that the available CHT options are limited, have relatively low response rates and are associated with only a short PFI (see adjuvant and palliative CHT). Therefore, instead of primary palliative CHT, with its significantly shorter PFI, maximal or at least optimal cytoreduction should currently be regarded as the method of choice. Whether this aim can be achieved needs to be ascertained in advance via optimal imaging diagnostic procedures. CHT should be kept in reserve as an option for palliative systemic therapy that will be necessary later anyway. There are currently no data that serve as an argument against such a course of action. If the required preconditions for surgical therapy are not met or if there are general contraindications, systemic therapy must be considered.

Due to the very poor prognosis with which extensive intraperitoneal dissemination is associated, performing ultra-radical surgery and both anterior and posterior exenterations should be avoided to the benefit of the patient's quality of life. Such practices can, however, be considered in cases of tumors that are without doubt confined to the pelvis. In these rare cases, administering pre-operative PET-CT would be beneficial. There are currently no respective valid data on ultra-radical surgery.

For carcinosarcomas that are confined to the uterus, the NCCN Guidelines recommend (2A recommendation) performing staging surgery involving total hysterectomy with bilateral salpingo-oophorectomy, pelvic and para-aortic lymphadenectomy, omentectomy, peritoneal biopsies and peritoneal cytology. It has yet to be substantiated with reliable data that performing surgical procedures that go beyond total hysterectomy plus salpingo-oophorectomy has a beneficial impact on overall and recurrence-free survival. Notwithstanding, there is overall consensus that the aforementioned additional surgical options should be performed if doing so can be reasonably expected of the patient given her overall condition. They currently only serve as means of forecasting patient prognosis without any consequences in terms of adjuvant therapy, so that they cannot be deemed standard practice. Likewise, refraining from these measures cannot be classified as malpractice. Total hysterectomy plus salpingo-oophorectomy thus currently constitutes a justifiable therapeutic option. There are no data to suggest that performing an extended or radical hysterectomy impacts on survival.

For carcinosarcomas that have spread to involve the pelvis and the abdominal cavity, and for which the results of imaging diagnostics suggest that maximal, but at the very least optimal cytoreduction (debulking) appears to be achievable, opting for said course of action must currently be regarded as the therapeutic route of choice. In this context, it can be sensible to remove any enlarged lymph nodes as well.

7.1.8 Adjuvant and additive radio-, chemo- and hormone therapy

In retrospective studies (93) conducted in the 1990s, subjecting patients with uterine sarcomas, including UCS, to postoperative RT was still associated with improvements in DFS and OS. The first randomized phase III study (EORTC 55874) on adjuvant RT and uterine sarcoma included 91 UCS in stages I and II. The findings are congruent to those from a randomized study investigating the administration of adjuvant RT in cases of intermediate and high-risk EC (15). OS remained unchanged in both studies. Just as was the case for EC, the local recurrence rate in the RT group was reduced for UCS as well, while the number of distant metastases was elevated. In numerous retrospective surveys with larger sample sizes, standalone RT yielded no benefits for survival, but the number of local recurrences could in fact be reduced, by up to 100 % in some instances (32, 49, 60, 81, 89, 165, 211, 212, 276). Further retrospective analyses have compared patients who received CHT with or without RT to patients who underwent RT alone, and found that considerably more extravaginal pelvic recurrences occurred (80 or 90.9 %) in RT only patients compared to the two CHT arms (149, 150). The conclusion was drawn from the EORTC 55874 study that – the reduced rates of recurrence notwithstanding – subjecting patients with UCS to ERT is not routinely indicated due to the toxicity of the measure and the fact that doing so has no impact on OS (202). The authors also state that there is no evidence to prove that performing RT without prior LNE yields any benefits. However, they go on to state that VBT could be advisable in cases of cervical stromal invasion. Extensive retrospective SEER data (272) on adjuvant RT in 1,819 UCS in stages I and II stand somewhat in contradiction to the results from the aforementioned randomized EORTC 55874 study (202). According to the SEER data, receiving RT was associated with a 21 % reduction in cancer-specific mortality. The reduction was particularly considerable (25 %) in patients who had not undergone LNE. At the same time, for patients who underwent LNE, adjuvant RT conferred only a modest survival advantage. The data could be interpreted as being supportive of the notion that an LNE could possibly improve survival or that LNE can be replaced by ERT. The results from the EORTC 55874 study, the findings from a randomized study on postoperative RT and EC (15) and numerous biases in the SEER analysis are counterarguments against such considerations. Aware of the many biases in the SEER analysis, the authors formulated no recommendations for administering adjuvant ERT on the basis of their data. A very recent analysis of 10,609 UCS contained in the National Cancer Database (USA) revealed that standalone postoperative RT has no impact on OS (210). The apparent failure of RT to impact on survival is likely due to the fact that between 26 and 50 % of patients present with distant metastasis at the time of primary diagnosis, compared to only 17 % who exhibit "only" nodal involvement (4, 165), and that recurrences are initially manifested outside the lesser pelvis in a majority of cases (147, 214, 231). OS is, therefore, apparently not decided in the pelvic region. This is further exacerbated by the fact that pelvic ERT will be unable to reach nodal metastases located higher up in the body. Interestingly, in another retrospective study (56), the DFI and OS among patients who underwent standalone RT or standalone CHT did not differ substantially from those of patients who did not undergo such measures. The GCIG consensus (21) also assumes the stance that standalone RT is unlikely to impact favorably on survival. According to the current NCCN recommendations (175), postoperative therapy can be entirely dispensed with in cases of stage IA disease without myometrial invasion and in which no disease is found in the hysterectomy specimen. This recommendation has been subject to critical scrutiny in light of the fact that disease recurs in up to 18 % of such cases (34). Therefore, the guidelines state (2A recommendation) that CHT or (!) pelvic ERT are options that can be considered. The German guidelines (54) state that RT should be indicated for patients with stage I and II disease as a means for reducing the rate of local relapse, albeit without becoming more specific as regards the precise form such RT should take. Congruent to modern overviews, the NCCN Guidelines do not recommend performing whole abdomen ERT with or without VBT (175, 203). The Japanese guidelines allow for such a course of action to be considered (169). In making such decisions, the fact that this measure is highly toxic and that known patient deaths (260) are associated with it needs to be borne in mind. A review of all the data allows the conclusion that there is currently no indication for administering standalone postoperative ERT in cases of UCS limited to the uterus. Where a patient insists on such treatment, she must be unequivocally and comprehensively informed of the possible complications that can arise, and that the benefits of the procedure on OS have not been scientifically proven.

Overall, analogous to the results of a randomized study on EC (180), the randomized EORTC study (202) could not resolve the question whether administering standalone VBT (which is low on side effects) is enough to reduce local recurrence. A recent analysis (95) did in fact reveal that undergoing standalone VBT can serve to significantly reduce the rate of vaginal recurrence. VBT even achieved better results than standalone ERT. According to a recent analysis of SEER data, OS was independent from the type or mode of irradiation applied (192), making standalone VBT without ERT an option to consider seriously. Overall, there are no data that go against applying VBT alone. However, it must be borne in mind that the high risk of local relapse or developing metastases appears to remain, even when VBT is combined with an LNE (30). Moreover, it has yet to be scientifically substantiated whether administering intraoperative RT to patients with R1/2 resections has a favorable impact. As was to be expected, DFS and OS were only dependent on the extent of residual disease (73). In the USA, 20.7 % of patients undergo standalone RT (201).

While reductions in rates of local recurrence can be achieved, there are no data to suggest that subjecting patients with carcinosarcomas confined to the uterus to standalone adjuvant external radiotherapy has a beneficial impact on overall survival. The same applies to combining it with vaginal brachytherapy. Standalone postoperative percutaneous radiotherapy is therefore generally not indicated, not least in light of the side effects. The NCCN Guidelines make the 2A recommendation to consider subjecting stage IA patients without myometrial invasion to percutaneous irradiation instead of chemotherapy or only clinical observation. More recent analyses confirm that, analogous to endometrioid carcinoma, standalone vaginal brachytherapy can be sufficient to reduce rates of local recurrence. Standalone vaginal brachytherapy is not categorically ruled out by any of the authoritative recommendations and guidelines. Therefore, if additional chemotherapy is not planned, standalone brachytherapy can be opted for whenever irradiation is being considered. There are no data that go against choosing such course of action.

To date, there have been no randomized studies that have focused specifically on the use of adjuvant CHT in patients with R0 resected stage I/II UCS. According to the UCS-specific data yielded from the only applicable randomized study that covered all types of uterine sarcoma, adjuvant CHT apparently had no significant effect on OS (186). To be fair, it needs to be highlighted that doxorubicin was the cytostatic agent used, one that is regarded as being not very effective when used in a monotherapeutic context in CS. However, numerous retrospective analyses, the majority of which covered all types of uterine sarcoma, have failed to prove that adjuvant CHT has a real positive impact (72, 121, 130, 254, 274).

Regarding adjuvant CHT, reference is often made in the literature to the randomized phase III study (GOG 150). In advance, it should be noted that said study does not constitute a truly adjuvant (!) therapeutic study per se, since it encompassed stage I through IV with an eligible residual disease of ≤ 1 cm. The study compared whole abdomen ERT to a CHT regimen consisting of three cycles of ifosfamide and cisplatin, independent of LN status (269). The recurrence rate and mortality rate in the CHT group were 21 % resp. 29 % lower than in the RT arm, though this advantage was not statistically significant. The data according to which postoperative RT does not improve OS in UCS patients already suggested that CHT could indeed be potentially effective in the adjuvant context. However, since there was no control group, it cannot be ruled out that whole abdomen ERT might well have effected less favorable outcomes than might have been achieved via observation alone, not least if one considers the two toxicity-associated deaths that occurred within the RT arm. The authors concluded that administering CHT for longer (more than three cycles) and/or including other substances (e.g. paclitaxel) in the regimen might serve to amplify the minor benefit for survival revealed in their study.

Only few retrospective studies have concentrated on the application of adjuvant CHT to patients with stage I and II disease. In studies of UCS exclusively, undergoing standalone CHT was found to yield only insignificant improvements in DFS and OS (see below) (147, 273). In one extensive study on women aged > 65 years, applying adjuvant CHT to patients with stage I disease did not improve survival, not even when combined with RT. For stage II patients, there was only a statistically insignificant reduction in mortality risk (82). In one single arm study, applying adjuvant CHT consisting of ifosfamide plus cisplatin to stage I/II disease achieved a 5-year OS of 62 %, though the study lacked a control group (235). A multicenter retrospective study (34) covered 111 UCS in stages I and II in 4 arms – RT, CHT, CHT-RT and observation. Ifosfamide plus cisplatin and carboplatin plus paclitaxel were the most frequently used CHT regimens. RT consisted of pelvic ERT in 63 %, ERT plus VBT in 20 %, and only VBT in 17 % of cases. Overall, CHT was associated with better DFS and (weakly associated) with longer OS compared to the RT and observation arms. The data pertaining to CHT-RT could not be evaluated as the subsample was too small. Another retrospective study (149), designed in accordance to the GOG 150 study (269), compared CHT (usually 6 cycles with carboplatin plus paclitaxel, or in some cases ifosfamide plus cisplatin) with and without sequential ERT to standalone ERT in patients with stage I–IV. CHT with and without ERT achieved longer DFS and OS compared to standalone ERT, though the association was not statistically significant. Another study with the same design (150) covered cases of completely resected heterologous UCS with a sarcomatous RMS component. The analysis revealed that CHT with and without RT was associated with an (albeit statistically insignificant) improvement in DFS and 3-year OS (total group 20.7 % vs. 16.7 %). The results for stages I and II were more promising than for patients with higher stages of disease. In a further study (153) covering 38 stage I/II UCS, administering "sandwich therapy" using 4 (stage I) or 6 cycles (stage II) of cisplatin plus epirubicin along with intermediary RT achieved an OS of 78 % (stage I) and 100 % (stage II) within a median of 55 mo. Two further studies (160, 270) compared a CHT regimen of 3–6 cycles of ifosfamide plus cisplatin combined with subsequent RT (CHT-RT) to observation, standalone CHT, and standalone RT. Pelvic or whole abdomen RT were administered with a dosage of between 45 and 54 resp. 45 and 50 Gy in 20–30 fractions, and included VBT in some cases. Overall, when adjusted for stage of disease, the results suggest that sequential CHT-RT was associated with a beneficial impact on survival, without the additional RT causing noticeably more morbidity. These results notwithstanding, it must be critically noted that the relatively small samples (49 and

43 UCS, resp.) included patients in all stages of disease, and that there were recognizable selection biases at play in these two studies. In a recent retrospective comparison (88), sequential CHT-RT (n 20) was associated with significantly superior DFS and OS compared to RT (n 14) and CHT (n 3) in patients in stages I and II on univariate analysis. However, besides its small sample size, the study is also marred by (in part substantial) biases, and the results could not be confirmed in multivariate analyses.

In another more recent study (54) with a relatively small sample, patients with stage I/II disease who were subjected merely to observation had a fourfold mortality rate compared to patients who underwent standalone CHT. Compared to standalone CHT, CHT-RT improved DFS, but had no impact on OS. An extensive analysis by the National Cancer Database (USA) (201) covering 10,604 cases of stage I–IV UCS found that adjuvant CHT and CHT-RT are associated with improved OS.

Overall, the data situation pertaining to standalone adjuvant CHT is confusing. It has yet to be reliably scientifically substantiated that adjuvant CHT significantly improves DFS and OS in patients whose uterus-confined UCS have been primarily R0 resected. Accordingly, administering standalone adjuvant CHT currently cannot be defined or classified as the standard (226). This stance is also adopted in the current GCIG Consensus (21), according to which there are insufficient data to justify regarding adjuvant CHT as standard procedure. According to the German guidelines, decisions for or against CHT should be made on a case-by-case basis, though without providing any recommendations or information that can be of assistance for the decision-making process (54). Not applying CHT, regardless of LN status, can currently not be regarded as erroneous practice. This notwithstanding, when taken together, the literature does signify or suggest that adjuvant CHT is likely to improve survival, so there are no hard data that go against such practice. Accordingly, the current NCCN Guidelines make the 2A recommendation, even without a verified scientific basis, to consider administering adjuvant CHT with or without RT to stage I/II patients with myometrial invasion or more advanced disease (175). They also make the 2A recommendation to subject stage IA patients with myometrial invasion to CHT with or without ERT (see below). It needs to be repeated here that these recommendations are merely based on consensus and not on scientific evidence. In light of a relapse/metastasization rate of 18 % (34), the exclusion of stage IA disease without myometrial invasion from the recommendation must be critically scrutinized. The Japanese guidelines state that both CHT and RT can be considered, both with equal levels of recommendation (169).

While randomized studies are still lacking, both older and more recent analyses do consistently suggest that CHT-RT achieves the best results in the adjuvant setting (56, 88, 95, 201).

CHT-RT comes at the price of increased toxicity, especially when combined with ERT. Therefore, analogous to the approach adopted for CHT in primarily advanced and metastasized UCS, it would indeed be sensible to replace the highly toxic combination of ifosfamide plus cisplatin with carboplatin plus paclitaxel in the adjuvant CHT-RT setting. A recent study has revealed that CHT with carboplatin plus paclitaxel is not only significantly less toxic, but also more effective in stages I–IV than ifosfamide plus cisplatin (median DFS 11.6 vs. 16.6, med. OS 17.1 vs. 35.1 mo) (144). In the meantime, paclitaxel plus carboplatin has been found to be less toxic than, and equally effective to ifosfamide plus paclitaxel or ifosfamide plus cisplatin with or without additional epirubicin. Accordingly, the former is currently the most frequently applied or recommended combination (56, 95, 132, 147, 149, 150, 203). Comparable retrospective, prospective and randomized studies on high-risk EC serve to support such an approach (100, 155, 167, 168). Ifosfamide monotherapy "sandwiched" with RT is another option for UCS. Compared to a combination with cisplatin, ifosfamide monotherapy was equally effective but significantly less toxic (62).

In the EORTC 55874 study (201), a reduction in the rate of local recurrence was observed following percutaneous RT, though there were no apparent benefits for survival. By analogy to EC (180), this could indeed imply that the local effect might also be achievable via VBT. Against this backdrop, combining CHT with VBT seems to be a sensible option. A small retrospective study (266) and a more recent publication (55) have shown that doing so can yield results (DFS and OS) identical to those achieved by administering a CHT-ERT combination. Since the period until postoperative relapse is often only very short, it is important to begin CHT-RT as soon as possible after surgery (55).

One advantage of doing so lies in the fact that VBT can be incorporated into the CHT schedule – the duration of treatment does not increase, nor does its level of toxicity (168). When CHT is contraindicated, VBT can be opted for instead as a minimum option for reducing the likelihood of local recurrence.

Overall, the NCCN Guidelines (175) allow CHT-RT to be taken into consideration in the adjuvant context. This recommendation is echoed in the GCIG Consensus (21), albeit with reference to the current lack of substantiated benefits. However, ultimately there are no hard reliable data that go against adjuvant CHT-RT. Most of the available analyses are based on very small samples, and there are no randomized studies in which statistically significant benefits for survival have been scientifically substantiated. This state of affairs is insufficient to be able to declare CHT-RT the postoperative standard. When CHT-RT is nonetheless opted for, the patients must be unequivocally informed of the toxicity involved, and that the procedure has not yet been proven to achieve more favorable outcomes, at least in terms of OS. After all, the broad DFS bandwidth revealed in the literature strongly suggests that disease often even progresses while CHT-RT is still ongoing. Deciding against adjuvant CHT-RT or opting for "mere" observation can thus not be classified as erroneous practice, regardless of LN status. In the USA, 39.9 % of patients receive no form of adjuvant therapy (201).

In stage III patients, assuming a purely observational stance is associated with poorer PFS and OS compared to standalone CHT. CHT-RT prolonged PFS only to an insignificant degree, and did not improve OS at all (54). A further larger analysis (201) concludes that postoperative CHT-RT is associated with longer OS.

Standalone adjuvant chemotherapy has not yet been proven to be prognostically beneficial when applied to patients with uterine carcinosarcoma who have undergone adequate surgery. Accordingly, it cannot be recommended as standard practice. Current (retrospective) studies do, however, suggest that adjuvant sequential radiochemotherapy can have a favorable impact on relapse free interval and overall survival in patients with carcinosarcoma confined to the uterus, regardless of nodal status. More recent data also suggest that combining chemotherapy with brachytherapy can achieve the same results as chemotherapy combined with percutaneous radiotherapy. However, the effectiveness of radiochemotherapy has yet to be reliably scientifically verified, so that it, too, cannot be recommended as standard practice. At the same time, not administering radiochemotherapy cannot be classified as erroneous practice. Patients who desire such therapy must be unequivocally informed of the lack of scientifically proven benefits and of the side effects that all forms of adjuvant therapy can involve.

According to retrospective studies, administering postoperative CHT or CHT-RT to patients who have undergone debulking surgery with or without complete tumor resection is associated with a longer PFI and improved OS (see above). Due to numerous biases and inexplicable findings, however, the authors of the respective studies themselves conclude that the observed benefits are far from proven, even when there is residual disease, and recommend that the results should not be overvalued (241).

The randomized GOG 150 study (269) compared the effects of postoperative CHT using ifosfamide plus cisplatin to those of whole abdomen ERT in stage I–IV UCS patients who had undergone optimal debulking leaving < 1 cm residual disease. The results suggest that CHT achieved superior results in terms of survival. However, the difference was not statistically significant. The downside is that the study lacks a nihil arm, and that two women in the ERT group died of irradiation-associated toxicity. Moreover, in each treatment arm, 4 patients with residual disease (4/5, 4/6) relapsed within a very short period of time, though it should be noted that only 3 cycles of CHT had been administered. This might have been insufficient to yield a measurable effect. The statistically unsubstantiated finding that applying postoperative CHT after cytoreductive surgery has a positive impact on survival can therefore at least be questioned. In a further study, 11 of 49 women underwent standalone pelvic or whole abdomen ERT with or without VBT, while the rest received CHT with or without RT. In 60.5 % of cases, patients received 6 cycles of paclitaxel plus carboplatin, or 4–6 cycles of ifosfamide plus cisplatin (as in the GOG 150 study) or another CHT schedule (149). CHT with and without RT achieved a 3-year PFI and 3-year OS of 35 % and 66 %, respectively, while the figures for the standalone RT arm were 9 % and 34 %. CHT with or without RT was thus superior to standalone RT, however not to a degree that was statistically significant. The study failed to clarify whether adding RT to CHT had a favorable impact in itself. Likewise, it remains unknown whether VBT had a therapeutic effect.

Against the backdrop of the retrospective and randomized EORTC 55874 and GOG 150 studies, it cannot be assumed that applying standalone postoperative RT to patients with advanced UCS, and who have undergone debulking surgery with and without residual disease, will be beneficial in terms of survival. However, the literature tends to lean in favor of the notion that postoperative CHT could potentially have a favorable impact on survival. Taking into consideration all available data pertaining to UCS and EC, and despite some contradictory statements and assumptions (241), postoperative CHT-RT could possibly be expected to yield the most beneficial results (100, 155, 160, 270).

The current NCCN Guidelines (175) state (2A recommendation) that performing postoperative CHT with or without targeted (!) RT can indeed be considered. There is major disagreement (category 3 recommendation) whether whole abdomen ERT, either alone or in combination with CHT, constitutes an adequate measure. Therefore, in light of the high toxicity of the measure and the fact that it has not yet been proven to have a beneficial prognostic impact, combining whole abdomen ERT with CHT would currently not be justifiable.

Targeted ERT with or without VBT appears to be a sensible option especially for localized tumors or patients who have undergone R1/2 resection on localized tumors. Standalone postoperative systemic therapy is indicated for patients who have undergone R1/2 resection for extensive disease, or for patients in whom multiple organs are metastatically involved, though it needs to be noted that, for these scenarios, too, adopting such a course of action has not yet been proven to be beneficial.

Since significant survival benefits have yet to be scientifically substantiated for all of the aforementioned measures, administering postoperative CHT or CHT-RT to patients who have undergone surgery on advanced CS cannot be deemed standard practice or procedure. Refraining from postoperative CHT or CHT-RT can thus not be regarded as erroneous practice, not least because doing so serves to maintain the few applicable chemotherapeutic options available for later use in the palliative context. This applies in particular when the resection margins are clinically or even microscopically free of residual disease (R0 resection).

At the same time, there are currently no data which definitively militate against postoperative CHT or CHT-RT. Given the lack of alternatives and the very poor prognosis with which UCS are generally associated, drawing on postoperative CHT or CHT-RT in adherence to the aforementioned restrictions would be a justifiable decision. However, patients must be unequivocally informed of the absence of proven benefits and the relatively high level of toxicity with which such treatment is unavoidably linked. Applicable regimens and schedules for CHT and CHT-RT correspond to those used in the adjuvant or palliative contexts.

In contrast, systemic therapy – if need be in combination with targeted RT – is clearly indicated when tumor residuals remain in threatening or risky locations.

The effect of performing ERT with or without VBT on PFI in the lesser pelvis as reported in all RT studies suffices as grounds for subjecting patients with residual disease in the lesser pelvis to targeted ERT and/or VBT, depending on the exact localization. The swift progression that such findings usually exhibit necessitates that

RT be administered as soon as possible once the surgical wounds have healed. If CHT-RT is planned, RT should be administered before CHT in these special cases (276).

The data situation is extremely poor regarding the use of adjuvant HT in patients with HR positive UCS. In the few accounts that have been described in the literature, adjuvant HT was not superior to "mere" observation in terms of median DFS and OS (265). Analogous to EC, adjuvant HT is not even indicated in cases of HR positive tumors. Administering tamoxifen therapy, as still sometimes occurs in practice, must be deemed obsolete, not least in light of the non-negligible role that tamoxifen plays in the etiology and pathogenesis of CS (cf. pathogenesis).

There are also no data available and no indications that pertain to the postoperative application of additive HT to patients with receptor positive advanced UCS.

Therapy proposal: standalone chemotherapy

Paclitaxel 175 mg/m^2 i.v. (day 1) + Carboplatin AUC 5–6 i.v. (day 1)	q 4 wk
Ifosfamide 1.5 g/m^2 i.v. (day 1–5) + Cisplatin 20 mg/m^2 i.v. (day 1–5)	q 3 wk
Ifosfamide 1.6 g/m^2 i.v. (day 1–3) + Paclitaxel 135 mg/m^2 i.v. (day 1)	q 3 wk

Therapy proposal: sequential radiochemotherapy

Paclitaxel 175 mg/m^2 i.v. (day 1) + Carboplatin AUC 5–6 i.v. (day 1) q 4 wk

Ifosfamide 1.2–1.5 g/m^2 i.v. (day 1–5) + Cisplatin 20 mg/m^2 i.v. (day 1–4) or 60 mg/m^2 i.v. (day 1), q 3–4 wk over 3 to maximum 6 cycles, reduction to 4 days ifosfamide in case of myelotoxicity, q 3–4 wk

Subsequent pelvic ERT with 45–54 Gy (or whole abdomen RT 45–50 Gy) with/without VBT of the vaginal stump with 3 × 5 Gy in 0.5 cm tissue depth or standalone VBT of the vaginal stump with 7 × 3 to 6 × 4 Gy in 0.5 cm tissue depth.

Therapy proposal: "Sandwich" radiochemotherapy

Ifosfamide 1.2 g/m^2 i.v. (day 1–5) q 3 wk over 3 cycles each before and after RT

There is no indication for subjecting patients with advanced CS who have undergone cytoreductive surgery to standalone additive pelvic or whole abdomen radiation therapy. Standalone radiotherapy or sequential radiochemotherapy could be adequate for cases in which localized tumors have been subjected to R1/2 resection. Radiotherapy must take the form of targeted (!) percutaneous radiation and/or brachytherapy in such cases. For patients who have undergone R1/2 resection on disseminated disease or multiorgan metastasization, standalone postoperative systemic therapy is indicated at most. No postoperative measures have yet been proven to yield significant improvements in survival. Therefore, administering chemotherapy or radiochemotherapy to patients who have undergone surgery on advanced uterine carcinosarcomas cannot be defined as standard practice, though there are no definitive data that militate against such an approach. Moreover, there is no evidence to suggest that assuming an observant stance until symptoms or threatening metastases arise impacts negatively on survival. Applicable treatment schedules are identical to those for chemotherapy or radiochemotherapy in an adjuvant or palliative setting. The rules pertaining to palliative therapy apply when metastases are in threatening or risky locations, or when tumor-associated symptoms arise. In cases in which there is residual disease in the pelvis, radiation therapy, if even planned, should be administered without undue delay.

There is no indication for adjuvant or additive hormone therapy, even when the hormone receptors are positive.

7.1.9 Primary radio-, chemo- and hormone therapy, approach in case of general inoperability

OS is distinctly poorer in patients with stage I UCS who undergo standalone RT than in those who undergo surgery (202). The most fundamental reasons for this difference are that recurrences of UCS are almost exclusively localized outside of the pelvis, that OS is determined by the distant metastases, and that there is usually already occult metastatic dissemination at the time of primary diagnosis. Therefore, there is no indication for performing primary RT on generally operable patients with operable UCS. Should a patient refuse surgery, the case should be treated as though the patient was generally inoperable. However, in such cases, patients must be insistently and unequivocally informed of the fact that subjecting operable UCS to primary RT has not yet been proven to be beneficial.

The therapeutic effect that can be expected from subjecting advanced UCS to primary RT is even poorer than that in cases of UCS that are confined to the uterus. No usable data exist in this regard to our knowledge. Therefore, there is no indication for administering standalone primary RT to patients with advanced tumors. Should the patient insist on primary RT, treatment should be approached as though she were generally inoperable.

Barely any information has been published on the use of neoadjuvant CHT or CHT-RT in patients with primarily inoperable UCS. Analogous to postoperative CHT, CHT-RT and palliative CHT, carboplatin plus paclitaxel or ifosfamide plus cisplatin would be the most suitable combinations for such an indication as well. There are accounts of cases in which neoadjuvant CHT effected remissions in advanced UCS, thus making them accessible to subsequent optimal debulking. Carboplatin plus paclitaxel (187), paclitaxel plus ifosfamide (185) and irinotecan plus cisplatin (239) were the combinations used. Accordingly, neoadjuvant CHT can be applied as a “therapy attempt” to achieve operability in exceptional cases, so long as the patient is in a good general state of health. CHT-RT would be another justifiable alternative in this regard. In light of the rapid rate of growth that UCS generally exhibit, and the short amount of time this leaves for further therapeutic intervention, applying neoadjuvant CHT could well turn out to have been too time-consuming if the tumor shows no response to systemic or actinic therapy. This risk should not be underestimated, given the generally low response rates. While doing so might well effect a remission, it remains questionable whether it has a favorable impact on prognosis. Studies have in fact revealed that undergoing neoadjuvant therapy prior to debulking surgery has no or only marginal influence on subsequent prognosis for UCS and OCS (187, 232). If neoadjuvant therapy is opted for regardless, the patient must be unequivocally and comprehensively informed of the potential side effects and that the measure has yet to be proven to be beneficial.

If there is a general contraindication against surgery in a case in which UCS is confined to the uterus or the pelvis, administering sequential CHT-RT (regimen see adjuvant CHT-RT) as a "therapy attempt" seems to be the most adequate alternative.

For cases in which CHT is also contraindicated, standalone RT consisting of pelvic ERT and VBT can be opted for instead. The question, whether or not subjecting advanced tumors that extend beyond the pelvis to whole abdomen ERT would be justified, currently remains unresolved. Such intervention can, however, be considered for cases in which the tumor has spread beyond the lesser pelvis, but remains confined to the abdominal cavity. Effects on OS have yet to be proven, but cannot be reliably ruled out entirely. Whole abdomen ERT might possibly achieve a temporary arrest of growth. Substantial gastrointestinal and hepatic toxicity needs to be reckoned with in the field of irradiation, which can ultimately result in death (269). For this reason, whole abdomen ERT should not be combined with CHT. The current NCCN recommendations classify said combination as inadequate therapy (174). Systemic therapy will most likely be the strategy of choice for generally inoperable patients with abdominally disseminated disease. The rules for palliative therapy apply in such cases.

As described below, palliative HT only achieves very poor results, which makes it seem unlikely from the outset that treatment with hormones will be effective in the neoadjuvant situation or in cases with contraindication against surgery. No data are in fact available to this end. Therefore, there is no indication for administering neoadjuvant or primary HT to patients with advanced disease or in inoperable UCS, even when their tumors test positive for hormone receptors.

Subjecting patients with operable, entirely uterine carcinosarcomas to primary radiotherapy is not indicated. Nor is primary standalone radiotherapy indicated for advanced tumors.

Neoadjuvant chemotherapy could be a conceivable option for reducing tumor size or for establishing local operability, though no survival-related benefits have yet been seen to result from such an approach, even when operability is indeed achieved by it. In light of the particularly poor prognosis with which advanced carcinosarcomas are generally associated, patients should rather be dissuaded from opting for neoadjuvant chemotherapy.

Applying sequential radiochemotherapy could be an option for cases of generally inoperable tumors that are confined to the uterus and the pelvis. Standalone percutaneous irradiation can be applied instead when chemotherapy is contraindicated. Whole abdomen radiation therapy can be considered for advanced tumors that extend beyond the pelvis without extraabdominal dissemination, but should not be combined with chemotherapy due to its high levels of toxicity. Alternatively, chemotherapy can be administered in accordance with the criteria and principles that pertain to the palliative situation. There are currently no data which suggest that the aforementioned measures impact on survival in any way whatsoever.

There is no indication for administering neoadjuvant or primary hormone therapy.

7.1.10 Aftercare, recurrences, metastases

Analogous to EC, aftercare and follow-up should be clinically guided by symptomatology via gynecological and general examination. Follow-up examinations should be scheduled every 3 mo in the first 2 years, every 6 mo for the next 3 years, and every 12 mo thereafter. TVS should be among the examinations routinely performed in this context, not least because it serves to identify local recurrences relatively early on. TVS should be complemented with color Doppler sonography when it yields ambiguous or suspicious findings, as the latter is well suited for visualizing whether a recurrent lesion is well vascularized (Fig. 7.1.18 (C)). The NCCN Guidelines recommend (2A recommendation) performing a CT of the abdomen and the thorax at the same intervals. It has not yet been proven that these measures serve to improve survival. The same applies for complex and laborious laboratory-chemical and technical examinations. More intensive diagnostic procedures, like PET-CT or MRI, should only be opted for when there is a respective clinical indication, when the aforementioned methods have revealed ambiguous or suspicious findings, or when the patient presents with symptoms (175). While PET-CT is indeed a meaningful and convincing method when indicated (203, 204), the benefits it can offer in terms of survival have still yet to be sufficiently validated.

It is contested whether measuring CA-125 levels should constitute an element of follow-up, not least because rising levels are not associated with any immediate therapeutic consequences. However, analogous to OCS, measuring CA-125 is deemed adequate for cases in which surgery is regarded as the primary option for treating recurrences and/or metastases (262). CA-125 is a well-suited means for monitoring palliative therapy (28). Overall, measuring the N/L ratio has also proven to be an appropriate measure for the aforementioned indications for measuring CA-125 (125). The N/L ratio is said to more accurately reflect recurrence and progression compared to CA-125 levels, and is generally a less laborious method (125). The cut-off value is at 2.12. Higher values could be suggestive of the presence of recurrence. Our own analyses (128) suggest that a cut-off value of 2.3 would be more appropriate. Notwithstanding, it still remains entirely unclear what the therapeutic consequences should be when asymptomatic patients are found to have positive CA-125 values or an elevated N/L ratio.

HRT with estrogens should be entirely refrained from in the very rare cases in which UCS are both ER and PGR positive. Patients with UCS that are receptor negative can be approached analogous to receptor negative EC and thus administered

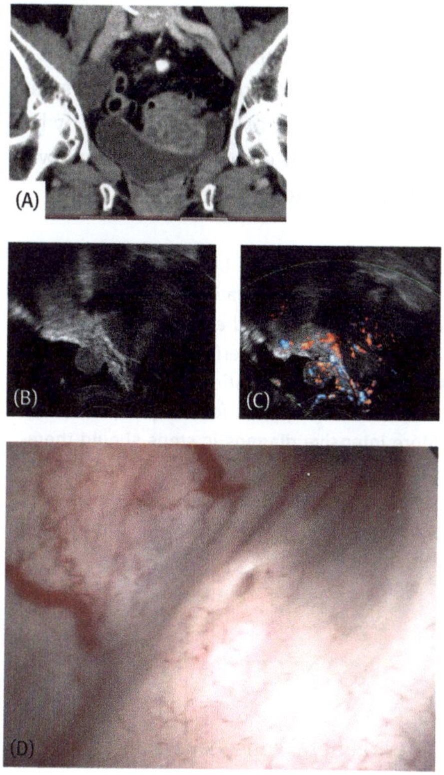

Fig. 7.1.18: (A) Coronal CT reveals a pelvic recurrence four months after radical hysterectomy with bilateral ovarectomy, pelvic and para-aortic lymphadenectomy and omentectomy in stage pT1b, N0, R0. The tumor has noticeably breached the bladder wall, predominantly on the left side; (B) said breach of the bladder wall is also nicely depicted in gray-scale sonography; (C) color Doppler sonography confirms both strong profusion in the tumor and that the bladder wall has ruptured. The strongly anechoic area at 12 o'clock, also visible as such in gray-scale sonography, is entirely without vasculature and corresponds to an area of necroses; (D) the superficial atypical vessels visualized in Doppler sonography were also clearly visible in cystoscopy, to the right of the left ureteral orifice.

HRT. There have as of yet been no accounts of negative consequences arising from doing so. Tamoxifen therapy must be deemed contraindicated, not least due to the non-negligible role that tamoxifen plays in the genesis of CS. In cases in which tamoxifen treatment is indicated due to synchronous or metachronic breast carcinoma, said treatment can be replaced with aromatase inhibitor therapy or treatment with GnRH analogues (in cases of younger patients) with the usual dosages.

Essential data pertaining to the diagnostic pitfalls and challenges associated with recurrences and metastases have already been presented and discussed in the context of macroscopic appearance and prognosis (see above). Overall, it must be reckoned with that recurrences and metastases will develop relatively swiftly after primary therapy. Distant metastases are already found at the time of primary diagnosis in 24–45 % of cases (4, 25, 107, 165, 274). Therefore, it is not rarely the case that the primary diagnosis is made on the basis of a metastasis. Dissemination into the entire abdominal cavity as well as to the lungs and liver is common. There is an account in which port site metastasis was the first verifiable indicator of disseminated metastatic disease in a patient who had undergone endoscopic HE (51). As is also the case for EC, metastatic dissemination to the vagina is not rare (Fig. 7.1.20 (A), (C)), while metastases are only exceptionally found in cerebrum and cerebellum (120). Brain metastases occur less frequently than they do in cases of endometrioid EC (173), which is likely a result of the fact that UCS are generally associated with shorter OS compared to EC.

CT (lungs in particular) and MRI are suitable imaging methods for diagnosing metastatic disease and its spread. Metastatic lesions in the liver are characterized by low attenuation in CECT and are thus easily discernible. They often present as lesions with weak overall attenuation surrounded by a strongly enhancing margin (113).

Analogous to endometrioid carcinoma, aftercare and follow-up should be clinically guided by symptoms via gynecological and general examination. Follow-up examinations should be scheduled every 3 mo in the first 2 years, every 6 mo for the next 3 years, and every 12 mo thereafter. Transvaginal sonography should be among the examinations routinely performed in this context. CT of the abdomen and the thorax can also be performed at the aforementioned intervals, though doing so has yet to be proven to improve survival. The same applies for complex, laborious laboratory-chemical and technical examinations. More intensive diagnostic steps should therefore only be taken when ambiguous or suspicious findings or symptoms present themselves. Measuring CA-125 levels and the neutrophil-lymphocyte ratio can be helpful in this regard.

Carcinosarcomas usually recur and metastasize very early. Extrapelvic dissemination is very frequent. CT and MRI are adequate diagnostic tools in this regard.

7.1.11 Surgical and postoperative additive treatment for recurrences and metastatic disease

For all of the measures described hereafter, there is general consensus that they constitute adequate therapeutic interventions that are based only on clinical experience or "lower-level evidence", except for some individual exceptional forms of intervention that are based on randomized studies. Since there are only few effective substances, response rates are poor, and PFI under or following palliative CHT is usually only short, it is sensible to first consider surgical therapeutic procedures. A good general condition and state of health is the fundamental precondition in this regard. Localized recurrences in the lesser pelvis and the abdominal cavity are the most common indication for surgery. Isolated pulmonary and liver metastases are also suitable for resection, so long as the abdominal cavity is free of disease. The Japanese guidelines also envisage that such an approach can be considered (169). A minimally invasive approach is a further option when there is more than one but fewer than five pulmonary or liver metastases. LITT, SIRT or chemoembolization are adequate options in such cases.

Only three cases of brain metastases have been reported in the literature. One patient survived for 25 mo following surgery plus RT, another who only underwent surgery died 38 days later, and the third woman died 2 mo upon initial presentation after having undergone no form of treatment at all (126). These experiences do not allow any therapeutic recommendations to be deduced. Notwithstanding, surgery plus RT might be an adequate strategy for patients with brain metastases when there are no other sites of metastatic involvement.

Subjecting patients with recurrent UCS to pelvic exenteration is apparently not associated with improved survival. Median OS for such cases is only 6 mo (123). In light of the fact that postoperative complaints only begin to decline after 3 mo, and that baseline quality of life is only returned to after 12 mo (205), the short OS of 6 mo with which pelvic exenteration is associated does not appear to suffice to constitute a beneficial effect.

There are currently no data that pertain to surgery in two compartments, for example lung and abdomen, on CS patients. Analogous to LMS for example, the preconditions that need to be fulfilled for such an approach would be that the patient is in a good general condition/state of health, that at least 6 mo have passed since previous surgery, and that it is probable that there will be no gross residual disease. In light of these factors, patients should first be subjected to extensive and precise imaging consisting at least of full body CT, preferably even PET-CT.

These restrictions do not apply to lifesaving symptomatic or palliative operations, for example such for alleviating ileus or facilitating urinary drainage.

Performing surgery on recurrent disease or metastases has the advantage that it puts off the onset of systemic therapy which itself is usually only effective for a short period of time. Essentially, however, there are no valid or reliable data which suggest that surgery achieves superior results to systemic therapy. Accordingly, CHT is bestowed the same degree of recommendation as cytoreductive surgery in the Japanese guidelines (169). Given the fact that such tumors are highly malignant and aggressive, surgery must ultimately also be understood as a highly palliative measure. Patients must be unequivocally informed of this state of affairs before undergoing any surgical intervention (Fig. 7.1.19).

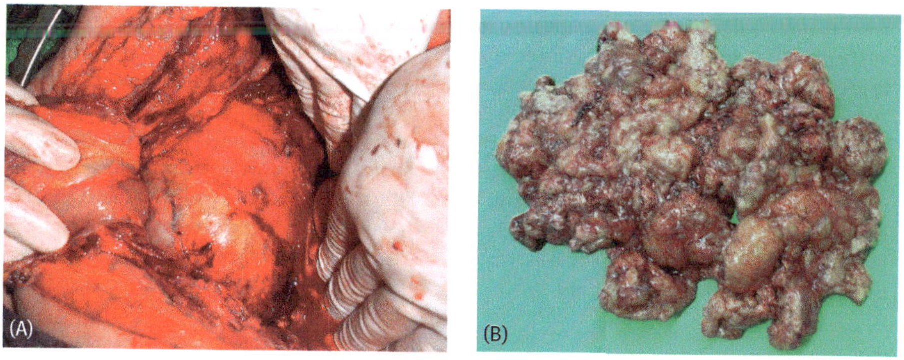

Fig. 7.1.19: (A) Encapsulated recurrence of carcinosarcoma that fills the whole pelvis, primary hysterectomy with pelvic and para-aortic lymphadenectomy performed 12 months prior; (B) Decomposing tumor depicted in (A), that was successfully fully clinically resected (max. cytoreduction); new recurrence after 4 months despite having been grossly disease-free and undergoing subsequent irradiation.

Subsequent targeted ERT can be administered in cases in which localized recurrences have been subjected to R1/2 resection. For patients who have undergone surgery on recurrences in the vaginal region, RT can take the form of standalone VBT.

The current data situation pertaining to RT and UCS gives rise to the assumption that additive RT will not have a beneficial impact on survival. The current NCCN Guidelines make the 2A recommendation to administer targeted RT with or without CHT, while there is major NCCN disagreement that additive whole abdomen ERT is appropriate (category 3 recommendation) (175).

The NCCN Guidelines make the category 2A recommendation to consider standalone postoperative CHT for patients with R1/R2 resection margins following surgery on large tumors.

No adequate literature has yet been published regarding the use of postoperative HT. At most, it could be considered for justifiable cases in which ER and PGR are positive. For all postoperative options and steps for patients who have undergone surgery on metastatic disease, please refer to what is stated in the context of surgery for primarily advanced UCS.

All of the interventions described above must be regarded as highly palliative modes of treatment. No data are available that could give insight into potential effects on survival. None of the aforementioned postoperative measures can be classified as standard practice, and refraining from them can thus not be deemed erroneous.

Since the effectiveness of palliative chemotherapy is very limited, a surgery-based strategy should be prioritized when there is localized recurrence/metastasis, under the precondition that the patient will be clinically disease-free thereafter. Surgery in two compartments can only be considered exceptionally. This equally applies to minimally invasive interventions in the vicinity of the lung and the liver. It has yet to be reliably and validly proven that surgery is in fact superior to palliative systemic therapy. Large recurrences, multiple organ metastasization and diffuse metastasization are all contraindications. The limitations do not apply to palliative or symptom guided operations used to alleviate acutely threatening situations (ileus, facilitating urine drainage) at short notice, so long as the patient's general condition allows it.

Patients who have undergone R1/2 resection on localized recurrences/metastases can undergo targeted (!) postoperative percutaneous radiotherapy, standalone brachytherapy, or a combination of the two. CHT can be considered when large parts of the surgical margins have residual disease (R1/2 resection), as can hormone therapy when there is estrogen and progesterone receptor positivity, though only in exceptional (!) cases. None of the stated measures can be defined as standard practice due to a lack of reliable data.

7.1.12 Palliative radio-, chemo- and hormone therapy, therapy with small molecules, supportive therapy

Barely any experiences have been reported that pertain to the application of standalone RT to recurrences and metastases of UCS. Standalone targeted RT is most likely indicated for localized (!) recurrences and distant metastases that are accessible to irradiation but not to surgery. Standalone VBT might possibly be sufficient for metastases in the vaginal region.

Analogous to carcinomas and pure sarcomas, severe pain from bone metastasis constitutes an important indication for the application of highly palliative ERT.

Notwithstanding, the patient must be informed that such course of action will only achieve a temporary remission or an alleviation of symptoms, without having any impact on OS.

Palliative CHT is indicated for cases of extensive recurrence, diffuse metastasization or findings that are not surgically accessible. No definitive statements can be made as to whether systemic therapy can be held in reserve when metastases diagnosed via imaging diagnostics are asymptomatic and in noncritical locations. Analogous to other malignancies of the female genital tract and the breast, due to the low response rates and the relatively short PFI that can be achieved during or after palliative CHT, as well as the fact that further chemotherapeutic options are limited, it appears to be a sensible option to put off systemic therapy until symptoms arise and/or until recurrences are localized in threatening or critical sites. In light of the generally poor prognosis, quality of life is the defining factor to which all interventions must be geared at this stage, and the toxicity of systemic therapy has a major impact on said quality of life. In any case, there are no valid and reliable data which suggest that beginning treatment immediately will offer any benefits in terms of OS. The authors of a systematic review on the use of palliative therapy in patients with uterine sarcomas and malignant mixed tumors appear to agree to such an approach, in that they only recommend CHT for symptomatic patients with inoperable disease (116). It is indispensable that patient to whom these circumstances apply are given comprehensive and informed counseling to this end.

The results from one study suggest that the sarcomatous component may be primarily responsible for the high degree of chemoresistance with which UCS are generally associated (188). These data could help to explain why UCS with a predominating epithelial component behave more like EC in terms of their chemotherapeutic response, while the chemotherapeutic behavior of UCS with a predominating sarcomatous component more closely resembles that of pure sarcoma.

Only very few cytostatic drugs are said to be effective for treating UCS in the palliative context. While effective when applied to patients with pure sarcoma, doxorubicin is rather not adequate for treating UCS in the palliative setting, neither alone (RR of 10–19 %) nor in combination with cyclophosphamide (116). Topotecan has been shown to achieve an RR of only 10 % (161). Ifosfamide, paclitaxel and cisplatin are regarded as the most effective monotherapeutic cytostatic agents, with RR of up to 36 %, 19 % and 18 %, respectively (49, 248). Ifosfamide is among the most rigorously researched cytostatic substances. A randomized GOG study compared a combination of ifosfamide plus cisplatin to a monotherapeutic ifosfamide regimen (234). Ifosfamide/cisplatin therapy was associated with an RR of 54 % and a median PFI of 6 mo, while the respective figures for the ifosfamide monotherapy arm were 36 % and

4 mo OS was identical in both arms, but ifosfamide/cisplatin had substantially higher toxicity. In a further phase II trial, alongside a high degree of toxicity, cisplatin plus ifosfamide achieved a median PFI of only 2–4 mo and an RR of only 33 % (198). In light of the substantial levels of toxicity observed, the authors of both studies recommend that this regimen should be used only in select individual cases (198, 234).

Another phase III study compared a combination of ifosfamide plus paclitaxel to ifosfamide monotherapy. With an RR of 45 %, a median PFI of 5.8 mo and an OS of 13.5 mo, combined CHT was clearly superior to monotherapy (RR 29 %, PFI 3.6 and OS 8.4 mo), though the rate of neutropenia and alopecia was higher (101). On the basis of these results, the ifosfamide-paclitaxel combination came to be declared the standard arm for future comparative studies at the time.

In one study, weekly administration of docetaxel plus gemcitabine as second-line treatment only achieved a PR of 8 %, but a CBR of almost 42 %. Median PFI was only 1.8 mo, with an OS of 4.9 mo (162). Bringing its high toxicity into the equation, docetaxel plus gemcitabine is an inadequate regimen for palliatively treating UCS.

Two studies examined the effectiveness of carboplatin plus paclitaxel in treating patients with advanced, metastasized and recurring UCS. This regimen achieved an RR of 54 % resp. 55 %, with tolerable toxicity levels. An additional 24 % of patients had SD, resulting in a CBR of 76 % (102, 196). However, while the 12 women covered in the smaller study (102) had a PFI of 12 mo, for the 46 patients in the larger study (196), PFI was lower, at only 7.6 mo, with an OS of 14.7 mo. Similar remission rates have been reported to have been achieved in recurrent and metastasized EC (156). In another study, administering carboplatin plus paclitaxel to patients with measurable advanced UCS achieved an RR of 62 %, a PFI of 7.9 mo and median OS of 21.1 mo Toxicity-related reductions in dosage were not necessary (132). Alopecia and fatigue are the most important toxicities associated with the carboplatin plus paclitaxel combination.

This combination has a number of advantages compared to ifosfamide plus paclitaxel or ifosfamide plus cisplatin. PFI and OS are superior, regimen-associated toxicity is less severe and easier to manage, and ultimately, carboplatin plus paclitaxel is used much more widely in practice (132, 196). More recent data suggest that, for stages I–IV, carboplatin plus paclitaxel is not only less toxic than ifosfamide plus cisplatin, but also achieves superior responses (median PFI 16.6 vs. 11.6 mo, med. OS 35.1 vs. 17.1 mo) (144). These results served to establish the carboplatin-paclitaxel combination as the gold standard in palliative therapy (102, 132, 203). Even heterologous UCS with a sarcomatous component consisting of RMS, deemed highly malignant, do not appear to respond any worse to paclitaxel plus carboplatin than homologous and other heterologous UCS do (150). If this treatment option is not available or applicable, treatment should first consist of ifosfamide monotherapy, especially when there is no acute pressure to achieve disease remission or when symptoms are only mild to moderate.

Primary application of the highly toxic combinations ifosfamide plus paclitaxel or ifosfamide plus cisplatin should only be considered when there is acute pressure to achieve disease remission, and only when administering carboplatin plus paclitaxel is contraindicated in the case at hand.

A feasibility study of sequential doublet chemotherapy consisting of 4 cycles each of carboplatin/doxorubicin followed by carboplatin/paclitaxel (carboplatin AUC 5, doxorubicin 50 mg/m^2, paclitaxel 175 mg/m^2) at 21 day intervals achieved remarkable results: the RR was 66.7 %, median PFI was 12 mo and OS was 19.6 mo, though the sample was rather small (11). The primary problem in the study was the incidence of neurotoxicity that sometimes made dosage reductions or the use of longer intervals necessary. No cardiac toxicity was observed. Some patients also underwent additional RT between the different CHT regimens. While the sample of patients to whom RT was applied was too small (within a small total sample as it is) to be able to assess its impact, interestingly, toxicity did not increase.

The promising RR mentioned above should not obscure the fact that median PFI for UCS usually does not exceed 2–8 mo, or up to 12 resp. 14 mo according to two retrospective studies. Accordingly, even when tumors do respond to CHT (sometimes impressively), they usually reprogress while still under CHT, or shortly thereafter (Fig. 7.1.20 (A)–(F))

More recent analyses suggest that UCS with a predominating epithelial component respond better to a combination of paclitaxel plus carboplatin (analogous to EC), while those in which the sarcomatous component is predominant show better responses when treated with cisplatin plus ifosfamide (188). Taking into account which tumor component is predominant in the individual case at hand can be helpful when faced with deciding between the two combinations when there is urgent pressure to achieve remission.

More recently, the combination of liposomal doxorubicin plus carboplatin has entered the focus of initial research studies and testing. A PR was observed in 57 % of the 7 women with recurrent UCS in two prospective phase II trials, with tolerable levels of toxicity. The studies yielded no assessable data regarding PFI (59, 134). In the DKSM database (128), a PR of at least 7 mo (end of follow-up) was achieved in 3 patients. Adding paclitaxel to this combination even yielded an RR of 62 % with a PFI of 8.2 mo and tolerable toxicity (193). If these results are confirmed in further trials, then liposomal doxorubicin plus carboplatin with and without paclitaxel should be preferred to therapy with ifosfamide plus cisplatin. Administering carboplatin plus liposomal doxorubicin served to achieve a further remission in some DKSM cases in which patients had undergone prior palliative CHT with carboplatin plus paclitaxel (128). Another study recounts an isolated case in which a temporary CR was achieved under liposomal doxorubicin monotherapy (40 mg/m^2 every 4 wks) (87). The DKSM (128) has had several cases of UCS in which the application of trofosfamide in a highly palliative context served to effect a long-lasting arrest in tumor growth. In one case (194), a relatively long period of SD was observed upon administration of trabectedin to a patient with OCS in whom prior CHT using paclitaxel plus carboplatin had failed. It can be assumed that this cytostatic agent will also be effective in UCS. Therefore, when tried and tested,

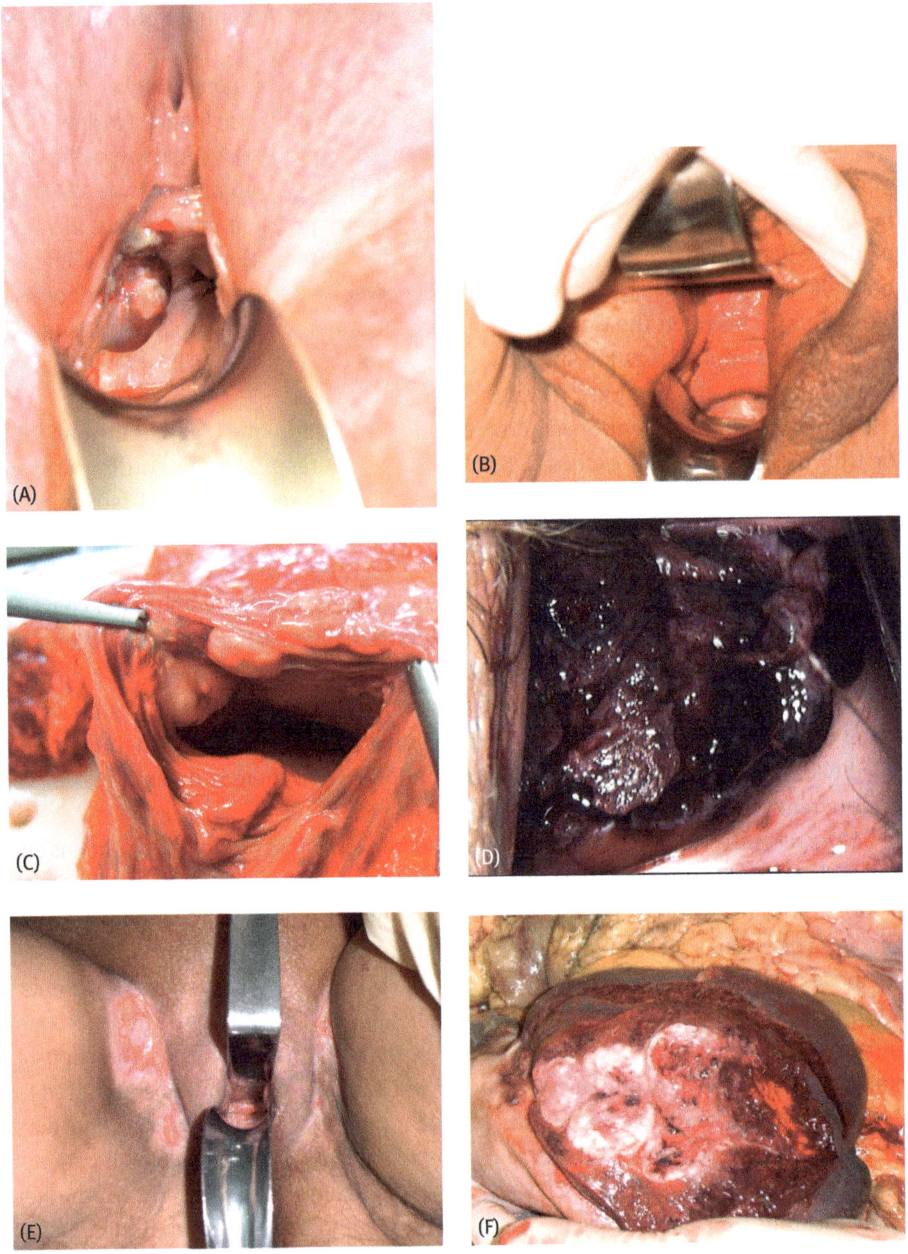

Fig. 7.1.20: (A) Vaginal metastases of a heterologous carcinosarcoma; (B) complete remission of the vaginal metastases depicted in (A) after 3 cycles of paclitaxel plus carboplatin; (C) a new vaginal recurrence with diffuse metastasization 5 months after complete remission, autopsy findings; (D) further case of carcinosarcoma that has infiltrated the vagina and that fills the entire lesser pelvis; (E) complete remission of the findings in (D) after 3 cycles of radiochemotherapy with severe skin- and hematotoxicity; (F) splenic metastases in the same patient, findings from autopsy 10 months after onset of palliative radiochemotherapy.

established CHT combinations have failed, therapeutic attempts using trofosfamide, liposomal doxorubicin or trabectedin (1.5 mg/m² over 24 h day 1, q 3 wk) can be opted for (see also OCS).

Therapy proposal

Monotherapy	Ifosfamide 2 g/m² i.v. (day 1–3)	q 3 wk
Polychemotherapy	Paclitaxel 175 mg/m² i.v. (day 1) + Carboplatin AUC 5 (day 1)	q 4 wk
	Ifosfamide 1.6 g/m² (day 1–3) + Paclitaxel 135 mg/m² i.v. (day 1)	q 3 wk
	Ifosfamide 1.5 g/m² i.v. (day 1–5) + Cisplatin 20 mg/m² i.v. (day 1–5)	q 3 wk
	PegLiposomal Doxorubicin 30–40 mg/m² 1 h i.v. + Carboplatin AUC 5–6 i.v. (day 1)	q 4 wk

Up to 44 % of UCS express ER, up to 19 % are PGR positive, and up to 24 % of UCS are both ER and PGR positive (cf. microscopic findings) (108, 265). Unfortunately, only very little is known about the exact distribution of the receptors between/in the epithelial and the sarcomatous components. Palliative HT would be at its most feasible if both the epithelial and the sarcomatous component expressed HR positivity. In any case, receptor status would need to be re-evaluated and positivity confirmed prior to palliative HT actually being administered. Where this precondition is met, when disease is not in a threatening or critical location, and when symptoms are mild to moderate, undertaking a "therapy attempt" using progestins can be considered (analogous to EC). Experiences with the use of MGA and MPA have been somewhat disappointing. In a study that also investigated the effects of palliative HT using MGA, within the sample of 6 UCS patients albeit with unknown receptor status, 3 patients showed no remission and 2 patients had a PFI of 3 mo. The last patient was treated with both MGA and tamoxifen and had a PFI of 37 mo (108). In contrast, a different, smaller study observed no response whatsoever (265). One publication recounts a case in which marked tumor shrinkage was achieved in a tamoxifen-associated UCS with unknown receptor status under letrozole treatment (2.5 mg daily) (267). These findings cannot be interpreted as constituting a recommendation to primarily subject recurrent tamoxifen-induced UCS to AI therapy. However, AI therapy could be adequate for treating a new progression in patients in whom progestin treatment had achieved an initial response. Analogous to EC (76, 99), administering the estrogen receptor blocker fulvestrant could be a sensible option in applicable cases. AI and/or fulvestrant are only used "off-label" in some countries. Nonresponsivity to HT constitutes an indication for CHT.

One study reports two cases in which a PFI of just over one year was observed under treatment with GnRH analogues, though it should be noted that hormone receptor status had not been assessed (117). The regulatory mechanism of GnRH analogues for tumor cells is apparently not dependent on the presence of steroid hormone receptor expression (71). Therefore, analogous to endometrioid EC and OC, GnRH analogues could be applied as ultima ratio when HT using steroid hormones or CHT has failed to achieve a response. This equally applies when the options mentioned above are contraindicated.

Therapy proposal

Progestins	Medroxyprogesterone acetate	150–200 mg/d oral
	Megestrol acetate	80–160 mg/d oral
AI	Letrozole	2.5 mg/d oral
	Anastrozole	1 mg/d oral
Estrogen receptor blocker	Fulvestrant	250 mg monthly i.m.
GnRH analogues	Zoladex	3.6 mg monthly

Joint expression of VEGF and EGFR in both the epithelial and the mesenchymal component of UCS qualify this neoplasm for treatment with antibodies that antagonize VEGF or with TKI. In a phase II study, administering the TKI pazopanib to pretreated women achieved no remissions at all, and SD for ≥ 6 mo with a median PFI of only 2 mo in 15.8 % of corresponding patients in the study (33). Better results could possibly be expected from combining pazopanib with CHT. Administering sorafenib, an inhibitor of multiple tyrosine protein kinases including VEGFR, to patients with advanced UCS, of whom some had already undergone prior treatment, yielded disappointing results (178). Verification of PDGFR expression in CS (2) provided the foundation for a phase II study with the TKI imatinib (106). With a median PFI of 1.8 mo and median OS of 5 mo, imatinib had practically no effect whatsoever on advanced UCS. In vitro analyses of Her-2/neu overexpressing uterine and ovarian cancer cell lines give rise to hopes that targeted immunotherapies could be developed for chemoresistant Her-2 positive tumors (96, 199). While thalidomide is known for its anti-angiogenetic activity (159), in one study, administering it to patients with UCS who have undergone prior CHT only yielded an RR of 4.4 % and a 6 month PFI of only 18 % (157). According to the authors, among other factors, selection biases and a too short treatment period were responsible for the poor results. A study initiated in 2008 (GOG-0232C) (5) on paclitaxel plus carboplatin and the PARP inhibitor iniparib had not yet been concluded at the time of writing.

Analogous to the other types of uterine sarcoma, given the very poor prognosis with which UCS is generally associated, opting for best supportive care instead of CHT or RT is a justifiable strategy that is also supported in the current NCCN Guidelines in the form of a 2A recommendation (175). Rendering supportive therapy appears to be the most adequate approach for cases of general dissemination with brain metastases.

Primary targeted radiotherapy is most likely to be indicated in cases in which local recurrences and distant metastases are surgically inaccessible. Since systemic therapy only has a limited effect, it could be sensible to administer it in the context of a "therapy attempt" before applying chemotherapy. Severe pain from bone metastasis constitutes an important indication for applying highly palliative radiotherapy.

There are no valid data which would suggest that undergoing systemic therapy is beneficial when tumor marker levels are elevated or when imaging has reliably revealed asymptomatic metastases at noncritical locations. In light of the short progression free interval with which all chemotherapeutic regimens and schedules are associated when applied to UCS, patients with mildly to moderately symptomatic noncritical recurrences/metastases should first undergo monochemotherapy. Disease progression during ongoing monochemotherapy and/or primarily severe or critical symptoms and/or acute pressure to achieve disease remission imply a need for polychemotherapy. Bearing the remission rate, levels of toxicity and progression free interval in mind, a combination of paclitaxel plus carboplatin should be regarded as the therapeutic regimen of choice.

Due to the very poor response rates that palliative hormone therapy achieves, it should only be considered exceptionally, for patients with receptor positive CS who are mildly symptomatic or whose recurrences are limited to non-threatening/noncritical locations. Administering progestins should be given consideration first. If progestin therapy is ineffective or if there is renewed disease progression, applying aromatase inhibitors or fulvestrant can be considered. GnRH analogues can be considered as ultima ratio if all other options have failed or when progestins, aromatase inhibitors or CHT are contraindicated. The results achieved by applying targeted substance-based therapies to carcinosarcomas have been disappointing overall.

Merely rendering best supportive treatment is a widely accepted therapeutic option when there is diffuse metastatic dissemination.

7.2 Extrauterine carcinosarcoma

7.2.1 Carcinosarcoma of the ovary

General, pathogenesis, pathologico-anatomical features

It is estimated that OCS account for no more than 4 % of ovarian carcinomas or 1 % of all malignant ovarian tumors (44, 86, 124). Within the DKSM materials database, the ovaries are the most common site of extrauterine CS (65 %), and 68.8 % of all ovarian sarcomas are CS (128). The majority of presenting women are postmenopausal, only 10.6 % are aged under 50 years, and 58.6 % are over 65 years of age. Average age is higher compared to patients with high-grade serous OC (82), but is slightly lower than for UCS (80). In contrast to UCS, white women are considerably more frequently affected than black women.

As is also the case for UCS, there appears to be a possible association with previous history of breast carcinoma and/or tamoxifen exposure (133). Genetic analyses have verified that OCS, like UCS, have a monoclonal histogenesis (112), which lends strength to the assumption that OCS generally result from a transdifferentiation of OC. Cases have been recounted in which OCS developed from a serous OC (78). This theory is further underlined by the concordant expression of p53 (78), or absence of such expression, in both tumor components. So-called collision tumors appear to be the exception among OCS. According to WHO Classification, OCS belongs to the endometrioid epithelial stromal tumors (136). Generally, staging for ovarian carcinoma is applied for OCS as well (268).

The ovaries constitute the most frequent extrauterine localization of carcinosarcoma. Sarcomatous dedifferentiation of a malignant ovarian carcinoma is the most likely pathogenesis.

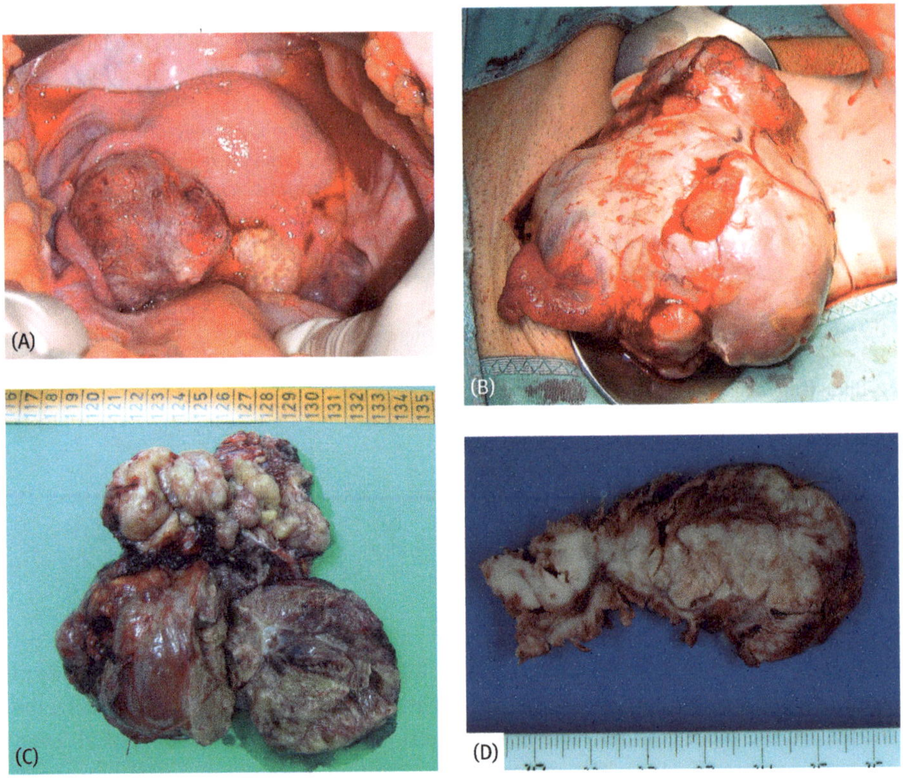

Fig. 7.2.1: (A), (B) Laparotomy findings of two ovarian carcinosarcomas with capsule ruptures; (C) opened specimen of (B). The solid components predominate macroscopically; (D) the ovary is almost entirely filled with a whitish-gray solid tumor, the numerous tissue-free voids are cysts and vessels that correlate to the anechoic regions in sonography.

About one third of OCS occur bilaterally (53). Macroscopically, they are not distinguishable from OC at first. The tumor capsule is usually breached relatively early on. Solid or cystic components can each predominate, though the former most frequently does so in practice (Fig. 7.2.1 (A)–(D)).

The microscopic aspect is that typical of CS. Hemorrhaging and necroses commonly occur. OCS and serous OC are also similar in terms of their early peritoneal dissemination. Like UCS, OCS can be homologous or heterologous, with a ratio of about 1 : 2–3 (7, 29, 98, 231). RMS or chondrosarcoma are the leading heterologous components; osteosarcoma and LS can also occur. In homologous OCS, LG-ESS and FS are most common. The epithelial component consists of endometrioid carcinoma in the majority of OCS. Further variations include serous, nondifferentiated, squamous cell, clear cell and in rare cases mucinous or neuroectodermal differentiations (183, 231). P53 mutations can sometimes be verified in both components (112). In one study, 66 % of examined OCS were ER positive, while all were PGR negative (79). Another research group found no hormone receptors at all (281). IHC findings pertaining to CK7, CK20, vimentin, CA-125 and CEA expression are consistent with the findings for UCS (131).

In OCS, one of the components – epithelial or sarcomatous – can be predominant. Serous and undifferentiated OC can metastasize as CS (7). Where both the primary tumor and the metastases express the same p53 mutation, either the primary diagnosis as OC might have been wrong, or the metastases might have transformed into OCS (77). Analogous to UCS, OCS metastases can be entirely sarcomatous or carcinomatous, so that it is not always possible to correctly deduce the primary tumor from them. Occasionally, only carcinomatous metastases are present. LN and intraperitoneal metastases are carcinomatous in 66 %, carcinosarcomatous in 32 %, and purely sarcomatous in 2 % of cases (7). Synchronous and metachronous OCS and UCS have already been discussed in the respective section on UCS above.

> Macroscopically, ovarian carcinosarcomas are practically undiscernible from ovarian carcinoma. The epithelial component usually consists of endometrioid carcinoma; the sarcomatous component can be homologous or heterologous. Ovarian carcinosarcoma can metastasize as sarcoma or carcinoma.

Clinical presentation, diagnostics, imaging, differential diagnostics

OCS can be difficult to discern from OC in terms of symptoms and clinical presentation. Depending on tumor size, relatively nonspecific symptoms include abdominal pain, nausea, dyspepsia, early satiety, constipation, and sometimes increased mictional frequency and weight loss (19). The features encountered in palpatory examination can be equally suggestive of OC. The diagnostic approach is the same as in cases in which OC is suspected. OC thus constitutes the most important DD.

A lower proportion of patients with OCS are found to have ascites compared with patients with OC (28), but when it is found, it has a higher incidence of being hemorrhagic than in carcinoma patients (40). The elevated CA-125 levels found in the majority of OCS (7, 28, 39, 40) could equally point to OC.

The pretherapeutic approach is laid out in the NCCN Guidelines Ovarian Cancer (174). As with OC, no effective screening methods exist for OCS.

Ovarian carcinosarcoma and ovarian carcinoma do not differ substantially in terms of symptoms, clinical features and diagnostics.

As with the macroscopic appearance of OCS, its sonographic appearance, too, does not appear to differ from OC in any particular or characteristic fashion. Therefore, when it comes to assessing a tumor's aggressiveness, it is generally adequate to orient oneself towards the characteristics of OC. Against this backdrop, the macroscopic and sonographic appearance can be highly pleomorphic, with larger cysts, solid elements with parietal papillary proliferations, hemorrhages and larger areas of necroses (Fig. 7.2.2 (A)–(E)). In OCS, however, the solid structures appear to be predominant, both clinically and in sonography (Fig. 7.2.2 (D), (E)). They are largely hyperechoic, though numerous anechoic cystic sections or voids remain, generating a pattern reminiscent of Swiss cheese. The ample small anechoic voids usually correspond to dilated vessels that are often characterized by hyperechoic margins or edges.

Doppler sonography shows increased irregular vascularization in the solid sections (Fig. 7.2.2 (F)). In addition to this high degree of vascularity, power Doppler imaging reveals low RI and pulsation index levels (210). Values of < 0.4 resp. < 1.0 are regarded as indicators for malignant activity. Due to their poor specificity, RI and pulsation index levels should not be the sole basis on which clinical discernments between malignancy and benignity are made (244). Ultimately, it is the summation of all of these sonographic findings that points to OCS, though without ruling OC out entirely. Solid structures with central arterial blood flow – also within individual nodules – are among the most consistent findings (14, 75, 250). A combination of the stated sonographic characteristics with little ascites, very rapid growth and a medical history of prior tamoxifen exposure can be a further indicator for OCS (Fig. 7.2.2 (A)–(C)).

CT is inappropriate for diagnosing histological types. Its primary purpose in this context is to determine disease spread. The CT image corresponds to the sonographic image, showing irregularly distributed solid and cystic elements and wide septa. In CECT, quick contrast agent absorption and subsequent homogeneous enhancement in the solid components, strong enhancement in the tumor wall and in the septa, and no enhancement in the necrotic tissue, are typical characteristics. These findings are, however, not exactly distinctive and can also be observed in OC (Fig. 7.2.3). It is interesting to note that, compared to OC, staging often reveals that metastases have already spread to the liver and the lungs (14).

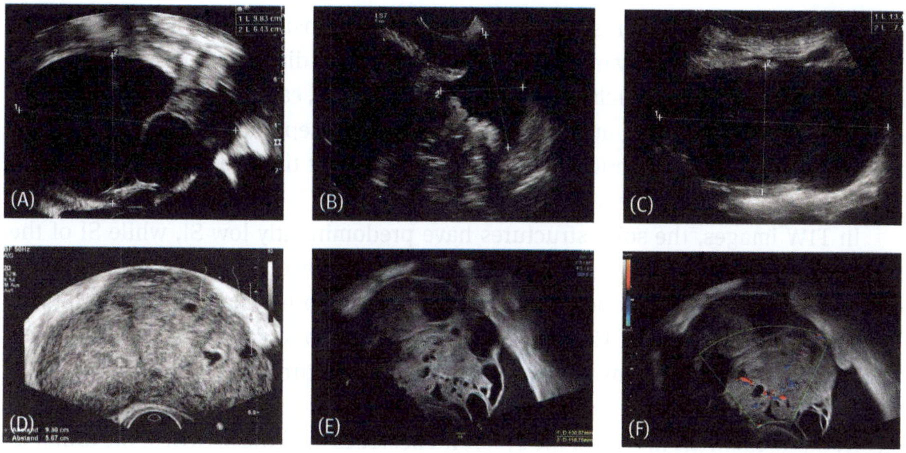

Fig. 7.2.2: Ovarian carcinosarcomas in sonography. (A)–(C) This tumor, that was equally pleomorphic on gross observation, exhibits all of the distinguishing features of carcinosarcoma in the different sectional planes, that can however also be found in ovarian carcinoma: predominantly cystic elements with septa of differing thickness (A), solid components with papillary growth into the cysts (B), extensive necroses with dull/weak echogenicity (C); (D) predominantly solid hyperechoic ovarian carcinosarcoma; (E) mixed solid-cystic carcinosarcoma, the solid components are hyperechoic, some of the anechoic voids constitute vessels, the cysts were also easy to discern macroscopically; (F) color Doppler sonography of (E) with noticeably irregular perfusion of the solid tumor components/septa.

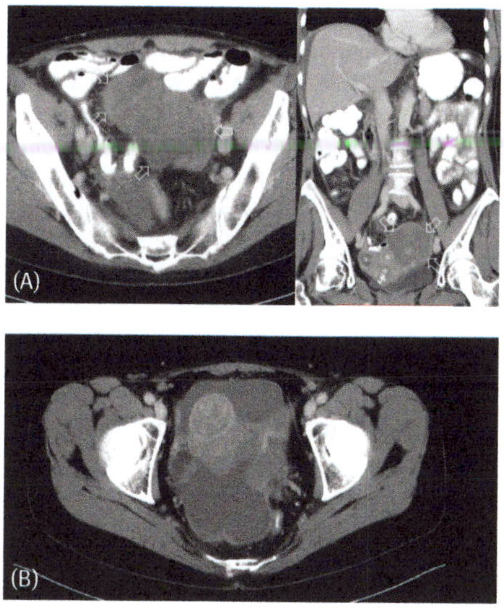

Fig. 7.2.3: (A) 60-year-old patient with ovarian carcinosarcoma. Abdominal CECT in the portal venous phase in the axial (left) and coronal (right) planes shows a nodular tumor (9 × 6 × 6 cm) with inhomogeneous enhancement originating from the left ovary (open arrows). The tumor ranges across the pelvic midline to the opposite side. The predominantly hypodense tumor components corresponded to extensive necroses in the surgical specimen. An incidental uterine myoma (stars) is recognizable in the right image; (B) this image of a further caudally located axial plane shows an ovarian tumor that fills the entire lesser pelvis, together with the myomatous uterus.

MRI can be indicated when sonographic findings are insufficient for predicting benignity or malignancy in ovarian tumors. A specific OCS diagnosis, and the definitive delineation from OC that such a diagnosis would require, cannot be achieved through MRI. Differently sized solid masses, cystic regions with septations exceeding 3 mm in thickness, necroses and noticeable invasion of adjacent tissue are regarded as morphologic criteria suggestive of a malignancy (75).

In T1W images, the solid structures have predominantly low SI, while SI of the fluid in the multilocular cysts can range from hypointense to variable intermediate, depending on its protein content. Hemorrhages on the other hand are characterized by high SI. By contrast, in T2W images, the SI of the solid components is predominantly high, which makes invasions of neighboring structures and tissues more visibly discernible than in CT images. T1WC images are often necessary in order to be able to clearly distinguish the high SI of the cysts and necroses from the high SI of the tumor in T2W images. T1WC shows a quick heterogeneous enhancement in the tumor wall, the solid components and the septa. Enhancement in the peritoneal metastases is delayed due to their slower absorption of the contrast agent. In T2W images, homogeneous hyperintensity makes ascites easy to distinguish (14, 191, 237).

PET-CT can be helpful for deciding whether or not to perform surgery for recurrent disease. It is not suitable for detecting small peritoneal implants, because respective findings can be concealed by intestinal metabolic activity (14). For individual cases, it appears to be more appropriate than CT for monitoring the efficacy of palliative therapy (87).

Ovarian carcinosarcoma barely differs from ovarian carcinoma in terms of its sonographic appearance and features. Solid structures with central arterial blood flow, also in the wide septa and individual nodules, are the most consistent findings. Likewise, there are no specific characteristics or findings in CT and MRI that allow ovarian carcinosarcoma to be reliably discerned from ovarian carcinoma. Likewise, the malignancy criteria that are characteristic for ovarian carcinoma also apply to ovarian carcinosarcoma. PET-CT can be useful as a means for monitoring palliative therapy.

OC is the most important clinical DD. In large tumors, one of the components might be overlooked entirely under histological examination, resulting in the OCS being misdiagnosed as carcinoma or pure sarcoma. Since OCS metastases can consist only of sarcomatous or only of carcinomatous cells, it is not always possible to correctly deduce the primary tumor from them. This risk is particularly pertinent when the diagnosis is based on a frozen section analysis. This is a typical pitfall, one for which the pathologists are not to blame as the sample they have to base their decision on is very small.

Histologically, immature teratoma and poorly differentiated Sertoli–Leydig cell tumors are possible DD. These, however, more typically occur in children and younger women. The latter are also often accompanied by signs of androgenization. Positive inhibin and/or calretinin expression is a clear indication for a Sertoli–Leydig cell tumor (42). Ovarian LG-ESS with sex cord-like elements and endometrioid carcinoma with reactive spindle cell stroma can have a histologic appearance similar to that of OCS (183). In endometrioid spindle cell carcinoma, the epithelial component is usually better differentiated, and there is a clear boundary between the epithelial and supposed sarcomatous components (42).

Ovarian carcinoma is the most important clinical differential diagnosis. The risk of histologically misdiagnosing carcinosarcoma as carcinoma or pure sarcoma is particularly great when diagnosis is based on a small amount of tissue (frozen section) or on the metastases only. Immature teratomas and poorly differentiated Sertoli–Leydig cell tumors exhibit a similar histologic picture.

Course, prognosis, operative, systemic and radiogenic therapy

Analogous to UCS, patient age and stage of disease are unfavorable prognostic factors for OCS (80, 189, 200). OCS is a highly aggressive malignancy – 61.6 % of patients present with stage III and stage IV at initial presentation (86). Advanced stage of disease at the time of primary diagnosis can partially be explained by the fact that many patients remain asymptomatic for a long time (80). Five-year OS among all OCS is only between 15–28.2 %, median OS has been measured to range from 6.4–18 mo (28, 80, 200). Stage I OCS have a 5-year OS of 73.4–83 %, while for stage III, it is 0–24.6 % (28, 200).

Median stage-specific OS periods are 75 mo, 5.1 mo, 8.5 mo and 5.5 mo for stages I, II, III and IV, respectively (28). The mortality risk for OCS patients is 76 % higher than for patients with high-grade serous OC (37, 200). Five-year and median OS in all OCS are significantly poorer compared to UCS (80). In 72.3 % of OCS patients, the abdominal cavity has already been affected at the time of initial diagnosis. However, stratification according to disease spread (e.g. to the abdominal cavity) shows that prognosis is worse for the uterine entities. Other studies suggest that prognosis is largely identical (189). Prognoses for heterologous and homologous OCS appear to be identical (28, 39, 40, 91, 98, 138).

LN were involved in 18–38.8 % of all cases under examination (80, 145). Systematic LNE in early stages and optimal cytoreduction in advanced stages are said to be associated with a more promising prognosis. In a recent study (145), pelvic LN involvement, but not para-aortic LN involvement, was found to be associated with poorer survival, while LNE had no impact on survival.

Metastatic spread is usually primarily intraperitoneal. The lymph nodes are less frequently involved (231). Contrary to OC and analogous to UCS, metastases do not remain limited to the peritoneum for long, instead also infiltrating the deeper structures early on. Therefore, extensive invasion of the abdominal wall is not uncommon (Fig. 7.2.4).

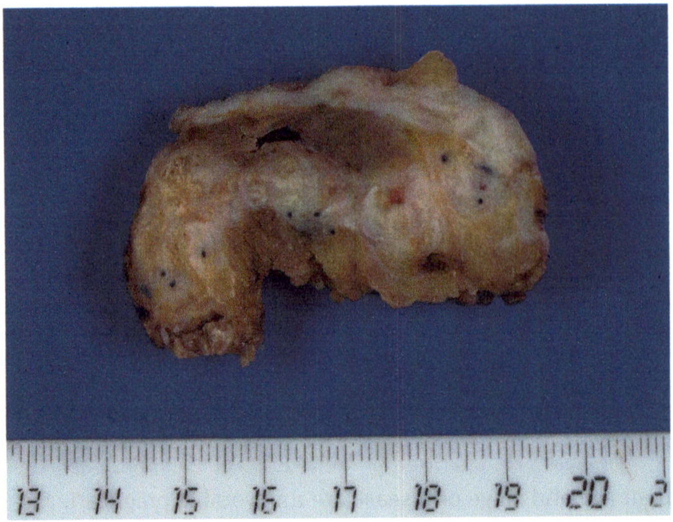

Fig. 7.2.4: Infiltration of the abdominal wall by an ovarian carcinosarcoma. Such findings are also often made pertaining to uterine carcinosarcomas.

Pulmonary metastases appear to occur more frequently than with OC (14, 39). Analogous to UCS, in OCS patients, too, the metastases are predominantly carcinomatous, and only rarely consist of the sarcomatous component (7, 231). Performing a frozen section procedure on intraperitoneal metastases can therefore result in a primary misdiagnosis. Normal preoperative CA-125 values (230) and positive ER expression (83) are said to be associated with a more promising prognosis.

The mortality risk for patients with ovarian carcinosarcoma is 76 % higher than for patients with serous ovarian carcinoma. Ovarian carcinosarcomas have a prognosis even worse than that of uterine carcinosarcomas. Nodal involvement worsens prognosis even further, and lymphadenectomy does not serve to improve the situation. Pulmonary metastasization apparently occurs more frequently than in patients with ovarian carcinoma.

Most OCS are clinically diagnosed as OC at the time of primary surgery. Accordingly, a definitive diagnosis is regularly only reached postoperatively or following frozen section diagnostics. The obstacles and problems associated with frozen section diagnostics have already been referred to in the context of UCS. When OCS has been definitively diagnosed as such, the current GCIG Consensus (21) and NCCN Guidelines Ovarian Cancer (174) recommend (2A recommendation) the same surgical approach as for OC, namely complete staging via vertical midline laparotomy. The abdominal cavity is opened, thoroughly visualized and palpated, and present ascites removed for cytological testing. If no ascites are found, administering peritoneal lavage is the most suitable method for gathering cellular material. Where there is no extraovarian metastasization, multiple proper biopsies should be performed on the peritoneum of the pelvis, the paracolic gutters and the diaphragm. TAH should then subsequently be performed together with BSO. In doing so, the uterus (including the cervix) and the adnexa should be removed as a self-contained specimen. Perforation of the tumor must be avoided at all costs. After at least infracolic omentectomy, systematic para-aortic and pelvic LNE constitute the final steps. The German S3 Guidelines (140) OC (deutsche S3-Leitlinien Ovarialkarzinom) recommend the same approach, albeit without making explicit reference to OCS.

The NCCN recommendation (174) is a product of consensus and is based only on lower-level evidence. The benefits of performing complete staging have yet to be proven, so following the recommended approach cannot be defined as standard practice. For OCS that are confined to the ovaries, performing TAH with BSO, and an omentectomy where appropriate, is widely accepted as the minimal surgical option. Additionally, selective LNE should be performed and the diaphragm and paracolic gutters should be biopsied (204). In practice, randomized studies have yet to verify beyond doubt that surgical measures beyond TAH with BSO can be beneficial in cases in which OCS are limited to the adnexa. Currently, no further consequences can be deduced from positive intraperitoneal cytological findings.

Studies suggest that, in early OC, complete surgical staging is associated with more favorable DFS and OS than incomplete staging (5-year PFI 79 % vs. 61 %, 5-year OS 89 % vs. 71 %) (249, 252). For OC confined to the ovaries, the necessary extent of the LNE procedure remains uncertain so that, currently, removing at least 10 LN through selective LNE is recommended (253). Whether or not these data also apply to OCS remains unclear. SEER analyses suggest that an LNE is associated with a significant improvement in OS in OCS patients, and the risk of mortality was 34 % lower than without an LNE (80, 200). Due to uncertainties pertaining to their collection of the data, the authors refrained from making any definitive statement as to whether or not this is in fact a therapeutic effect (80). In a recent study, pelvic and para-aortic LNE apparently had no impact on survival (145). The GCIG Consensus, too, is also rather vague when it comes to pinpointing the advantages of LNE (21). LN findings play a rather subordinate role in decisions pertaining to adjuvant therapy. In this context, reference should be made to the discussion about the benefits of LNE for UCS patients in this context. Interestingly, LNE is only performed on 41 % of OCS patients, while THE is carried out in virtually all cases (80, 200).

The NCCN Guidelines recommend that, where an OCS is detected after TAH with BSO or exclusive BSO, complete staging should be performed retroactively (174). Doing so is, however, not indicated due to the lack of a corresponding scientific basis.

Minimally invasive techniques are not categorically ruled out in cases in which OCS is limited to the adnexa, so long as they pose no hindrance to staging (174). For aggressive OCS, the NCCN Guidelines make no indication regarding fertility-preserving surgery (like unilaterally retaining a tumor-free adnexa, for example). Contrary to OC, this also applies to stage IA disease (21, 174). The minimal option should at least entail

TAH and resection of the remaining adnexa. SAH can be deemed appropriate under certain exceptional circumstances (174). Patients who choose organ-sparing surgery must be informed of the extremely high risk of recurrence that needs to be understood against the backdrop of an already very poor prognosis.

Maximal (or at least optimal) cytoreduction/debulking is recommended for stages II to IIIC (39, 174, 204). Depending on the patient's general condition, the following operations can be performed to achieve this goal: pelvic exenteration, bowel resection, peritoneal surface stripping (including diaphragm), splenectomy, partial liver resection, cholecystectomy, partial gastrectomy, partial resection of the urinary bladder and the uterus, distal pancreatectomy and appendectomy. For patients with extrapelvic tumor nodules smaller than 2 cm in diameter, undergoing additional bilateral pelvic and para-aortic LNE is recommended (174).

Definitions of what constitutes optimal debulking vary in the literature – no visible residual tumor (39), a largest residual tumor nodule with a maximum diameter equal to or less than 1 cm (138, 200, 223) or than 2 cm (28, 40, 50). This state of affairs severely complicates any analysis or joint evaluation of these entirely retrospective studies. Nonetheless, debulking in accordance with the latter two definitions is associated with a significant improvement in OS, and is regarded as the most important prognostic factor (28, 50, 98, 145, 200, 223, 229). Patients with only microscopic residual disease had a median OS of 47 mo. By comparison, patients with optimal debulking and microscopic residual tumor had an OS of 18 mo, and in patients with suboptimal cytoreduction, OS was 8 mo (200). In a different study, patients with residual tumors < 2 cm had a median OS of 14.8 mo and a 2-year OS of 39 %, while for patients whose residual tumors exceeded 2 cm, the figures were 3.1 mo ($P < 0.001$) and 0 %, respectively (28). Due to the generally poor prognosis for OCS in stages II and III, whether or not debulking to < 1 cm in fact leads to better results than < 2 cm, remains a disputed issue. Further research and studies have shown that a cytoreduction to < 2 cm had no positive effects on OS in 5 of 16 cases (40, 50, 53), or there was only an association with OS but not with PFI (40). A recent study covered tumors in stages II–IV and differentiated between patients with no visible residual disease, with ≤ 1 cm of residual disease, and > 1 cm of residual disease. Median PFI (29, 21 and 2 mo) and median OS (57, 32 and 11 mo) varied significantly between the groups (58). These differences remained when only stage III was considered.

In many cases, however, achieving maximal or optimal cytoreduction is not technically possible (138). Maximal debulking is achieved in 55 % of stage I/II and in 45 % of stage III/IV patients, and optimal debulking in 57–81 % of cases across all stages (39, 40, 138).

Upon critical review and assessment of all of these studies, many questions remain unanswered and there are numerous biases. In some cases, there was no stratification into the prognostically differing stages II and III or within stage III. Stage IIIC covered cases ranging from a single 2 cm large epicenter to massive dissemination. Therefore, it cannot be ruled out that optimal cytoreduction was primarily achieved in those cases with a smaller tumor burden and a corresponding more favorable initial prognosis. In some cases, there were no recognizable benefits for higher staged disease (222). The studies also fail to consider the type and duration of postoperative CHT sufficiently (if at all), and no reference is made to additional LNE and its respective benefits in terms of PFI and OS. Only one study (40) has given at least partial consideration to these issues. Stage I/II patients had a post-debulking PFI of 9.7 mo and median OS of 50 mo, compared to only 2.7 and 25 mo, respectively, in patients with advanced stage disease (stages III/IV). Postoperative CHT with paclitaxel and carboplatin resulted in a statistically longer PFI and OS compared to other regimens. Taking all studies together, it can currently be concluded that being aged over 60, advanced stage disease (III/IV), submaximal debulking (and suboptimal debulking with reservations), and omitting consecutive paclitaxel-platinum CHT are factors that result in poorer PFI and OS (39, 110).

For stage IIIB disease, the current NCCN Guidelines recommend systematic para-aortic and pelvic LNE in addition to cytoreduction. When there are extrapelvic metastases > 2 cm in their greatest dimension, only the enlarged LN should be resected if technically possible (174).

In summary, despite numerous unresolved questions, patients with stage II disease or higher should undergo maximal debulking (at the very least optimal debulking) and LN sampling, so long as this course of action can be reasonably expected of the patient and is justifiable in light of disease spread. This approach cannot, however, be defined as standard practice, as the effects on PFI and OS have not yet been substantiated through validated scientific studies. Due to the poor overall prognosis for OCS, extreme surgical operations (exenteration) should be subject to thorough prior consideration.

> For ovarian carcinosarcoma, right from stage IA, total abdominal total hysterectomy with bilateral salpingo-oophorectomy, pelvic and para-aortic lymphadenectomy, omentectomy, peritoneal biopsies and peritoneal cytology are recommended as an NCCN 2A recommendation. The advantages, in terms of overall and remission-free survival, of performing surgeries beyond total hysterectomy and salpingo-oophorectomy in patients with entirely ovarian carcinosarcoma, have not yet been confirmed through valid data. There is, however, consensus that the aforementioned additional surgical methods should nonetheless be performed so long as they can be expected of the patient given her overall condition. They cannot, however, be declared standard procedure as their recommendation is based solely on retrospective data. Therefore, following a minimalist strategy involving total abdominal hysterectomy with bilateral salpingo-oophorectomy and selective lymphadenectomy, where appropriate, can be regarded as a justifiable therapeutic option.
>
> There is consensus that patients with stage II disease and above should undergo maximal cytoreductive surgery (at least no gross residual disease), if need be in combination with selective lymphadenectomy of enlarged lymph nodes. While maximal debulking with and without lymphadenectomy is likely to have a favorable impact on overall survival, said impact has not been reliably substantiated beyond doubt in adequate studies. Therefore, such course of action cannot be defined as standard practice. Due to the lack of alternatives, it should nonetheless be opted for if it can be reasonably expected of the patient.

There are as of yet no significant or scientifically meaningful studies that investigate the application of postoperative RT with OCS patients (221). The NCCN Guidelines make no such recommendation (174) and, according to the GCIG Consensus (21), no benefits can be expected from RT. Whether or not applying tumor-directed RT to tumor residuals within the pelvis has an influence on PFI is not known. It is, however, thinkable that tumor-directed RT could well have an effect on delimited, localized tumors (as for UCS as well), so that tumor-directed ERT or VBT can be considered in exceptional cases (152).

Where a decision is made in favor of postoperative RT, the patient must be unequivocally informed of the lack of scientifically proven benefits that this course of action has for PFS and OS.

The benefits of applying adjuvant CHT in cases of stage I OCS in which R0 resection has been performed are as of yet unclear, or, put differently, could not yet be confirmed in randomized studies. The core problem in this regard is that, analogous to UCS, the response rates for all tested cytostatic drugs and their different combinations have been shown to be poor (see palliative therapy). Consequently, an ideal CHT regimen could not yet be defined (28, 80, 86, 110). The case samples covered in research studies on postoperative CHT almost unanimously include OCS of all stages (36, 98, 222, 243) or only advanced stages (28, 40, 50, 138, 223). According to the respective authors, this limits the degree to which one can conclude without any doubt that the suggested benefits of postoperative CHT also apply to OCS that have been completely resected. Nor have the authors of the most recent SEER analyses (80, 85, 200) been able to make any statement on the effectiveness of adjuvant CHT, even despite the large volume of data at their disposal. The current Cochrane review also comes to the conclusion that positive effects of adjuvant or postoperative CHT, RT or CHT-RT on life expectancy or quality of life have yet to be substantiated in adequate studies (221). This opinion is also mirrored in the current GCIG Consensus (21). The current NCCN Guidelines recommend (2A recommendation) applying postoperative CHT using chemotherapeutic agents that are also used in cases of EC, at all stages of disease. Overall, there is wide agreement that, in any case, a platinum-based CHT should be applied – combinations of platinum-based compounds with paclitaxel appear to be most promising (28, 39, 40, 53, 110, 145). It currently cannot be definitively pinpointed whether combining a platinum-based drug (usually carboplatin) with paclitaxel, or a combination of cisplatin plus ifosfamide is more favorable in terms of survival. There is, however, agreement that the latter combination is associated with higher levels of toxicity (145).

No data are available regarding the use of adjuvant HT in the context of OCS, so that – as is the case with UCS as well – it is not indicated even when the HR are positive.

The NCCN Guidelines generally recommend postoperative chemotherapy right from stage I. The data situation is particularly bleak regarding completely resected stage I tumors, and provides no evidence of beneficial effects. Though there is consensus that adjuvant chemotherapy be administered to patients with stage I disease, doing so cannot be defined as standard practice. Accordingly, refraining from adjuvant chemotherapy cannot be regarded as erroneous. There is also consensus, both in the NCCN Guidelines and in numerous retrospective studies, that any form and degree of cytoreductive surgery performed on patients with stage II disease and above should be followed up with postoperative chemotherapy. However, neither chemotherapy nor chemoradiotherapy in this context can be defined as standard practice, because respective adequate studies are still lacking. Thus, omitting such interventions cannot be deemed erroneous practice. Any chemotherapy schedule in this context should be platinum-based. A combination of carboplatin plus paclitaxel is most likely recommendable.

No data are available pertaining to the use of primary or neoadjuvant RT in patients with OCS.

Some publications have reported that primary or neoadjuvant CHT achieved disease remissions that allowed subsequent interval debulking surgery. Carboplatin plus paclitaxel (88, 187), paclitaxel plus ifosfamide (185) or irinotecan plus cisplatin (239) were the combinations administered. A randomized study on neoadjuvant platinum-based CHT and OC, which also included some cases of OCS, found that women presenting in stage IIIC with low tumor burden were more likely to benefit from primary cytoreductive surgery. For patients with stage IV and extensive stage IIIC disease, the outcomes following prior neoadjuvant CHT were more favorable (259, 261). Whether these data also apply to the small sample of OCS covered in the study cannot be definitively stated. Even where remission occurred, it remains questionable whether or not it had any positive effects on prognosis. In fact, neoadjuvant therapy prior to debulking surgery has been shown to have little to no influence on subsequent prognosis (187, 241). Moreover, poor responsivity of CS to CHT could well worsen the operative situation even further. The histological pattern of metastatic spread after neoadjuvant CHT (with combinations that are also effective with EC) indicates that the epithelial component was more responsive to the CHT (7) and that further prognosis is dictated by the remaining sarcomatous component. Neoadjuvant CHT should, therefore, only be considered as a means for achieving operability in exceptional cases. When this form of treatment is nonetheless opted for, the patient has to be unequivocally informed of the possible side effects and of the fact that benefits for survival have not yet been proven to result. The CHT combinations that should be considered are the same as those that are primarily used in the adjuvant and palliative contexts.

There is no indication for administering primary or neoadjuvant HT.

Primary or neoadjuvant chemotherapy as a means for achieving optimal cytoreduction should only be considered in exceptional cases in which the tumor and/or the patient are inoperable. These measures are unlikely to improve prognosis. There is no indication for primary or adjuvant radiotherapy or hormone therapy.

Aftercare, recurrences, metastases and their treatment

In general, regarding aftercare and follow-up, the same criteria apply as for UCS, as do the surgical therapeutic measures already described in the context of UCS and advanced OCS. The very poor overall prognosis with which OCS are associated is inevitably connected with the fact that recurrence and metastasization occur very early.

Validated research data suggest that rising CA-125 levels are not to be treated as an indication for administering palliative therapy for OC, as there are no data which suggest that such a therapeutic approach has a positive influence on OS (207). There is no reason to assume that these findings should not be considered for OCS as well. Measuring CA-125 is deemed sensible when surgery is regarded as the primary option for treating recurrences or metastases (262). Measuring CA-125 can also be a suitable means of palliative therapy control in cases that are difficult to assess and evaluate radiologically and clinically (28). Generally, measuring the N/L ratio, too, has proven to be appropriate for this purpose (cf. aftercare UCS) (125).

No particular surgical or postoperative additive therapeutic approaches or methods have yet been validated as adequate for treating patients with recurrent and/or metastasized OCS. The poor prognosis with which recurrent and metastasized OCS are associated, as well as the very rapid growth such tumors exhibit, serve to make respective surgical interventions largely inadequate or inapplicable. Generally, one can refer to the data that pertain to UCS in this context.

Regarding surgery and postoperative additive therapy for recurrences and metastases, reference can be had to the criteria and data presented for uterine carcinosarcoma in this context.

While effective in cases of pure sarcoma, doxorubicin has been shown to achieve a very low RR of only 4.7 % in OCS (164). At 17.9 % (233) and 20 % (243), respectively, the RR achieved with ifosfamide monotherapy and cisplatin monotherapy barely differ from those for UCS. A larger study investigated the effects of platinum-based CHT combinations on measurable lesions, and measured an RR of 25 % (CR 8 %, PR 17 %), an NC rate of 17 % and a PD rate of 58 %. OCS showed no response to nonplatinum-based CHT regimens (28). Further studies have mostly covered fewer patients, and found slightly higher RR for platinum-based CHT up to 40 % (median OS 8.7 mo) (98) and 33 % (median OS 8 mo) (36). An analysis (152) of all CHT studies known at the time found that RR for platinum-based regimens were clearly higher than for nonplatinum-based CHT. A case control study measured a surprisingly high RR of 62 % (CR 56 % and PR 6 %) for first-line platinum- and taxane-based CHT. However, the RR was lower than was measured for papillary serous OC (RR 83 %, CR 75 % and PR 8 %) (200).

The fact that the RR remains unfavorable overall can likely be attributed to the sarcomatous tumor component, as pure sarcoma are poorly responsive to CHT in general. This assumption is further supported by the pattern of metastatic spread following neoadjuvant CHT. As a matter of fact, in one study (7), interval debulking after CHT uncovered considerably fewer carcinomatous metastases than are usually found, but at the same time more metastases consisting of carcinosarcoma or purely sarcomatous metastases. This suggests that CHT first and foremost affects the carcinomatous component.

Overall, the combinations carboplatin plus paclitaxel or platinum plus ifosfamide achieve the best results in terms of remission and survival (40, 53, 146, 214, 234). Median PFI and OS are practically identical for both of these schedules (223). Generally, it is safe to assume that CHT in cases of OCS should always include a platinum compound, while the toxicity of carboplatin/paclitaxel is lower overall than for other platinum-based combinations.

One fundamental problem is that nearly all patients with recurring and/or metastatic OCS have already been treated with a platinum-based combination, and the alternatives are limited. One study recounts a patient with recurring OCS with multiple prior courses of platinum-based CHT, for whom a remission of more than 41 mo could be achieved under liposomal doxorubicin (104). Combining carboplatin with liposomal doxorubicin, as described in the context of UCS, is also a conceivable option. Trabectedin has also proven to be effective in OCS patients where paclitaxel plus carboplatin has not been successful, achieving a 13 mo PR in one study (194). Trabectedin is considered to be particularly effective at achieving responses in sarcoma. This could serve to explain both its effectiveness when used after CHT with paclitaxel plus platinum has failed, and also the microscopic pattern of sarcomatous metastasization following neoadjuvant CHT. Regarding dosage, reference should be made to the section on palliative CHT in the context of UCS. The DKSM (128) has several reports of cases of UCS in highly palliative situations, in which the use of trofosfamide was followed by longer periods of SD. Overall, it appears logical to focus on chemotherapeutic agents in second-line therapy that are particularly effective against sarcoma.

There are no meaningful data that pertain to treatment with small molecules.

Providing best supportive care is widely accepted for cases of advanced disease or cases in which there is diffuse metastasization.

In general, reference can be made to the summary on palliative chemotherapy and uterine carcinosarcoma above. Experience to date suggests that any palliative chemotherapeutic schedule or regimen should include a platinum-based agent. The remission rates that have been achieved using carboplatin plus paclitaxel and paclitaxel plus cisplatin do not differ from each other substantially. However, bringing toxicity and progression free interval into the equation makes paclitaxel plus carboplatin the more recommended option. There are no recommendations pertaining to second-line therapy. The experiences in some individual cases suggest that administering a combination of carboplatin plus liposomal doxorubicin, or monochemotherapy with ifosfamide or trabectedin (as a "therapeutic attempt" in all three of these cases) might be a conceivable option. There is no indication for palliative hormone therapy. Nor have any therapeutic measures involving the use of small molecules yet been established in practice.

7.2.2 Carcinosarcoma of the fallopian tube

TCS are staged in accordance with the criteria that apply to tubal carcinoma. TCS occur much less frequently than OCS, accounting for only 10 % of all cases of CS of the pelvis or the extrauterine genitalia in the DKSM database (128). In total, fewer than 100 cases have been described in case histories or surveys. According to reviews (94, 275), patients are aged between 29 and 80 years, with mean and median ages of 59.7 and 62 years, respectively. 62.7 % of TCS are heterologous tumors with sarcomatous components consisting of chondrosarcoma, RMS, osteosarcoma and LS. LMS and FS are the most common homologous components. The carcinomatous component can consist of adenocarcinoma, clear cell carcinoma, squamous cell carcinoma, endometrioid carcinoma and adenosquamous carcinoma (275). As is also the case with peritoneal CS, TCS occasionally occur with concomitant OC (171). Metastases and peritoneal disseminations are largely carcinomatous (275). It often occurs that TCS are initially subjected to surgery under the assumed diagnosis of OC based on the clinical findings and the results from frozen section analysis.

The behavior of TCS bears close resemblance to that of OCS, OC or tubal carcinoma, both clinically and in terms of the symptoms they present with. In early disease, TCS predominantly grows within the tubal lumen, causing the fallopian tube to dilate. Analogous to OCS, TCS relatively quickly invade the peritoneum. The ovaries must be unambiguously tumor-free in order for a TCS to be diagnosed as such.

In contrast to OCS, AUB (34.2 %) (275) or bloody, serous discharge present as symptoms more frequently, as do pelvic pains likely caused by the dilation of the tubal lumen caused by the tumor. Accordingly, tubal CS are discovered at a much earlier stage than OC and OCS on average. At the time of initial diagnosis, 54.2 % are in stage I or II (275). TCS can be clinically confused with a hydrosalpinx or tubo-ovarian abscesses. TCS and carcinoma cannot be reliably discerned from each other in sonography. An unsuspicious uterus and normal ovaries in sonography suggest that a correspondingly localized lesion could well be a tubal malignancy.

In CT, TCS have attenuation equal to that of other nonspecific soft tissue. In CECT, enhancement is weaker than that of normal myometrium. The tumor is usually hypointense in T1W-MR images, and homogeneously hyperintense in T2W (119).

Overall, prognosis and prognostic factors appear to be identical to those of OCS (145). Analogous to EC, OC, UCS and OCS, CA-125 expression is often elevated in TCS as well (40, 275).

Poorly differentiated endometrioid carcinoma with spindle cell features is the most important histological DD (258).

Median 3-year OS is 34.5 mo; 3-year OS is 54.8 %. OS is generally poorer than that in patients with tubal carcinoma (275).

The surgical approach corresponds to that for OCS (145). Retrospective data from a total of 59 cases suggest that surgery followed by CHT or CHT-RT is significantly superior to surgery alone in terms of survival, especially when platinum-based agents are administered. Polychemotherapy using ifosfamide, epirubicin and cisplatin (ifosfamide 1 g/m^2 d 1–3, epirubicin 40 mg/m^2 d 1, cisplatin 60 mg/m^2 d 1, q 4 wk) has achieved the best results to date, though the number of cases on which these experiences are based is rather small. While highly promising results have been seen under additive CHT-RT, they, too, are only based on a small sample (275). Generally speaking, CHT-RT should really only be considered when disease has spread within the pelvis.

Therapy, including surgery and postoperative measures, otherwise corresponds to that recommended for OCS.

Surgical treatment for the very rare carcinosarcomas of the fallopian tube is analogous to that for ovarian carcinosarcoma. Retrospective studies that cover small numbers of cases suggest that additive chemotherapy can possibly have favorable effects on survival. Chemotherapy should definitely include a platinum-based agent. Carboplatin plus paclitaxel or ifosfamide plus epirubicin plus cisplatin appear to be preferred combinations. There are no recommendations for second-line therapy. In general, reference can be made to the recommendations that relate to uterine and ovarian carcinosarcoma in this context.

7.2.3 Peritoneal carcinosarcoma

CS occasionally originate in the peritoneum. They are more frequent than TCS, accounting for 20 % of all CS of the pelvis and extrauterine genitalia. They are staged in accordance with the criteria that apply to OCS (see above). Peritoneal CS are normally localized in the vicinity of the pelvic peritoneum or the pouch of Douglas (247). What is decisive is that these tumors occur without involvement of the ovaries or tubes and that – when the tumor has spread in the pelvis – the surface of the ovaries is affected less than the surrounding surfaces. According to a case history analysis of 43 cases that included an extensive review of the literature (146), CS can also originate in the peritoneum of the abdominal cavity, the intestines and the mesentery. The median age of affected women is 64 years (33–87). Over 90 % of the tumors are heterologous CS. In one third of cases, they occur synchronously with carcinoma of the fallopian tubes, the ovaries, the endometrium and the cervix (146, 232). In principle, in these cases, they could also in fact constitute transdifferentiated carcinoma metastases. Peritoneal CS do not differ from OCS or OC in terms of symptoms, palpation and their macroscopic appearance. Diagnostics and both primary and palliative therapy are congruent to the approach followed for OCS and TCS (145). Almost without exception, peritoneal CS of the lesser pelvis are operated on under the assumed diagnosis of OC (115), and the prognoses for these two entities are virtually the same.

Primary peritoneal carcinosarcomas are the exception. Regarding clinical features, diagnostics and treatment, reference can be made to the ovarian and tubal carcinosarcomas.

7.2.4 Extraperitoneal carcinosarcoma

Extraperitoneal CS of the lesser pelvis are extremely rare. Only five cases have been described in the literature (230). They account for 5 % of all CS of the extrauterine genitalia and of the pelvis (128). Abdominal pains, often in connection with an obstruction of the urinary tract, are particularly fundamental symptoms.

CS can also occasionally occur in the abdominal walls of the lower abdomen (141). It is probable that at least some of these tumors arise from an endometriosis (26, 141, 230). Reliable R0 resection is generally the most common form of surgical therapy. Primary or postoperative ERT is to be dismissed in cases of CS of the abdominal walls due to the risk of necrosis to the skin. All other therapeutic measures correspond to the approach followed for OCS and UCS.

Extraperitoneal carcinosarcomas are rare and are virtually always diagnosed incidentally. In terms of clinical features, diagnostics, and treatment, reference can be made to the extrauterine carcinosarcomas. Carcinosarcomas of the abdominal wall should generally not be subjected to postoperative radiotherapy.

References

(1) Abidi A, Men K, Sherman A, Konia T, Azodi M. Cervical carcinosarcoma: A case report. J Reprod Med 2008; 53: 138–140
(2) Adams SF, Hickson JA, Hutto JY, Montag AG, Lengyel E, Yamada SD. PDGFR-alpha as a potential therapeutic target in uterine sarcomas. Gynecol Oncol. 2007; 104: 524–528
(3) Akahira J, Tokunaga H, Toyoshima M, Takano T, Nagase S, Yoshinaga K, Tase T, Wada Y, Ito K, Niikura H, Yamada H, Sato A, Sasano H, Yaegashi N. Prognoses and prognostic factors of carcinosarcoma, endometrial stromal sarcoma and uterine leiomyosarcoma: A comparison with uterine endometrial adenocarcinoma. Oncology 2006; 71: 333–340
(4) Albrektsen G, Heuch I, Wik E, Salvesen HB. Prognostic impact of parity in 493 uterine sarcoma patients. Int. J. Gynecol. Cancer 2009; 19: 1062–107
(5) Alvarez R. Gynecologic Oncology Group Report, Gynecol Oncol 2009; 113: 14–15
(6) Amant F, de la Rey M, Dorfling CM, van der Walt L, Dreyer G, Dreyer L, Vergote I, Lindeque BG, Van Rensburg EJ. PTEN mutations in uterine sarcomas. Gynecol Oncol 2002; 85: 165–699
(7) Amant F, Vloeberghs V, Woestenborghs H, Moerman P, Vergote I. Transition of epithelial toward mesenchymal differentiation during ovarian carcinosarcoma tumorigenesis. Gynecol Oncol 2003; 90: 372–377
(8) Amant F, Vloeberghs V, Woestenborghs H, Debiec-Rychter M, Verbist L, Moerman P, Vergote I. ERBB-2 gene overexpression and amplification in uterine sarcomas. Gynecol Oncol 2004; 95: 583–587
(9) Amant F, Cadron I, Fuso L, Berteloot P, de Jonge E, Jacomen G, Van Robaeys J, Neven P, Moerman P, Vergote I. Endometrial carcinosarcomas have a different prognosis and pattern of spread compared to high-risk epithelial endometrial cancer. Gynecol Oncol 2005; 98: 274–280
(10) Anagnostopoulos A, Ruthven S, Kingston R. Mesonephric adenocarcinoma of the uterine cervix and literature review. BMJ Case Rep 2012: DOI: 10.1136/bcr.01.2012.5632

(11) Ang JE, Shah RN, Everard M, Keyzor C, Coombes I, Jenkins A, Thomas K, A'Hern R, Jones RL, Blake P, Gabra H, Hall G, Gore ME, Kaye SB. A feasibility study of sequential doublet chemotherapy comprising carboplatin-doxorubicin and carboplatin-paclitaxel for advanced endometrial adenocarcinoma and carcinosarcoma. Ann Oncol 2009; 20: 1787–1793

(12) Arenas M, Rovirosa A, Hernández V, Ordi J, Jorcano S, Mellado B, Biete A. Uterine sarcomas in breast cancer patients treated with tamoxifen. Int J Gynecol Cancer 2006; 16: 861–865

(13) Arend R, Bagaria M, Lewin SN, Sun X, Deutsch I, Burke WM, Herzog TJ, Wright JD. Long-term outcome and natural history of uterine adenosarcomas. Gynecol Oncol 2010; 119: 305–8

(14) Armstrong P, Wasti ML, Rockall AG. Diagnostik Imgaging – Female Genital Tract. 6th edn. Wiley-Blackwell, Oxford 2009, pp. 255–270

(15) ASTEC/EN.5 Study Group, Blake P, Swart AM, Orton J, Kitchener H, Whelan T, Lukka H, Eisenhauer E, Bacon M, Tu D, Parmar MK, Amos C, Murray C, Qian W. Adjuvant external beam radiotherapy in the treatment of endometrial cancer (MRC ASTEC and NCIC CTG EN.5 randomised trials): pooled trial results, systematic review, and meta-analysis. Lancet 2009; 373: 137–146

(16) ASTEC study group, Kitchener H, Swart AM, Qian Q, AmosC, Parmar MK. Efficacy of systematic pelvic lymphadenectomy in endometrial cancer (MRC ASTEC trial): A randomised study. Lancet 2009; 373: 97–99

(17) Aviram R, Ochshorn Y, Markovitch O, Fishman A, Cohen I, Altaras MM, Tepper R. Uterine sarcomas versus leiomyomas: gray-scale and Doppler sonographic findings. J Clin Ultrasound. 33: 2005; 10–13.

(18) Bagué S, Rodríguez IM, Prat J. Malignant mesonephric tumors of the female genital tract: A clinicopathologic study of 9 cases. Am J Surg Pathol 2004; 28: 601–607

(19) Bansal N, Herzog TJ, Seshan VE, Schiff PB, Burke WM, Cohen C J, Wright JD. Uterine carcinosarcomas and grade 3 endometrioid cancers: evidence for distinct tumor behavior. Obstet Gynecol 2008; 112: 64–70

(20) Bansal S, Lewin SN, Burke WM, Deutsch I, Sun X, Herzog TJ, Wright JD. Sarcoma of the cervix: natural history and outcomes. Gynecol Oncol 2010; 118: 134–138

(21) Berton-Rigaud D, Devouassoux-Shisheboran M, Ledermann JA, Leitao MM, Powell MA, Poveda A, Beale P, Glasspool RM, Creutzberg CL, Harter P, Kim JW, Reed NS, Ray-Coquard I. Gynecologic Cancer InterGroup (GCIG) Consensus Review for uterine and ovarian carcinosarcoma. Int J Gynecol Cancer. 2014; 24 (9 Suppl 3): S55–60

(22) Bharwani N, Newland A, Tunariu N, Babar S, Sahdev A, Rockall AG, Reznek RH. MRI appearances of uterine malignant mixed müllerian tumors. AJR Am J Roentgenol 2010; 195: 1268–1275

(23) Biscuola M, Van de Vijver K, Castilla MÁ, Romero-Pérez L, López-García MÁ, Díaz-Martín J, Matias-Guiu X, Oliva E, Palacios Calvo J. Oncogene alterations in endometrial carcinosarcomas. Hum Pathol 2013; 44: 852–859

(24) Bland AE, Stone R, Heuser C, Shu J, Jazaeri A, Shutter J, Atkins K, Rice L. A clinical and biological comparison between malignant mixed müllerian tumors and grade 3 endometrioid endometrial carcinomas. Int J Gynecol Cancer 2009; 19: 261–265

(25) Bodner-Adler B, Bodner K, Obermair A, Czerwenka K, Petru E, Leodolter S, Mayerhofer K. Prognostic parameters in carcinosarcomas of the uterus: A clinico-pathologic study. Anticancer Res 2001; 21: 3069–3074

(26) Booth C, Zahn CM, McBroom J, Maxwell GL. Retroperitoneal müllerian carcinosarcoma associated with endometriosis: A case report. Gynecol Oncol 2004; 93: 546–549

(27) Brooks SE, Zhan M, Cote T, Baquet CR. Surveillance, epidemiology, and end results analysis of 2677 cases of uterine sarcoma 1989–1999. Gynecol Oncol 2004; 93: 204–208

(28) Brown E, Stewart M, Rye T, Al-Nafussi A, Williams AR, Bradburn M, Smyth J, Gabra H. Carcinosarcoma of the ovary: 19 years of prospective data from a single center. Cancer 2004; 100: 2148–2153
(29) Brown J, Broaddus R, Koeller M, Burke TW, Gershenson DM, Bodurka DC. Sarcomatoid carcinoma of the cervix. Gynecol Oncol 2003; 90: 23–28
(30) Brown LC, Petersen IA, Haddock MG, Bakkum-Gamez JN, Lee LJ, Cimbak NC, Berkowitz RS, Viswanathan AN. Vaginal brachytherapy for early-stage carcinosarcoma of the uterus. Brachytherapy 2015; 14: 433–439
(31) Cacciatore B, Lehtovirta P, Wahlström T, Ylöstalo P. Ultrasound findings in uterine mixed müllerian sarcomas and endometrial stromal sarcomas. Gynecol Oncol 1989; 35: 290–293
(32) Callister M, Ramondetta LM, Jhingran A, Burke TW, Eifel PJ. Malignant mixed Müllerian tumors of the uterus: Analysis of patterns of failure, prognostic factors, and treatment outcome. Int J Radiat Oncol Biol Phys 2004; 58: 786–796
(33) Campos SM, Brady WE, Moxley KM, O'Cearbhaill RE, Lee PS, Disilvestro PA, Rotmensch J, Rose PG, Thaker PH, O'Malley DM, Hanjani P, Zuna RE, Hensley ML. A phase II evaluation of pazopanib in the treatment of recurrent or persistent carcinosarcoma of the uterus: A Gynecologic Oncology Group study. Gynecol Oncol 133; 2014: 537–541
(34) Cantrell LA, Havrilesky L, Moore DT, O'Malley D, Liotta M, Secord AA, Nagel CI, Cohn DE, Fader AN, Wallace AH, Rose P, Gehrig PA. A multi-institutional cohort study of adjuvant therapy in stage I–II uterine carcinosarcoma. Gynecol Oncol 2012; 127: 22–26
(35) Celik H, Kokcu A, Yildiz l. endometrial stromal sarcoma with coexistent endometrioid adenocarcinoma in a woman with previous breast cancer: A preliminary case report. Eur J Gynaecol cancer 33: 2012; 493–495
(36) Chang J, Sharpe JC, A'Hern RP, Fisher C, Blake P, Shepherd J, Gore ME Carcinosarcoma of the ovary: incidence, prognosis, treatment and survival of patients. Ann Oncol 1995; 6: 755–758
(37) Chiang YC, Chen CA, Chiang CJ, Hsu TH, Lin MC, You SL, Cheng WF, Lai MS. Trends in incidence and survival outcome of epithelial ovarian cancer: 30-year national population-based registry in Taiwan. J Gynecol Oncol 2013; 24: 342–51
(38) Chiyoda T, Tsuda H, Tanaka H, Kataoka F, Nomura H, Nishimura S, Takano M, Susumu N, Saya H, Aoki D. Expression profiles of carcinosarcoma of the uterine corpus – are these similar to carcinoma or sarcoma? Genes Chromosomes Cancer 2012; 51: 229–239
(39) Chun KC, Kim JJ, Kim DY, Kim JH, Kim YM, Nam JH, Kim YT. Optimal debulking surgery followed by paclitaxel/platinum chemotherapy is very effective in treating ovarian carcinosarcomas: A single center experience. Gynecol Obstet Invest 2011; 72: 208–214
(40) Cicin I, Saip P, Eralp Y, Selam M, Topuz S, Ozluk Y, Aydin Y, Topuz E. Ovarian carcinosarcomas: clinicopathological prognostic factors and evaluation of chemotherapy regimens containing platinum. Gynecol Oncol 2008; 108: 136–40
(41) Cimbaluk D, Rotmensch J, Scudiere J, Gown A, Bitterman P. Uterine carcinosarcoma: immunohistochemical studies on tissue microarrays with focus on potential therapeutic targets. Gynecol Oncol 2007; 105: 138–144
(42) Clement PB, Scully RE. Mullerian adenosarcoma of the uterus: A clinicopathologic analysis of 100 cases with a review of the literature. Hum Pathol 1990; 21: 363–381
(43) Clement PB, Zubovits JT, Young RH, Scully RE. Malignant mullerian mixed tumors of the uterine cervix: A report of nine cases of a neoplasm with morphology often different from its counterpart in the corpus. Int J Gynecol Pathol 1998; 17: 211–22
(44) Clement PB, Young RH. Atlas of Gynaecologic Surgical Pathology. Elsevier Saunders 2008
(45) Connor R. The contribution of diagnostic imaging in rare gynecological malignancies. In: Reed N, Green JA, Gershenon DM, Siddiqui N, Connor R (eds.). Rare and Uncommon Gynecological Cancers – A Clinical Guide. Springer, Berlin Heidelberg 2011, pp. 15–64

(46) Coosemans A, Van Calster B, Verbist G, Moerman P, Vergote I, Van Gool SW, Amant F. Wilms tumor gene 1 (WT1) is a prognostic marker in high-grade uterine sarcoma. Int J Gynecol Cancer 21: 2011; 302–308

(47) Cormio G, Loizzi V, Nardelli C, Fattizzi N, Selvaggi L. Non-puerperal uterine inversion due to uterine sarcoma. Gynecol Obstet Invest 2006; 61: 171–173

(48) Creasman WT, Mutch DE, Herzog TJ. ASTEC lymphadenectomy and radiation therapy studies: are conclusions valid? Gynecol Oncol 2010; 116:293–294

(49) Curtin JP, Blessing JA, Soper JT, DeGeest K. Paclitaxel in the treatment of carcinosarcoma of the uterus: A gynecologic oncology group study. Gynecol Oncol 2001; 83: 268–270

(50) Dai Y, Shen K, Lang JH, Huang HF, Pan LY, Wu M, Yang JX, Zhong DR. Primary sarcoma of the ovary: clinicopathological characteristics, prognostic factors and evaluation of therapy. Chin Med J 2011; 124: 1316–1321

(51) Dandapani M, Seagle BL, Chacho MS, Shahabi S. Delayed and clinically isolated port site carcinosarcoma recurrence as an early indicator of disseminated disease. Gynecol Oncol Rep 2015; 14: 12–15

(52) de Jong RA, Nijman HW, Wijbrandi TF, Reyners AK, Boezen HM, Hollema H. Molecular markers and clinical behavior of uterine carcinosarcomas: focus on the epithelial tumor component. Mod Pathol 2011; 24: 1368–1379

(53) del Carmen MG, Birrer M, Schorge JO. Carcinosarcoma of the ovary: A review of the literature. Gynecol Oncol 2012; 125: 271–7

(54) Denschlag D, Thiel FC, Ackermann S, Harter P, Juhasz-Boess I, Mallmann P, Strauss HG, Ulrich U, Horn LC, Schmidt D, Vordermark D, Vogl T, Reichardt P, Gaß P, Gebhardt M, Beckmann MW. Sarcoma of the Uterus. Guideline of the DGGG (S2k-Level, AWMF Registry No. 015/074, August 2015). Geburtshilfe Frauenheilkd 2015; 75: 1028–1042

(55) Desai NB, Kollmeier MA, Makker V, Levine DA, Abu-Rustum NR, Alektiar KM. Comparison of outcomes in early stage uterine carcinosarcoma and uterine serous carcinoma. Gynecol Oncol 2014; 135: 49–53

(56) Dickson EL, Vogel RI, Gehrig PA, Pierce S, Havrilesky L, Secord AA, Dottino J, Fader AN, Ricci S, Geller MA. A multi-institutional study of outcomes in stage I–III uterine carcinosarcoma. Gynecol Oncol 2015; 139: 275–82.

(57) Donner LR. Uterine carcinosarcoma with complete sarcomatous overgrowth mimicking pure embryonal rhabdomyosarcoma. Int J Gynecol Pathol 2003; 22: 89–91

(58) Doo DW, Erickson BK, Arend RC, Connerc MC, Huh WK, Leath CA III. Radical surgical cytoreduction in the treatment of ovarian carcinosarcoma. Gynecol Oncol 133: 2014; 234–237

(59) Du Bois A, Pfisterer J, Burchardi N, Loibl S, Huober J, Wimberger P, Burges A, Stähle A, Jackisch C, Kölbl H. Arbeitsgemeinschaft Gynäekologische Onkologie Studiengruppe Ovarialkarzinom; Kommission Uterus. Combination therapy with pegylated liposomal doxorubicin and carboplatin in gynecologic malignancies: A prospective phase II study of the Arbeitsgemeinschaft Gynäekologische Onkologie Studiengruppe Ovarialkarzinom (AGO-OVAR) and Kommission Uterus (AGO-K-Ut). Gynecol Oncol 2007; 107: 518–525

(60) Dusenbery KE, Potish RA, Argenta PA, Judson PL. On the apparent failure of adjuvant pelvic radiotherapy to improve survival for women with uterine sarcomas confined to the uterus. Am J Clin Oncol 2005; 28: 295–300

(61) Edge SB, Byrd DR, Compton CC. AJCC Cancer Staging Manual. 7th edn. New York, Springer 2010

(62) Einstein MH, Klobocista M, Hou JY, Lee S, Mutyala S, Mehta K, Reimers LL, Kuo DY, Huang GS, Goldberg GL. Phase II trial of adjuvant pelvic radiation “sandwiched” between ifosfamide or ifosfamide plus cisplatin in women with uterine carcinosarcoma. Gynecol Oncol 2012; 124: 26–30

(63) Ellenson LH, Ronnet BM, Soslow RA, Zaino RJ, Kurman RJ. Endometrial Carcinoma. In: Kurman RJ, Ellenson LH, Ronnett BM (eds.). Blustein's Pathology of the Female Genital Tract. 6th edn. Springer New York, Dodrecht, Heidelberg, London, 2011, pp. 393–452
(64) El Maalouf G, Duvillard P, Rey A, Morice P, Haie-Meder Ch, Lhommé C, Pautier P. Clinical features, recurrence patterns and treatment in endometrial stromal sarcomas: A thirty-year single-institution experience. J Clin Oncol 26 (15S) 2008; 26: Abstr. 10547
(65) Emoto M, Udo T, Kubota M, Ishiguro M, Iwasaki H, Kikuchi M, Kawarabayashi T. Neovascularization of uterine carcinosarcoma: report of two cases analyzed by color Doppler ultrasonography and microvessel density. J Ultrasound Med 1999; 18: 315–319
(66) Erickson BK, Doo DW, Zhang B, Huha WK, Leath CA III. Black race independently predicts worse survival in uterine carcinosarcoma. Gynecol Oncol 133: 2014, 238–241
(67) Emoto M, Charnock-Jones DS, Licence DR, Ishiguro M, Kawai M, Yanaihara A, Saito T, Hachisuga T, Iwasaki H, Kawarabayashi T, Smith SK. Localization of the VEGF and angiopoietin genes in uterine carcinosarcoma. Gynecol Oncol 2004; 95: 474–482
(68) Felix AS, Scott McMeekin D, Mutch D, Walker JL, Creasman WT, Cohn DE, Ali S, Moore RG, Downs LS, Ioffe OB, Park KJ, Sherman ME, Brinton LA. Associations between etiologic factors and mortality after endometrial cancer diagnosis: The NRG Oncology/Gynecologic Oncology Group 210 trial. Gynecol Oncol 2015; 139: 70–76
(69) Ferguson SE, Tornos C, Hummer A, Barakat RR, Soslow RA. Prognostic features of surgical stage I uterine carcinosarcoma. Am J Surg Pathol 2007; 31: 1653–1661
(70) 70 FIGO Committee on Gynecologic Oncology: Revised FIGO staging for carcinoma of the vulva, cervix, and endometrium. Int J Gynecol Obstet 2009; 105: 103–104
(71) Fister S, Günthert AR, Aicher B, Paulini KW, Emons G, Gründker C. GnRH-II antagonists induce apoptosis in human endometrial, ovarian, and breast cancer cells via activation of stress-induced MAPKs p38 and JNK and proapoptotic protein Bax. Cancer Res 2009; 69: 6473–81
(72) Fleming GF. Systemic chemotherapy for uterine carcinoma: metastatic and adjuvant. J Clin Oncol 2007; 2983–2989
(73) Foley OW, Rauh-Hain JA, Clark RM, Goodman A, Growdon WB, Boruta DM, Schorge JO, Del Carmen MG. Intraoperative radiation therapy in the management of gynecologic malignancies. Am J Clin Oncol 2014; DOI: 10.1097/COC.0000000000000063
(74) Fujiwara H, Shibahara H, Usui R, Takamizawa S, Kosuge S, Ohwada M, Suzuki M, Sato I. Unsuspected uterine carcinosarcoma (heterologous) diagnosed following conservative therapies with medroxyprogesterone acetate for presumed early-stage endometrial carcinoma. Am J Reprod Immunol 2002; 47: 129–131
(75) Funt SA, Hann LE. Detection and characterization of adnexal masses. Radiol Clin North Am 2002; 40: 591–608
(76) Gadducci A, Cosio S, Genazzani AR. Use of estrogen antagonists and aromatase inhibitors in breast cancer and hormonally sensitive tumors of the uterine body. Curr Opin Investig Drugs 2004; 5: 1031–1044
(77) Gadducci A, Cosio S, Romanini A, Genazzani AR. The management of patients with uterine sarcoma: A debated clinical challenge. Crit Rev Oncol Hematol 2008; 65: 129–142
(78) Gallardo A, Matias-Guiu X, Lagarda H, Catasus L, Bussaglia E, Gras E, Suarez D, Prat J. Malignant mullerian mixed tumor arising from ovarian serous carcinoma: A clinicopathologic and molecular study of two cases. Int J Gynecol Pathol 2002; 21: 268–272
(79) Gallup DG, Gable DS, Talledo OE, Otken LB. A clinical-pathologic study of mixed müllerian tumors of the uterus over a 16-year period—the Medical College of Georgia experience. Am J Obstet Gynecol 1989; 161: 533–538

(80) Garg G, Shah JP, Kumar S, Bryant CS, Munkarah A, Morris RT. Ovarian and uterine carcinosarcomas: A comparative analysis of prognostic variables and survival outcomes. Int J Gynecol Cancer 2010; 20: 888–894
(81) Garg G, Gao F, Wright JD, Hagemann AR, Mutch DG, Powell MA. Positive peritoneal cytology is an independent risk-factor in early stage endometrial cancer. Gynecol Oncol 2013; 128: 77–82
(82) Garg G, Yee C, Schwartz K, Mutch DG, Morris RT, Powell MA. Patterns of care, predictors, and outcomes of chemotherapy in elderly women with early-stage uterine carcinosarcoma: A population-based analysis. Gynecol Oncol 133: 2014; 242–249
(83) Geisler JP, Wiemann MC, Miller GA, Zhou Z, Geisler HE Estrogen and progesterone receptors in malignant mixed mesodermal tumors of the ovary. J Surg Oncol 1995; 59: 45–47
(84) Genever AV, Abdi S Can MRI predict the diagnosis of endometrial carcinosarcoma? Clin Radiol 2011; 66: 621–624
(85) George E, Lillemoe TJ, Twiggs LB, Perrone T. Malignant mixed müllerian tumor versus high-grade endometrial carcinoma and aggressive variants of endometrial carcinoma: A comparative analysis of survival. Int J Gynecol Pathol 1995; 14: 39–44
(86) George EM, Herzog TJ, Neugut AI, Lu YS, Burke WM, Lewin SN, Hershman DL, Wright JD Carcinosarcoma of the ovary: Natural history, patterns of treatment, and outcome. Gynecol Oncol 2013; 131: 42–45
(87) Gómez-Raposo C, López-Gómez M, Sereno M, Zambrana F, Casado E. Complete response with pegylated liposomal doxorubicin as a second-line therapy in metastatic ovarian carcinosarcoma. Significance of assessment of the response by FDG-PET. Gynecol Oncol Case Rep 2012; 4: 67–68
(88) Gungorduk K, Ozdemir A, Ertas IE, Gokcu M, Telli E, Oge T, Sahbaz A, Sayhan S, Sanci M, Harma M, Ozalp S. Adjuvant treatment modalities, prognostic predictors and outcomes of uterine carcinosarcomas. Cancer Res Treat 2015; 47: 282–289
(89) Gonzalez Bosquet J, Terstriep SA, Cliby WA, Brown-Jones M, Kaur JS, Podratz KC, Keeney GL. The impact of multi-modal therapy on survival for uterine carcinosarcomas. Gynecol Oncol 2010; 116: 419–423
(90) Gorai I, Yanagibashi T, Taki A, Udagawa K, Miyagi E, Nakazawa T, Hirahara F, Nagashima Y, Minaguchi H. Uterine carcinosarcoma is derived from a single stem cell: An in vitro study. Int J Cancer 1997; 72: 821–827
(91) Gourley C, Al-Nafussi A, Abdulkader M, Smyth JF, Gabra H Malignant mixed mesodermal tumours: biology and clinical aspects. Eur J Cancer2002; 38: 1437–46
(92) Guarino M, Giordano F, Pallotti F, Polizzotti G, Tricomi P, Cristofori E. Malignant mixed müllerian tumor of the uterus. Features favoring its origin from a common cell clone and an epithelial-to-mesenchymal transformation mechanism of histogenesis. Tumori 1998; 84: 391–397
(93) Guedea F, Rovirosa A, Anglada L, Delannes M, Marin S, DuBois JB, Daly-Schveitzer N. Impact of radiotherapy on local control and survival in uterine sarcomas: A retrospective study from the group oncologic català-occità. Int J Radiat Oncol Biol Phys 1999; 44: 47–52
(94) Gupta R, Jenison EL. A rare case of carcinosarcoma of the fallopian tube presenting with torsion, rupture and hemoperitoneum Gynecol Oncol Case Reports 2011; 2: 4–5
(95) Guttmann DM, Li H, Sevak P, Grover S, Jacobson G, Feldman A, Rubin S, Chu C, Bhatia S, Elshaikh MA, Lin LL. The impact of adjuvant therapy on survival and recurrence patterns in women with early-stage uterine carcinosarcoma: A multi-institutional study. Int J Gynecol Cancer 2016; 26:141–148
(96) Guzzo F, Bellone S, Buza N, Hui P, Carrara L, Varughese J, Cocco E, Betti M, Todeschini P, Gasparrini S, Schwartz PE, Rutherford TJ, Angioli R, Pecorelli S, Santin AD. HER2/neu as a

potential target for immunotherapy in gynecologic carcinosarcomas. Int J Gynecol Pathol 2012; 31: 211–221
(97) Hanprasertpong J, Wootipoom V, Hanprasertpong TJ. Non-puerperal uterine inversion and uterine sarcoma (malignant mixed müllerian tumor): report of an unusual case. Obstet Gynaecol Res 2004; 30: 105–108
(98) Harris MA, Delap LM, Sengupta PS, Wilkinson PM, Welch RS, Swindell R, Shanks JH, Wilson G, Slade RJ, Reynolds K, Jayson GC. Carcinosarcoma of the ovary. Br J Cancer 2003; 88: 654–657
(99) Hoffman MA, Khan A. Durable response of metastatic endometrial carcinoma to treatment with fulvestrant (Faslodex) after prior progestin and anastrozole therapy. Gynecol Oncol 2005; 100: 439–441
(100) Hogberg T, Signorelli M, de Oliveira CF, Fossati R, Lissoni AA, Sorbe B, Andersson H, Grenman S, Lundgren C, Rosenberg P, Boman K, Tholander B, Scambia G, Reed N, Cormio G, Tognon G, Clarke J, Sawicki T, Zola P, Kristensen G. Sequential adjuvant chemotherapy and radiotherapy in endometrial cancer—results from two randomised studies. Eur J Cancer 2010; 46: 2422–2331
(101) Homesley HD, Filiaci V, Markman M, Bitterman P, Eaton L, Kilgore LC, Monk BJ, Ueland FR. Phase III trial of ifosfamide with or without paclitaxel in advanced uterine carcinosarcoma: A Gynaecologic Oncology Group Study. J Clin Oncol 2007; 25: 526–531
(102) Hoskins PJ, Le N, Ellard S, Lee U, Martin LA, Swenerton KD, Tinker AV. Carboplatin plus paclitaxel for advanced or recurrent uterine malignant mixed mullerian tumors. The British Columbia Cancer Agency experience. Gynecol Oncol 2008; 108: 58–62
(103) Hoskins PJ, Le N. Preoperative tumor markers at diagnosis in women with malignant mixed müllerian tumors/carcinosarcoma of the uterus. Int J Gynecol Cancer 2008; 18: 1200–1201
(104) Hsieh CL, Chang TC, Lai CH, Jung SM, Chou HH. Excellent progression-free survival with liposomal doxorubicin for a patient with recurrent ovarian malignant mixed müllerian tumor: case report and literature review. Gynecol Oncol 2004; 94: 854–857
(105) Huang GS, Chiu LG, Gebb JS, Gunter MJ, Sukumvanich P, Goldberg GL, Einstein MH. Serum CA125 predicts extrauterine disease and survival in uterine carcinosarcoma. Gynecol Oncol 2007; 107: 513–517
(106) Huh WK, Sill MW, Darcy KM, Elias KM, Hoffman JS, Boggess JF, Alvarez RD, Long HJ, O'Malley DM, Birrer MJ. Efficacy and safety of imatinib mesylate (Gleevec) and immunohistochemical expression of c-Kit and PDGFR-beta in a Gynecologic Oncology Group Phase II Trial in women with recurrent or persistent carcinosarcomas of the uterus. Gynecol Oncol 2010; 117: 248–254
(107) Inthasorn P, Carte J, Valmadr S, Beale P, Russell P, Dalrymple C. Analysis of clinicopathologic factors in malignant mixed Müllerian tumors of the uterine corpus. Int J Gynecol Cancer. 2002; 12: 348–353
(108) Ioffe YJ, Li AJ, Walsh CS, Karlan BY, Leuchter R, Forscher C, Cass I. Hormone receptor expression in uterine sarcomas: prognostic and therapeutic roles. Gynecol Oncol 2009; 115: 466–471
(109) Ito E, Saito T, Suzuki T, Fujii M, Kudo R. Cytology of vaginal and uterine sarcomas. Acta Cytol 2004; 48: 601–7
(110) Jernigan AM, Fader AN, Nutter B, Rose P, Tseng JH, Escobar PF. Ovarian carcinosarcoma: effects of cytoreductive status and platinum-based chemotherapy on survival. Obstet Gynecol Int. 2013; 2013:490508. DOI: 10.1155/2013/490508
(111) Jha P, Chang ST, Rabban JT, Chen LM, Yeh BM, Coakley FV. Utility of the broccoli sign in the distinction of prolapsed uterine tumor from cervical tumor. Eur J Radiol 2012; 81: 1931–1936
(112) Jin Z, Ogata S, Tamura G, Katayama Y, Fukase M, Yajima M, Motoyama T. Carcinosarcomas (malignant mullerian mixed tumors) of the uterus and ovary: A genetic study with special reference to histogenesis. Int J Gynecol Pathol 2003; 22: 368–373

(113) Jung DC, Kim KH. Post–treatment changes and recurrence of uterine malignancies. In: Kim SH (ed.). Radiology Illustrated Gynecologic Imaging. 2nd edn. Springer 2012, pp. 299–348

(114) Kalluri R, Weinberg RA. The basics of epithelial-mesenchymal transition. J Clin Invest 2009; 119: 1420–1428

(115) Kanis M, Kesterson JP, Shroff S, Lele S, Mhawech-Fauceglia P. Malignant mixed müllerian tumor of primary peritoneal origin. Ann Diagn Pathol 2011; 15: 273–277

(116) Kanjeekal S, Chambers A, Fung MF, Verma S. Systemic therapy for advanced uterine sarcoma: A systematic review of the literature. Gynecol Oncol 2005; 97: 624–637

(117) Katesmark M, Lawton F. Gonadotrophin-releasing hormone (GnRH) analogues in the treatment of mixed mullerian tumours of the uterus: two case reports and review. Sarcoma 1998; 2: 197–200

(118) Kato H, Kanematsu M, Furui T, Imai A, Hirose Y, Kondo H, Goshima S, Tsuge Y. Carcinosarcoma of the uterus: radiologic-pathologic correlations with magnetic resonance imaging including diffusion-weighted imaging. Magn Reson Imaging 2008; 26: 1446–1450

(119) Kawakami S, Togashi K, Kimura I, Nakano Y, Koshiyama M, Takakura K, Konishi I, Mori T, Konishi J. Primary malignant tumor of the fallopian tube: Appearance at CT and MR imaging. Radiology 1993; 186: 503–508

(120) Kedzia W, Pruski D, Iwaniec K, Przybylski M, Friebe Z, Rajpert-Kedzia H. Carcinosarcoma (malignant mixed mesodermal tumor) of the uterus: clinicoimmunohistochemical and histogenetic characteristics. Folia Histochem Cytobiol 2012; 50: 513–518

(121) Kelly KL, Craighead PS. Characteristics and management of uterine sarcoma patients treated at the Tom Baker Centre. Int J Gynecol Cancer 2005; 15: 132–139

(122) Kenny SL, McBride HA, Jamison J, McCluggage WG. Mesonephric adenocarcinomas of the uterine cervix and corpus: HPV-negative neoplasms that are commonly PAX8, CA125, and HMGA2 positive and that may be immunoreactive with TTF1 and hepatocyte nuclear factor 1-β. Am J Surg Pathol 2012; 36: 799–807

(123) Khoury-Collado F, Einstein MH, Bochner BH, Alektiar KM, Sonoda Y, Abu-Rustum NR, Brown CL, Gardner GJ, Barakat RR, Chi DS. Pelvic exenteration with curative intent for recurrent uterine malignancies. Gynecol Oncol 2012; 124: 42–47

(124) Khunamornpong S, Suprasert P, Chiangmai WN, Siriaunkgul S. Metastatic tumors to the ovaries: A study of 170 cases in northern Thailand. Int J Gynecol Cancer. Suppl 1: 2006; 16: 132–138

(125) Kim HS, Han KH, Chung HH, Kim JW, Park NH, Song YS, Kang SB. Neutrophil to lymphocyte ratio for preoperative diagnosis of uterine sarcomas: A case-matched comparison. Eur J Surg Oncol 2010; 36: 691–698

(126) Kim JK, Lee SK, Myong NH, Kang YD. Biopsy-proven cerebellar metastasis from a malignant mixed mullerian tumor (MMMT) of the uterus: case report. Eur J Gynaecol Oncol 2009; 30: 196–198

(127) Kloos I, Delaloge S, Pautier P, Di Palma M, Goupil A, Duvillard P, Cailleux PE, L'homme C. Tamoxifen-related uterine carcinosarcomas occur under/after prolonged treatment: report of five cases and review of the literature. Int J Gynecol Cancer. 2002; 12: 496–500

(128) Köhler G, Belau A, Dennis K, Hesse J, Köller M, Krichbaum J, Kühnast M, Lehnhoff H, Lehr A, Linke L, Marcinek A, Müller S, Riechmann C, Schalitz S, Simon J, Spring P, Schädler J, Ständer C, Trojnarska D, Wilcke S, Witte N, Zygmunt M; Deutsches klinisches Kompetenzzentrum für genitale Sarkome und Mischtumoren an der Universitätsmedizin Greifswald (DKSM) und Kooperationspartner VAAO Deutschland und FK Frankfurt/Sachsenhausen. DKSM-Datenbank und Promotions- und Forschungsgruppe genitale Sarkome, Greifswald 2016, http://www.medizin.uni-greifswald.de/gyn/dksm/

(129) Koivisto-Korander R, Butzow R, Koivisto AM, Leminen A. Immunohistochemical studies on uterine carcinosarcoma, leiomyosarcoma, and endometrial stromal sarcoma: expression and prognostic importance of ten different markers. Tumour Biol 2011; 32: 451–459

(130) Kokawa K, Nishiyama K, Ikeuchi M, Ihara Y, Akamatsu N, Enomoto T, Ishiko O, Motoyama S, Fujii S, Umesaki N. Clinical outcomes of uterine sarcomas: results from 14 years worth of experience in the Kinki district in Japan (1990–2003). Int J Gynecol Cancer 2006; 16: 1358–1363

(131) Kondi-Pafiti A, Grapsa D, Hasiakos D, Gennatas K, Fotiou S. Carcinosarcomas of the uterus and ovary: A clinicopathologic and immunohistochemical study of 11 cases. Eur J Gynaecol Oncol 2009; 30: 93–7

(132) Lacour RA, Euscher E, Atkinson EN, Sun CC, Ramirez PT, Coleman RL, Brown J, Gano JB, Burke TW, Ramondetta LM. A phase II trial of paclitaxel and carboplatin in women with advanced or recurrent uterine carcinosarcoma. Int J Gynecol Cancer 2011; 21: 517–522

(133) Lavie O, Longacre T, Segev Y, Husain A. Ovarian carcinosarcomas associated with prolonged use of tamoxifen: case reports. Int J Gynecol Cancer 2009; 19: 1521–1523

(134) Lê LH, Swenerton KD, Elit L, Provencher DM, Stuart GC, LE T, Lee U, Rodgers A, Pond GR, Hu H, Oza AM. Phase II multicenter open-label study of carboplatin and pegylated liposomal doxorubicin in uterine and cervical malignancies. Int J Gynecol Cancer 2005; 15: 799–806

(135) Lee EJ, Joo HJ, Ryu HS. Malignant mixed Müllerian tumors of the uterus: sonographic spectrum. Ultrasound Obstet Gynecol 2012; 39: 348–353

(136) Lee KR, Tavassoli FA, Prat J, et al. Surface Epithelial-Stromal Tumors. In: Mesenchymal Tumours and Related Lesions. In: Tavassoli FA, Devilee P (eds.). Word Health Organization Classification of Tumours. Pathology and genetics of tumours of the breast and female genital organs. IARC Press: Lyon 2003, pp. 51–79

(137) Lee SH, Kim J, Kim JH, Lee KH, Park JS, Hur SY. Malignant mixed mullerian tumor of the cervix including components of a rhabdomyosarcoma: case report and literature review. Eur J Gynaecol Oncol 2010; 31: 462–466

(138) Leiser AL, Chi DS, Ishill NM, Tew WP. Carcinosarcoma of the ovary treated with platinum and taxane: The Memorial Sloan-Kettering Cancer Center experience. Gynecol Oncol 2007; 105: 657–661

(139) Leitao MM, Tornos C, Wolfson A, O'Cearbhaill R. Corpus: mesenchymal tumors. In: Barakat RR, Berchuk A, Markman M, Randall ME (eds.). Principles and Practice of Gynecologic Oncology. Sixth edn. Lippincott Williams & Wilkins, Philadelphia 2013, online ed. pos. 47172–74393

(140) Leitlinienprogramm Onkologie (Deutsche Krebsgesellschaft, Deutsche Krebshilfe, AWMF): S3-Leitlinie Diagnostik, Therapie und Nachsorge maligner Ovarialtumoren, Langversion 1.0, AWMF Registrierungsnummer: 032-035OL, http://leitlinienprogramm-onkologie.de/Leitlinien.7.0.html

(141) Leng J, Lang J, Guo L, Li H, Liu Z. Carcinosarcoma arising from atypical endometriosis in a cesarean section scar. Int J Gynecol Cancer 2006; 16: 432–435

(142) Long B, Liu FW, Bristow RE. Disparities in uterine cancer epidemiology, treatment, and survival among African Americans in the United States. Gynecol Oncol. 2013; 130: 652–659

(143) Lopez-Chardi L, González-Bosquet E, Rovira Zurriaga C, Laïlla Vicens JM. Mesonephric carcinosarcoma of the uterine cervix: A case report. Eur J Gynaecol Oncol 2013; 34: 336–338

(144) Lorusso D, Martinelli F, Mancini M, Sarno I, Ditto A, Raspagliesi F. Carboplatin-Paclitaxel versus Cisplatin-Ifosfamide in the treatment of uterine carcinosarcoma: A retrospective cohort study. Int J Gynecol Cancer 2014; 24: 1256–1261

(145) Lu CH, Chen IH, Chen YJ, Wang KL, Qiu JT, Lin H, Lin WC, Liou WS, Huang YF, Lin YS, Tee YT, Hung YC. Primary treatment and prognostic factors of carcinosarcoma of the ovary, fallopian

tube, and peritoneum: A Taiwanese Gynecologic Oncology Group study. Int J Gynecol Cancer. 2014; 24: 506–512.
(146) Ma CJ, Yang SF, Huang CC, Chai CY, Cheng KI, Tsai EM, Wang JY. Malignant mixed müllerian tumor of primary mesenteric origin associated with a synchronous ovarian cancer: case report and literature review. Eur J Gynaecol Oncol 2008; 29: 289–293
(147) Machida H, Takahashi K, Nomura H, Matoda M, Omatsu K, Kato K, Umayahara K, Takeshima N. Impact of multimodal therapy on the survival of patients with newly diagnosed uterine carcinosarcoma. Eur J Gynaecol Oncol 2013; 34: 291–295
(148) Major FJ, Blessing JA, Silverberg SG, Morrow CP, Creasman WT, Currie JL, Yordan E, Brady MF. Prognostic factors in early-stage uterine sarcoma. A Gynecologic Oncology Group study. Cancer 1993; 71 (Suppl 4): 1702–1709
(149) Makker V, Abu-Rustum NR, Alektiar KM, Aghajanian CA, Zhou Q, Iasonos A, Hensley MLA. Retrospective assessment of outcomes of chemotherapy-based versus radiation-only adjuvant treatment for completely resected stage I-IV uterine carcinosarcoma. Gynecol Oncol 2008; 111: 249–254
(150) Makker V, Kravetz SJ, Gallagher J, Orodel OP, Zhou Q, Iasonos A, Delair D, Aghajanian C, Hensley MLA. Treatment outcomes in completely resected stage I to stage IV uterine carcinosarcoma with rhabdomyosarcoma differentiation. Int J Gynecol Cancer 2013; 23: 1635–1641
(151) Manfredi R, Gui B, Maresca G, Fanfani F, Bonomo L. Endometrial cancer: magnetic resonance imaging. Abdom Imaging 2005; 30: 626–636
(152) Mano MS, Rosa DD, Azambuja E, Ismael G, Braga S, D'Hondt V, Piccart M, Awada A. Current management of ovarian carcinosarcoma. Int J Gynecol Cancer 2007; 17: 316–624
(153) Manolitsas TP, Wain GV, Williams KE, Freidlander M, Hacker NF. Multimodality therapy for patients with clinical Stage I and II malignant mixed Müllerian tumors of the uterus. Cancer 2001; 15; 91: 1437–1443
(154) Mariani A, El-Nashar SA, Dowdy SC. Lymphadenectomy in endometrial cancer: which is the right question? Int J Gynecol Cancer 2010; 20: 52–54
(155) Matsuura M, Suzuki T, Morishita M, Tanaka R, Ito E, Saito T. Chemotherapy (CT) with radiotherapy versus CT alone for FIGO Stage IIIc endometrial cancer. Eur J Gynaecol Oncol 2009; 30: 40–44
(156) Mazgani M, Le N, Hoskins PJ. Reuse of carboplatin and paclitaxel in patients with relapsed endometrial cancer – the British Columbia Cancer Agency experience. Gynecol Oncol 2008; 111: 474–477
(157) McMeekin DS, Sill MW, Darcy KM, Abulafia O, Hanjani P, Pearl ML, Rubin SC, Rose PG, Small L, Benbrook DM. A phase II trial of thalidomide in patients with refractory uterine carcinosarcoma and correlation with biomarkers of angiogenesis: A Gynecologic Oncology Group study. Gynecol Oncol 2012; 127: 356–361
(158) Meguro S, Yasuda M, Shimizu M, Kurosaki A, Fujiwara K. Mesonephric adenocarcinoma with a sarcomatous component, a notable subtype of cervical carcinosarcoma: A case report and review of the literature. Diagn Pathol. 2013; 7;8 (1):74. http://www.diagnosticpathology.org/content/8/1/74, published online
(159) Melchert M, List A. The thalidomide saga. Int J Biochem Cell Biol 2007; 39: 1489–1499
(160) Menczer J, Levy T, Piura B, Chetrit A, Altaras M, Meirovitz M, Glezerman M, Fishman A. A comparison between different postoperative treatment modalities of uterine carcinosarcoma. Gynecol Oncol 2005; 97: 166–170
(161) Miller DS, Blessing JA, Schilder J, Munkarah A, Lee YC. Phase II evaluation of topotecan in carcinosarcoma of the uterus: A Gynecologic Oncology Group study. Gynecol Oncol 2005; 98: 217–221

(162) Miller BE, Blessing JA, Stehman FB, Shahin MS, Yamada SD, Secord AA, Warshal DP, Abulafia O, Richards WE, Van Le L. A phase II evaluation of weekly gemcitabine and docetaxel for second-line treatment of recurrent carcinosarcoma of the uterus: A gynecologic oncology group study. Gynecol Oncol 2010; 118: 139–144
(163) Moinfar F, Azodi M, Tavassoli FA. Uterine sarcomas. Pathology 2007; 39: 55–71
(164) Morrow CP, Bundy BN, Hoffman J, Sutton G, Homesley H. Adriamycin chemotherapy for malignant mixed mesodermal tumor of the ovary. A Gynecologic Oncology Group Study. Am J Clin Oncol 1986; 9: 24–26
(165) Mourton SM, Xing GB, Leiserowitz GS. Survival of patients with uterine carcinosarcoma: Analysis of risk factors. Gynecol Oncol 2008; 108: S32–S33
(166) Murray SK, Clement PB, Young RH. Endometrioid carcinomas of the uterine corpus with sex cord-like formations, hyalinization, and other unusual morphologic features: A report of 31 cases of a neoplasm that may be confused with carcinosarcoma and other uterine neoplasms. Am J Surg Pathol 2005; 29: 157–166
(167) Mustea A, Koensgen D, Belau A, Sehouli J, Lichtenegger W, Schneidewind L, Sommer H, Markmann S, Scharf JP, Ehmke M, Ledwon P, Braicu I, Zygmunt M, Koehler G. Adjuvant sequential chemoradiation therapy in high-risk endometrial cancer: results of a prospective, multicenter phase-II study of the NOGGO (North-Eastern German Society of Gynaecological Oncology). Cancer Chemother Pharmacol 2013; 72: 975–83
(168) Nagar H, Boothe D, Parikh A, Yondorf M, Parashar B, Gupta D, Holcomb K, Caputo T, Chao KS, Nori D, Wernicke AG. Administration of concurrent vaginal brachytherapy during chemotherapy for treatment of endometrial cancer. Int J Radiat Oncol Biol Phys 2013; 87: 665–669
(169) Nagase S, Katabuchi H, Hiura M, Sakuragi N, Aoki Y, Kigawa J, Saito T, Hachisuga T, Ito K, Uno T, Katsumata N, Komiyama S, Susumu N, Emoto M, Kobayashi H, Metoki H, Konishi I, Ochiai K, Mikami M, Sugiyama T, Mukai M, Sagae S, Hoshiai H, Aoki D, Ohmichi M, Yoshikawa H, Iwasaka T, Udagawa Y, Yaegashi N; Japan Society of Gynecologic Oncology. Evidence-based guidelines for treatment of uterine body neoplasm in Japan: Japan Society of Gynecologic Oncology (JSGO) 2009 edition. Int J Clin Oncol 2010; 15:531–542.
(170) Nam JH. Surgical treatment of uterine sarcoma. Best Pract Res Clin Obstet Gynaecol 2011; 25: 751–760
(171) Nappi L, Indraccolo U, Matteo M, Rosenberg P, Greco P. Malignant mixed müllerian tumor of the fallopian tube coincident with a primary serous carcinoma of the ovary. Case report Eur J Gynaecol Oncol 2007; 28: 511–512
(172) Nasu K, Kawano Y, Hirota Y, Matsui N, Hayata T, Miyakawa I. Immunohistochemical study of c-erb B-2 expression in malignant mixed müllerian tumors of the female genital tract. J Obstet Gynaecol Res 1996; 22: 347–351
(173) Nasu K, Satoh T, Nishio S, Nagai Y, Ito K, Otsuki T, Hongo A, Hirashima Y, Ogura T, Shimada M. Clinicopathologic features of brain metastases from gynecologic malignancies: A retrospective study of 139 cases (KCOG-G1001s trial). Gynecol Oncol 128: 2013; 198–203
(174) National Comprehensive Cancer Network: NCCN Clinical Practice Guidelines in Oncology – Ovarian cancer including fallopian tube cancer and primary peritoneal cancer. Version 1.2016, NCCN.org
(175) National Comprehensive Cancer Network: NCCN Practice Guidelines in Oncology –Uterine neoplasms. Version 2.2016, www.nccn.org
(176) Naumann RW. The role of lymphadenectomy in endometrial cancer: was the ASTEC trial doomed by design and are we destined to repeat that mistake? Gynecol Oncol 2012; 126: 5–11

(177) Nemani D, Mitra N, Guo M, Lin L. Assessing the effects of lymphadenectomy and radiation therapy in patients with uterine carcinosarcoma: A SEER analysis. Gynecol Oncol 2008; 111: 82–88
(178) Nimeiri HS, Oza AM, Morgan RJ, Huo D, Elit L, Knost JA, Wade JL 3rd, Agamah E, Vokes EE, Fleming GF. A phase II study of sorafenib in advanced uterine carcinoma/carcinosarcoma: A trial of the Chicago, PMH, and California Phase II Consortia. Gynecol Oncol 2010; 117: 37–40
(179) Nordal RR, Kristensen GB, Stenwig AE, Nesland JM, Pettersen EO, Trope CG. An evaluation of prognostic factors in uterine carcinosarcoma. Gynecol Oncol 1997; 67: 316–321
(180) Nout RA, Putter H, Jürgenliemk-Schulz IM, Jobsen JJ, Lutgens LC, van der Steen-Banasik EM, Mens JW, Slot A, Stenfert Kroese MC, van Bunningen BN, Smit VT, Nijman HW, van den Tol PP, Creutzberg CL. Quality of life after pelvic radiotherapy or vaginal brachytherapy for endometrial cancer: first results of the randomized PORTEC-2 trial. J Clin Oncol 2009; 27: 3547–3556
(181) Nucci MR, Crum CP. Neuroendocrine Carcinoma, Mixed Epithelial/Mesenchymal and Mesenchymal Tumors, and Miscellaneous Lesions of the Cervix. In: Crum P C, Nucci MR, Lee KR (eds.). Diagnostic Gynecologic and Obstetric Pathology. 2nd edn. Elsevier-Saunders, Philadelphia 2011, pp. 379–406
(182) Nucci MR, Quade BJ. Uterine mesenchymal tumors. In: Crum PC, Lee KR (eds.). Diagnostic Gynecologic and Obstetric Pathology. Elsevier-Saunders, Philadelphia 2006, pp. 611–673
(183) Nucci MR, Crum CP, Lee KR. The Pathology of Pelvic-ovarian Epithelial (epithelial-stromal) Tumors. In: Crum CP, Nucci MR, Lee KR (eds). Diagnostic Gynecologic and Obstetric Pathology. Elsevier Saunders 2011, pp. 818–895
(184) Oguz A. Malignant Mixed Mesodermal Tumor. In: Hricak HH, Akin O, Sala E, Ascher SM, Levine D, Reinhold C (eds.). Diagnostic Imaging Gynecology. Amyrsis 2007, 2/172–2/175
(185) Okazawa M, Masuhara K, Miyoshi A, Fujiwara K, Ohta Y, Yoshino K, Kamiura S, Tomita Y. A rare case of ovarian carcinosarcoma successfully treated with the neoadjuvant chemotherapy of paclitaxel and ifosfamide. Obstet Gynaecol 2011; 31: 274–275
(186) Omura GA, Blessing JA, Major F, Lifshitz S, Ehrlich CE, Mangan C, Beecham J, Park R, Silverberg S. A randomized clinical trial of adjuvant adriamycin in uterine sarcomas: A Gynecologic Oncology Group Study. J Clin Oncol 1985; 3: 1240–1245
(187) Otsuka I, Takaya H, Takagi K, Tanaka A, Kaseki H, Izuta C, Sato M, Matsuura T, Suzuki [Carcinosarcoma of the ovary treated with paclitaxel and carboplatin chemotherapy – a report of 4 cases]. Gan To Kagaku Ryoho. 2013 Sep; 40(9): 1249–53 (Abstract).
(188) Ozguroglu M, Bilici A, Ilvan S, Turna H, Atalay B, Mandel N, Sahinler I. Determining predominating histologic component in malignant mixed müllerian tumors: is it worth it? Int J Gynecol Cancer 2008; 18: 809–812
(189) Pacaut C, Bourmaud A, Rivoirard R, Moriceau G, Guy JB, Collard O, Bosacki C, Jacquin JP, Levy A, Chauleur C, Magné N, Merrouche Y. Uterine and ovary carcinosarcomas: outcome, prognosis factors, and adjuvant therapy. Am J Clin Oncol 2013; DOI: 10.1097/COC.0b013e3182979b27
(190) Panici PB, Basile S, Maneschi F, Alberto Lissoni A, Signorelli M, Scambia G, Angioli R, Tateo S, Mangili G, Katsaros D, Garozzo G, Campagnutta E, Donadello N, Greggi S, Melpignano M, Raspagliesi F, Ragni N, Cormio G, Grassi R, Franchi M, Giannarelli D, Fossati R, Torri V, Amoroso M, Crocè C, Mangioni C. Systematic pelvic lymphadenectomy vs. no lymphadenectomy in early-stage endometrial carcinoma: randomized clinical trial. J Natl Cancer Inst 2008; 100: 1707–1716
(191) Park SB, Moon MH. Epithelial tumors of the ovary. In: Kim SH (ed.). Radiology Illustrated Gynecologic Imaging. 2nd edn. Springer 2012, pp. 527–619

(192) Patel N, Hegarty SE, Cantrell LA, Mishra MV, Showalter TN. Evaluation of brachytherapy and external beam radiation therapy for early stage, node-negative uterine carcinosarcoma. Brachytherapy 2015; 14: 606–612
(193) Pectasides D, Pectasides E, Papaxoinis G, Xiros N, Sykiotis C, Papachristodoulou A, Tountas N, Panayiotides J, Economopoulos T. Combination chemotherapy with carboplatin, paclitaxel and pegylated liposomal doxorubicin for advanced or recurrent carcinosarcoma of the uterus: clinical experience of a single institution. Gynecol Oncol 2008; 110: 299–303
(194) Petru E, Kolovetsiou V, Idris T. Prolonged response to trabectedin in a patient with ovarian carcinosarcoma refractory to adjuvant platinum-taxane. J Solid Tumors 2013; 3: 9–11
(195) Piscuoglio S, Burke KA, Ng CK, Papanastasiou AD, Geyer FC, Macedo GS, Martelotto LG, de Bruijn I, De Filippo MR, Schultheis AM, Ioris RA, Levine DA, Soslow RA, Rubin BP, Reis-Filho JS, Weigelt B. Uterine adenosarcomas are mesenchymal neoplasms. J Pathol 2016; 238: 381–388
(196) Powell MA, Filiaci VL, Rose PG, Mannel RS, Hanjani P, Degeest K, Miller BE, Susumu N, Ueland FR. Phase II evaluation of paclitaxel and carboplatin in the treatment of carcinosarcoma of the uterus: A Gynecologic Oncology Group study. J Clin Oncol 2010; 28: 2727–2731
(197) Pradhan TS, Stevens EE, Ablavsky M, Salame G, Lee YC, Abulafia O. FIGO staging for carcinosarcoma: can the revised staging system predict overall survival? Gynecol Oncol 2011; 123: 221–224
(198) Ramondetta LM, Burke TW, Jhingran A, Schmandt R, Bevers MW, Wolf JK, Levenback CF, Broaddus R. A phase II trial of cisplatin, ifosfamide, and mesna in patients with advanced or recurrent uterine malignant mixed müllerian tumors with evaluation of potential molecular targets. Gynecol Oncol 2003; 90: 529–536
(199) Raspollini MR, Susini T, Amunni G, Paglierani M, Castiglione F, Garbini F, Carriero C, Scarselli G, Taddei GL. Expression and amplification of HER-2/neu oncogene in uterine carcinosarcomas: A marker for potential molecularly targeted treatment? Int J Gynecol Cancer 2006; 16: 416–422
(200) Rauh-Hain JA, Growdon WB, Rodriguez N, Goodman AK, Boruta DM 2nd, Schorge JO, Horowitz NS, del Carmen MG. Carcinosarcoma of the ovary: A case-control study. Gynecol Oncol 2011; 121: 477–481
(201) Rauh-Hain JA, Starbuck KD, Meyer LA, Clemmer J, Schorge JO, Lu KH, Del Carmen MG. Patterns of care, predictors and outcomes of chemotherapy for uterine carcinosarcoma: A National Cancer Database analysis. Gynecol Oncol 2015; 139: 84–89
(202) Reed NS, Mangioni C, Malmström H, Scarfone G, Poveda A, Pecorelli S, Tateo S, Franchi M, Jobsen JJ, Coens C, Teodorovic I, Vergote I, Vermorken JB. Phase III randomised study to evaluate the role of adjuvant pelvic radiotherapy in the treatment of uterine sarcomas stages I and II: An European Organisation for Research and Treatment of Cancer Gynaecological Cancer Group study (protocol 55874). Eur J Cancer 2008; 44: 808–818
(203) Reed NS. The management of uterine sarcomas. Clin Oncol 2008; 20: 470–478
(204) Reed N. Ovarian carcinomasarcomas. In: Reed N, Green JA, Gershenon DM, Siddiqui N, Connor R. Rare and uncommon gynecological cancers. A Clinical Guide. Springer Heidelberg New York 2011, pp. 135–142
(205) Rezk YA, Hurley KE, Carter J, Dao F, Bochner BH, Aubey JJ, Caceres A, Einstein MH, Abu-Rustum NR, Barakat RR, Makker V, Chi DS. A prospective study of quality of life in patients undergoing pelvic exenteration: interim results. Gynecol Oncol 2013; 128: 191–197
(206) Rovirosa A, Ascaso C, Arenas M, Ríos I, Del Pino M, Ordi J, Morales J, Gascón M, Pahisa J, Biete A. Pathologic prognostic factors in stage I-III uterine carcinosarcoma treated with postoperative radiotherapy. Arch Gynecol Obstet. 2014; 290: 329–334

(207) Rustin GJ, et 128 collaborators. Early versus delayed treatment of relapsed ovarian cancer (MRC OV05/EORTC 55955): A randomised trial. Lancet 2010; 376: 1155–1163
(208) Sadeghi R, Zakavi SR, Hasanzadeh M, Treglia G, Giovanella L, Kadkhodayan S. Diagnostic performance of fluorine-18-fluorodeoxyglucose positron emission tomography imaging in uterine sarcomas: systematic review and meta-analysis of the literature. Int J Gynecol Cancer 2013; 23: 1349–1356
(209) Sagae S, Yamashita K, Ishioka S, Nishioka Y, Terasawa K, Mori M, Yamashiro K, Kanemoto T, Kudo R. Preoperative diagnosis and treatment results in 106 patients with uterine sarcoma in Hokkaido, Japan. Oncology 2004; 67: 33–39
(210) Sala E. Mixed mullerian tumor, ovary. In: Hricak HH, Akin O, Sala E, Ascher SM, Levine D, Reinhold C (eds.). Diagnostic Imaging Gynecology. Amyrsis 2007, 7/146–7/149
(211) Salazar OM, Bonfiglio TA, Patten SF, Keller BE, Feldstein ML, Dunne ME, Rudolph JH. Uterine sarcomas: analysis of failures with special emphasis on the use of adjuvant radiation therapy, natural history, treatment and prognosis. Cancer 1978; 42: 1161–1170
(212) Sampath S, Schultheiss TE, Ryu JK, Wong JY. The role of adjuvant radiation in uterine sarcomas. Int J Radiat Oncol Biol Phys 76: 2010; 728–734
(213) Sawada M, Tsuda H, Kimura M, Okamoto S, Kita T, Kasamatsu T, Yamada T, Kikuchi Y, Honjo H, Matsubara O. Different expression patterns of KIT, EGFR, and HER-2 (c-erbB-2) oncoproteins between epithelial and mesenchymal components in uterine carcinosarcoma. Cancer Sci 2003; 94: 986–991
(214) Scott McMeekin D. Sarcoma of the Uterus. In: DiSaia PJ, Creasman WT (eds.). Clinical Gynecologic Oncology. 7th edn. Mosby Elsevier 2007, pp. 185–199
(215) Seidman JD, Chauhan S. Evaluation of the relationship between adenosarcoma and carcinosarcoma and a hypothesis of the histogenesis of uterine sarcomas. Int J Gynecol Pathol 2003; 22: 75–82
(216) Semczuk A, Skomra D, Chyzyńska M, Szewczuk W, Olcha P, Korobowicz E. Immunohistochemical analysis of carcinomatous and sarcomatous components in the uterine carcinosarcoma: A case report. Pathol Res Pract 2008; 204: 203–207
(217) Shah SH, Jagannathan JP, Krajewski K, O'Regan KN, George S, Ramaiya NH. Uterine sarcomas: then and now. Am J Roentgenol 2012; 199: 213–223
(218) Sharma NK, Sorosky JI, Bender D, Fletcher MS, Sood AK. Malignant mixed mullerian tumor (MMMT) of the cervix. Gynecol Oncol 2005; 97: 442–445
(219) Shibata R, Umezawa A, Takehara K, Aoki D, Nozawa S, Hata J. Primary carcinosarcoma of the vagina. Pathol Int 2003; 53: 106–110
(220) Shin YR, Rha SE. Miscellaneous Tumors of the Uterus. In: Kim SH (ed.). Radiology Illustrated Gynecologic Imaging. 2nd edn. Springer 2012, pp. 249–297
(221) Shylasree TS, Bryant A, Athavale R. Chemotherapy and/or radiotherapy in combination with surgery for ovarian carcinosarcoma. Cochrane Database of Systematic Reviews 2013, Issue 2. Art. No. CD006246. DOI: 10.1002/14651858.CD006246.pub2
(222) Signorelli M, Chiappa V, Minig L, Fruscio R, Perego P, Caspani G, Battistello M, Colombo N. Platinum, anthracycline, and alkylating agent-based chemotherapy for ovarian carcinosarcoma. Int J Gynecol Cancer 2009; 19: 1142–1146
(223) Silasi DA, Illuzzi JL, Kelly MG, Rutherford TJ, Mor G, Azodi M, Schwartz PE. Carcinosarcoma of the ovary. Int J Gynecol Cancer 2008; 18: 22–29
(224) Silverberg SG, Major FJ, Blessing J, Fetter B, Askin FB, Liao SY, Miller A. Carcinosarcoma (malignant mixed mesodermal tumor) of the uterus. A Gynecologic Oncology Group pathologic study of 203 cases. Int J Gynecol Pathol 1990; 9: 1–19
(225) Sinha A, Sinha D, Aslam M, Fitzgibbon MN. Non-puerperal complete uterine inversion caused by malignant mixed mullerian tumour of the uterus. Gynecol Surg 2007; 4: 123–125

(226) Sleijfer S, Seynaeve C, Verweij J. Gynaecological sarcomas. Curr Opin Oncol 2007; 19: 492–496
(227) Sobin IH, Gospodaroricz MK, Wittekind CH (eds.). TNM Classification of Malignant Tumors. 7th edn. Wiley & Sons, Weinheim 2010
(228) Song T, Choi CH, Lee YY, Kim TJ, Lee JW, Kim BG, Bae DS. Which is worse: uterine papillary serous carcinomas or carcinosarcomas? J Gynecol Oncol 2011; 22: 83–88
(229) Sood AK, Sorosky JI, Gelder MS, Buller RE, Anderson B, Wilkinson EJ, Benda JA, Morgan LS. Primary ovarian sarcoma: analysis of prognostic variables and the role of surgical cytoreduction. Cancer 1998; 82: 1731–1737
(230) Sparks D, Chase D, Forsyth M, Ghani A. A rare case of primary extragenital retroperitoneal carcinosarcoma with review of the literature. Gynecol Surg 2010; 7: 259–262
(231) Sreenan JJ, Hart WR. Carcinosarcomas of the female genital tract. A pathologic study of 29 metastatic tumors: further evidence for the dominant role of the epithelial component and the conversion theory of histogenesis. Am J Surg Pathol 1995; 19: 666–674
(232) Sumathi VP, Murnaghan M, Dobbs SP, McCluggage WG. Extragenital müllerian carcinosarcoma arising from the peritoneum: report of two cases. Int J Gynecol Cancer 2002; 12: 764–767
(233) Sutton GP, Blessing JA, Homesley HD, Malfetano JH. A phase II trial of ifosfamide and mesna in patients with advanced or recurrent mixed mesodermal tumors of the ovary previously treated with platinum-based chemotherapy: A Gynecologic Oncology Group study. Gynecol Oncol 1994; 53: 24–26
(234) Sutton G, Brunetto VL, Kilgore L, Soper JT, McGehee R, Olt G, Lentz SS, Sorosky J, Hsiu JG. A phase III trial of ifosfamide with or without cisplatin in carcinosarcoma of the uterus: A Gynecologic Oncology Group study. Gynecol Oncol 2000; 79: 147–153
(235) Sutton G, Kauderer J, Carson LF, Lentz SS, Whitney CW, Gallion H. Adjuvant ifosfamide and cisplatin in patients with completely resected stage I or II carcinosarcomas (mixed mesodermal tumors) of the uterus: A Gynecologic Oncology Group study. Gynecol Oncol 2005; 96: 630–634
(236) Swerdlow AJ, Jones ME. British Tamoxifen Second Cancer Study Group: Tamoxifen treatment for breast cancer and risk of endometrial cancer: A case-control study. J Natl Cancer Inst 2005; 97: 375–384
(237) Szklaruk J, Tamm EP, Choi H, Varavithya V. MR imaging of common and uncommon large pelvic masses. Radiographics 2003; 23: 403–424
(238) Szukala SA, Marks JR, Burchette JL, Elbendary AA, Krigman HR. Co-expression of p53 by epithelial and stromal elements in carcinosarcoma of the female genital tract: An immunohistochemical study of 19 cases. Int J Gynecol Cancer 1999; 9: 131–136
(239) Takami M, Idei T, Nakayama Y, Ohta H, Fukai H, Matsumoto H, Togo Y, Sakamoto H, Yamamoto T, Satoh K. [A case of advanced ovarian carcinosarcoma that responded remarkably to neoadjuvant chemotherapy of combined CPT-11 and CDDP] (Abstr.). Gan To Kagaku Ryoho. 2002; 29: 305–308
(240) Tanaka YO, Tsunoda H, Minami R, Yoshikawa H, Minami M. Carcinosarcoma of the uterus: MR findings. J Magn Reson Imaging 2008; 28: 434–439
(241) Tanner EJ, Leitao MM Jr, Garg K, Chi DS, Sonoda Y, Gardner GJ, Barakat RR, Jewell EL. The role of cytoreductive surgery for newly diagnosed advanced-stage uterine carcinosarcoma. Gynecol Oncol 2011; 123: 548–552
(242) Tasic L, Vasiljevic M, Prorocic M, Jurisic A, Dragojevic-Dikic S, Jankovic-Raznatovic S. Carcinosarcoma of the uterus in advanced stage: A case report. Eur J Gynaecol Oncol 2013; 34: 343–346

(243) Tate Thigpen J, Blessing JA, DeGeest K, Look KY, Homesley HD; Gynecologic Oncology Group. Cisplatin as initial chemotherapy in ovarian carcinosarcomas: A Gynecologic Oncology Group study. Gynecol Oncol 2004; 93: 336–339
(244) Tekay A, Jouppila P. Controversies in assessment of ovarian tumors with transvaginal color Doppler ultrasound. Acta Obstet Gynecol Scand 1996; 75: 316–329
(245) Temkin SM, Hellmann M, Lee YC, Abulafia O. Early-stage carcinosarcoma of the uterus: the significance of lymph node count. Int J Gynecol Cancer 2007; 17: 215–219
(246) Teo SY, Babagbemi KT, Peters HE, Mortele KJ. Primary malignant mixed mullerian tumor of the uterus: findings on sonography, CT, and gadolinium-enhanced MRI. AJR Am J Roentgenol 2008; 191: 2782–2783
(247) Terada T. Carcinosarcoma in the pouch of Douglas. Arch Gynecol Obstet 2010; 281: 345–348
(248) Thigpen JT, Blessing JA, Beecham J, Homesley H, Yordan E. Phase II trial of cisplatin as first-line chemotherapy in patients with advanced or recurrent uterine sarcomas: A Gynecologic Oncology Group study. J Clin Oncol 1991; 9: 1962–1966
(249) Timmers PJ, Zwinderman K, Coens C, Vergote I, Trimbos JB. Lymph node sampling and taking of blind biopsies are important elements of the surgical staging of early ovarian cancer. Int J Gynecol Cancer 2010; 20: 1142–1147
(250) Timor-Tritsch I E, Goldstein St: Ultraschalldiagnostik in der Gynäkologie. München Jena, Urban & Fischer, 2008
(251) Tirumani SH, Ojili V, Shanbhogue AK, Fasih N, Ryan JG, Reinhold C. Current concepts in the imaging of uterine sarcoma. Abdom Imaging 2013; 38: 397–411
(252) Trimbos B, Timmers P, Pecorelli S, Coens C, Ven K, van der Burg M, Casado A. Surgical staging and treatment of early ovarian cancer: long-term analysis from a randomized trial. J Natl Cancer Inst 2010; 102: 982–987
(253) Trimbos JB. Lymphadenectomy in ovarian cancer: standard of care or unnecessary risk. Curr Opin Oncol 2011; 23: 507–511
(254) Tsikouras P, Liberis V, Galazios G, Savidis A, Grapsa A, Grapsas X, Teichmann AT, Maroulis G. Uterine sarcoma: A report of 57 cases over a 16-year period analysis. Eur J Gynaecol Oncol 2008; 29: 129–134
(255) Uehara T, Onda T, Togami S, Amano T, Tanikawa M, Sawada M, Ikeda S, Kato T, Kasamatsu T. Prognostic impact of the history of breast cancer and of hormone therapy in uterine carcinosarcoma. Int J Gynecol Cancer 2012; 22: 280–285
(256) Vaida AP, Horowitz NS, Oliva E, Halpern EF, Duska LR. Uterine malignant mullerian tumors should not be included in studies of endometrial cancers. Gynecol Oncol 2006; 103: 684–687
(257) Van den Bosch T, Coosemans A, Morina M, Timmerman D, Amant F. Screening for uterine tumours. Best Pract Res Clin Obstet Gynaecol 2012; 26: 257–66
(258) Vang R, Wheeler JE. Diseases of the fallopian tube and paratubal region. In: Kurman R J, Ellenson RH, Ronnett M (eds.). Blaustein's Pathology of the Female Tract. Sixth edn. Springer 2011; 530–578
(259) van Meurs HS, Tajik P, Hof MH, Vergote I, Kenter GG, Mol BW, Buist MR, Bossuyt PM. Which patients benefit most from primary surgery or neoadjuvant chemotherapy in stage IIIC or IV ovarian cancer? An exploratory analysis of the European Organisation for Research and Treatment of Cancer 55971 randomised trial. Eur J Cancer 2013; 49: 3191–3201
(260) Varela-Duran J, Nochomovitz LE, Prem KA, Dehner LP. Postirradiation mixed müllerian tumors of the uterus: A comparative clinicopathologic study. Cancer 1980; 45: 1625–1631
(261) Vergote I, Tropé CG, Amant F, Kristensen GB, Ehlen T, Johnson N, Verheijen RH, van der Burg ME, Lacave AJ, Panici PB, Kenter GG, Casado A, Mendiola C, Coens C, Verleye L, Stuart GC, Pecorelli S, Reed NS; European Organization for Research and Treatment of

Cancer-Gynaecological Cancer Group; NCIC Clinical Trials Group. Neoadjuvant chemotherapy or primary surgery in stage IIIC or IV ovarian cancer. N Engl J Med 2010; 363: 943–953
(262) Verheijen RH, Cibula D, Zola P, Reed N; Council of the European Society of Gynaecologic Oncology. Cancer antigen 125: lost to follow-up?: A European Society of Gynaecological Oncology Consensus Statement. Int J Gynecol Cancer 2: 2012; 170–174.
(263) Vorgias G, Fotiou S. The role of lymphadenectomy in uterine carcinosarcomas (malignant mixed mullerian tumours): A critical literature review. Arch Gynecol Obstet 2010; 282: 659–664
(264) Wada H, Enomoto T, Fujita M, Yoshino K, Nakashima R, Kurachi H, Haba T, Wakasa K, Shroyer KR, Tsujimoto M, Hongyo T, Nomura T, Murata Y. Molecular evidence that most but not all carcinosarcomas of the uterus are combination tumors. Cancer Res 1997; 57: 5379–85
(265) Wade K, Quinn MA, Hammond I, Williams K, Cauchi M. Uterine sarcoma: steroid receptors and response to hormonal therapy. Gynecol Oncol 1990; 39: 364–367
(266) Wang H, Lin KY, Merl M, Higgins SA, Silasi D, Santin A, Azodi M, Rutherford T, Schwartz PE, Abu-Khalaf MM. Cisplastin (C) and ifosfamide (I) chemotherapy with vaginal cuff brachytherapy (VCBT) for treatment of uterine carcinosarcoma. J Clin Oncol 2010; 28: (Suppl.) Abstr 5123
(267) Wang X, Tangjitgamol S, Liu J, Kavanagh JJ. Response of recurrent uterine high-grade malignant mixed müllerian tumor to letrozole. Int J Gynecol Cancer 2005; 15: 1243–1248
(268) Wittekind Ch, Comptom CC. TNM-Supplement – a commentary on uniform use. UICC and John Wiley & Sons, Weinheim 2013
(269) Wolfson AH, Brady MF, Rocereto T, Mannel RS, Lee YC, Futoran RJ, Cohn DE, Ioffe OB. A Gynecologic Oncology Group randomized phase III trial of whole abdominal irradiation (WAI) vs. cisplatin-ifosfamide and mesna (CIM) as post-surgical therapy in stage I-IV carcinosarcoma (CS) of the uterus. Gynecol Oncol 2007; 107: 177–185
(270) Wong L, See HT, Khoo-Tan HS, Low JS, Ng WT, Low JJ. Combined adjuvant cisplatin and ifosfamide chemotherapy and radiotherapy for malignant mixed müllerian tumors of the uterus. Int J Gynecol Cancer 2006; 16: 1364–1369
(271) Wright JD, Rosenblum K, Huettner PC, Mutch DG, Rader JS, Powell MA, Gibb RK. Cervical sarcomas: An analysis of incidence and outcome. Gynecol Oncol 2005; 99: 348–351
(272) Wright JD, Seshan VE, Shah M, Schiff PB, Burke WM, Cohen CJ, Herzog TJ. The role of radiation in improving survival for early-stage carcinosarcoma and leiomyosarcoma. Am J Obstet Gynecol 2008; 199: 536.e1–8
(273) Wu TI, Hsu KH, Huang HJ, Hsueh S, Chou HH, Tsai CS, Ho KC, Chao A, Chang TC, Lai CH. Prognostic factors and adjuvant therapy in uterine carcinosarcoma. Eur J Gynaecol Oncol 2008; 29: 483–488
(274) Yamada SD, Burger RA, Brewster WR, Anton D, Kohler MF, Monk BJ. Pathologic variables and adjuvant therapy as predictors of recurrence and survival for patients with surgically evaluated carcinosarcoma of the uterus. Cancer 2000; 88: 2782–2786
(275) Yokoyama Y, Yokota M, Futagami M, Mizunuma H. Carcinosarcoma of the fallopian tube: report of four cases and review of literature. Asia Pac J Clin Oncol 8: 2012; 303–311
(276) Yu JI, Choi DH, Huh SJ, Park W, Oh D, Bae DS. The reasonable timing of the adjuvant radiotherapy in the treatment of uterine carcinosarcoma according to the surgical intent: suggestion based on progression patterns. Radiat Oncol J 2013; 31: 72–80
(277) Yue X, Utsunomiya H, Akahira JI, Suzuki F, Ito K, Nagase S, Sasano H, Yaegashi N. Expression of steroid and xenobiotic receptor in uterine carcinosarcoma, leiomyosarcoma and endometrial stromal sarcoma. Oncol Lett 2013; 5: 835–839
(278) Zafrakas M, Zepiridis L, Theodoridis TD, Venizelos ID, Papanicolaou A, Agorastos T, Bontis JN. ERBB2 (HER2) protein expression in uterine sarcomas. Eur J Gynaecol Oncol 2009; 30: 292–294

(279) Zeisberg M, Neilson EG. Biomarkers for epithelial-mesenchymal transitions. J Clin Invest 2009; 119: 1429–37
(280) Zhang C, Hu W, Jia N, Li Q, Hua K, Tao X, Wang L, Feng W. Uterine carcinosarcoma and high-risk endometrial carcinomas: A clinicopathological comparison. Int J Gynecol Cancer 2015; 25: 629–636
(281) Zorzou MP, Markaki S, Rodolakis A, Kastritis E, Bozas G, Dimopoulos MA, Papadimitriou CA. Clinicopathological features of ovarian carcinosarcomas: A single institution experience. Gynecol Oncol 2005; 96: 136–42

Image references

Bahmann R, Otto D. Ketteler Krankenhaus Offenbach, Radiologie, Offenbach. Fig. 7.1.18 (A)
Baier P. Wollensack S. Ketteler Krankenhaus Offenbach, Gynäkologie und Geburtshilfe, Offenbach. Figs. 7.1.18 (B)–(D); 7.2.2 (E), (F)
Enke E. Gynäkologisch-geburtshilfliche Abteilung, Collm Klinik Oschatz, Oschatz. Fig. 7.1.11 (A), (B)
Evert M, Evert K. Universitätsmedizin Greifswald, Institut für Pathologie, Greifswald. Figs. 7.1.1 (B); 7.1.2 (A); 7.1.4 (A), (B); 7.1.5 (A), (B); 7.1.6 (A)–(C); 7.1.7 (A)–(F); 7.1.8 (A)–(H); 7.1.9 (F), (I); 7.1.17 (A)–(G); 7.1.20 (C), (F); 7.2.1 (D)
Evert M, Evert K. Institut für Pathologie, Universität Regensburg, Regensburg. Figs. 7.1.11 (C); 7.2.4
Günther W. Mutterhaus der Borromäerinnen, Gynäkologisch-geburtshilfliche Abteilung, Trier. Fig. 7.1.12 (A)
Hegerfeld R. Mutter-Kind-Zentrum Ostholstein, Sana Kliniken, Klinik Eutin, Eutin. Fig. 7.2.2 (A)–(C)
Herz M, Adrian-Kasten S. Gemeinschaftspraxis Frauenärztinnen, Vechta. Fig. 7.1.12 (B), (C)
Heß TH, ST Vincenz-Krankenhaus Limburg, Abt. f. Diagnostische Radiologie und interventionelle Radiologie und Nuklearmedizin, Limburg. Fig. 7.1.13
Hosten N, Hegenscheid K. Universitätsmedizin Greifswald, Institut für Diagnostische Radiologie und Neuroradiologie, Greifswald. Fig. 7.1.14
Köhler G. Universitätsmedizin Greifswald, Klinik Frauenheilkunde und Geburtshilfe, Greifswald. Figs. 7.1.1 (A); 7.1.2 (B)–(F); 7.1.3 (A), (B); 7.1.5 (C); 7.1.9 (A)–(E), (G), (H); 7.1.15; 7.1.16 (A)–(C); 7.1.19 (A), (B); 7.1.20 (A), (B), (D), (E); 7.2.1 (A)–(C)
Schütte M, Knaack U. Gyncollegweserland, Lübecke. Fig. 7.1.12 (D)
Vestring, Th. Diakoniekrankenhaus Rotenburg (Wümme), Institut für diagnostische und interventionelle Radiologie/Neuroradiologie, Rotenburg. Fig. 7.2.3 (A), (B)
Weiss E. Klinikverbund Südwest, KKH Böblingen, Frauenklinik. Böblingen. Fig. 7.2.2 (D)
Zechlin T, Hegerfeld R. Sana Klinik Eutin, Klinik für Frauenheilkunde und Geburtshilfe. Eutin. Fig. 7.1.10

Marek Zygmunt, Matthias Evert, Katja Evert and Günter Köhler

8 Fertility and pregnancy and variants of leiomyoma, smooth muscle tumors of unclear malignant potential, stromal tumors, genital sarcomas, PEComas and mixed tumors

8.1 General, symptoms, clinical presentation, diagnostics, differential diagnostics, prognosis

Genital or pelvic retroperitoneal sarcomas and pregnancy only very rarely occur simultaneously. According to one review, up until 2009, only 41 such cases had been described for women aged between 17 and 39 years (54, 64). During pregnancy, larger uterine tumors or rapid growth can result in miscarriage, premature birth, positional changes of the fetus or a labor obstruction. For all uterine and retroperitoneal sarcomas, the rate of premature birth ranges from 13.3 % to 18.2 %, and the children born have an average weight of 2,843 ± 791 g. No accounts have yet been published in which uterine sarcoma has been passed over transplacentally. The majority of cases covered in the aforementioned review were uterine sarcomas (37.5 %), while vulvar and vaginal sarcomas accounted for 22.5 % and 12.5 %, respectively. Sarcomas of the fallopian tube and the ovaries were not observed (54).

LMS (33.5 %) and LG-ESS (26.7 %) were the types of genital sarcoma most commonly encountered during pregnancy. The aforementioned review (54) also reported two embryonal RMS, one AS, one LS, and one sarcoma NOS.

In most cases, the presence of uterine sarcoma in pregnant women became evident in the first or the third trimester (54). Tumors had an average size of 8.1 cm in their largest dimension. Of a total of 15 uterine sarcomas, two became evident because of postpartum bleeding, and a further two due to rapid growth in the 11th and 30th week of gestation, respectively (54). Two or more symptoms were present simultaneously in only 20 % of cases. Overall, symptoms in the form of pains, vaginal bleeding, and rapid tumor growth largely correspond to those encountered outside of pregnancy.

Clinical diagnosis of uterine sarcomas in pregnant women is inevitably complicated. In 20 % of cases, uterine sarcomas are first thought to be LM. In the aforementioned review (54), in total, 42.5 % of all genital sarcomas were not initially suspected to be malignancies, and 22.5 % were incidental diagnoses. In 20 % of cases, sarcomas were only diagnosed during cesarean sections, and the suspected diagnosis was in fact reached via sonography in only 1 of 15 cases (54). The greatest diagnostic problem is that LM have a prevalence of around 10 % in pregnant women (43). During gestation 71.4 % of ordinary LM also exhibit significant growth, though said growth is more rapid in the first trimester (18). Myxoid LM, a type of neoplasm that predominantly arises in connection with pregnancy anyway, have also been observed to exhibit particularly rapid growth during gestation (37). Therefore, “rapidly growing myomas” during pregnancy are only exceptionally in fact uterine sarcomas (54). To be certain, LM discovered during pregnancy should be quickly examined via vaginal and/or transabdominal sonography. If the cumulative context of anamnesis, current clinical findings and symptoms plus suspicious sonographic findings suggests the presence of a malignant mesenchymal tumor, performing Doppler sonography along with a measurement of the RI is indicated. Doing so helps to more precisely assess whether a lesion is potentially LMS or LG-ESS (26). Patients should undergo an MRI when there is doubt. However, for LMS, MRI alone has a positive predictive value of only around 83 % (27). In summary, during pregnancy, both LMS and ESS exhibit largely the same characteristics in terms of clinical presentation and imaging diagnostics as they do outside of gestation (cf. flowchart in Vol. 1, Chapter 6).

It is unclear whether performing transcervical punch biopsy (analogous to the soft tissue tumors) is adequate or sensible. On the one hand, the informative value and significance of a punch biopsy, and the results such practice will yield, is strongly limited for both LMS and LG-ESS (cf. Chapters 2 and 6, Vol. 1). On the other hand, the question whether this method could potentially cause intraperitoneal tumor cell dissemination remains unresolved. The potential risks associated with intraperitoneal needle or punch biopsies are discussed in more detail in Chapters 2 and 6 in Volume 1. Performing a transcervical punch biopsy can be considered in exceptional cases, if such a procedure is even technically feasible.

Determining whether smooth muscle tumors in pregnant women are malignant or benign is already significantly exacerbated by the fact that cellularity is high and mitotic activity is elevated in the gestational context, and that necroses can also potentially be present in regular LM. Such findings are an expression of the elevated level of progesterone production. Whether a smooth muscle tumor should be classified as STUMP or as LMS is a particularly difficult decision to make in cases in which the number of mitoses is right at the threshold between these two entities, the TCN are minimal, or questionable necroses are present. See Chapters 1 and 2 in Vol. 1 for more detail.

The greatest differential diagnostic challenge during pregnancy is myoma degeneration, which presents with lower abdominal pains, rapid growth and suspicious results from multiple consecutive sonographic examinations.

Pregnant patients with uterine sarcomas have a mean and median survival of 2.5 and 1.5 years, respectively. These comparably unfavorable survival data are not least the result of relatively short periods of follow-up (average of 2.8 years) as well as the fact that two patients were lost within one year. Since the three patients who died had advanced/metastasized disease at the time of initial presentation, it cannot be concluded that pregnancy impacts negatively on prognosis for patients with uterine sarcomas. This is true especially für LG-ESS.

In a literature review (54), pregnant women with extrauterine-genital and abdominopelvic intra- and retroperitoneal sarcomas were aged between 17 and 41 years. Of all sarcomas detected in pregnant women 27.5 % were retroperitoneal. Analogous to the uterine variants of sarcoma, any mass that is palpable in the genital region during pregnancy must be assumed to be extrauterine sarcoma, even though their incidence during gestation is so low. Extrauterine-genital sarcomas are usually not independent tumor variants specific to the affected organ, but rather constitute STS that are "merely" localized there. Data pertaining to tubal sarcomas are practically nonexistent. A case of tubal sarcoma with dramatic intrapartum hemorrhage was described more than 50 years ago (65). At the time, histological diagnoses were not immunohistochemically substantiated. Looking back, the diagnosis seems barely believable.

Of the vulvar sarcomas observed in the literature to date, 5 were LMS, 2 were epithelioid sarcomas, 1 was undifferentiated sarcoma, 1 was botryoid sarcoma and 1 was RMS. Patient age ranged from 19 to 41 years. The distribution of the different entities roughly corresponds to the distribution in nonpregnant women (5). Tumor diameter ranged from 2.5 to 10 cm (mean: 6 cm). Only 2 patients reported pains. Most of the reported vulvar tumors were primarily identified as such due to suspicious growth, two were initially thought to be Bartholin's cysts. Similar to the uterine variants, the majority of vulvar sarcomas are incidental findings exclusively made in the first or third trimester. Four out of 10 patients had distant metastatic disease at the time of initial diagnosis, and these are the only women who were lost during follow-up. Only one sarcoma was diagnosed postpartum, while 5 sarcomas were surgically removed after delivery. It cannot be concluded from the data whether vulvar sarcomas have any influence on fertility and pregnancy, nor whether gravidity has an unfavorable influence on prognosis.

In pregnant patients, retroperitoneal sarcomas are usually discovered incidentally during cesarean sections, because of rapid growth or because patients present with symptoms like pain and sensations of distention (35, 54). In some cases, retroperitoneal sarcomas become evident because of weight loss during pregnancy. Myxoid and pleomorphic LS are the most common retroperitoneal tumors during pregnancy, followed by LMS. Premature birth is the most important complication, arising in 13.3 % of uterine and 18.2 % of retroperitoneal sarcomas. The ample amount of space that the tumor comes to require is deemed the principal cause for such complications – retroperitoneal sarcomas are known to reach sizes of up to 25 cm in pregnant women. Only 12.5 % of the children born to term exhibited intrauterine growth retardation. Vaginal births and births via cesarean sections accounted for equal shares (50 % each).

Diagnostics and therapy are largely guided by the principles that apply to uterine sarcomas and STS.

The survival rates among pregnant women with uterine sarcomas and those with extrauterine sarcomas do not differ. Median and mean survival are 3.3 and 2.5 years, respectively, for all genital and pelvic retroperitoneal localizations and histological entities; the 2-, 3- and 5-year cumulative survival rates are 60 %, 38 % and 17 %, respectively (54). Chemotherapy and/or radiation therapy were almost exclusively reserved for patients who already presented with metastatic disease at the time of primary diagnosis.

Resection should be performed in any case of a malignant tumor in which it is suitably localized and resection is technically possible during pregnancy. Otherwise, therapeutic decisions should be made on an interdisciplinary basis, taking the respective neoplasms' prognosis and gestational age into account. Neoadjuvant CHT could be a sensible alternative when patients desire to preserve their fertility. Alternatively, terminating the pregnancy or adopting an observant approach would have to be considered.

Uterine, extrauterine-genital and pelvic-retroperitoneal sarcomas rarely occur during pregnancy. They are usually incidental findings, and are often initially assumed to be leiomyoma when localized in the genital region. Leiomyosarcomas and low-grade endometrial stromal sarcomas are the most common types of sarcomas to arise in the uterus during gestation.

The symptoms and clinical findings presented by uterine sarcomas during pregnancy largely correspond to those of respective sarcomas outside of gestation. Ample use should be made of MRI and Doppler sonography whenever there are suspicious or abnormal findings. For extrauterine sarcomas, surgery is generally both indicated and possible without needing to terminate gestation. The prognosis for pregnant women with intrauterine and extrauterine sarcomas does not appear to differ from that for nonpregnant women with the same neoplasms.

8.2 Disseminated (diffuse) peritoneal leiomyomatosis

In principle, one must differentiate between pregnancy and hormone-associated DPLM on the one hand, and metastasized DPLM on the other. In around half of all observed cases, DPLM is incidentally diagnosed either during or shortly after gestation. All the available data do suggest that disease occurs de novo or recurs during the respective pregnancy (see pathogenesis of DPLM, Vol. 1, Chapter 1). DPLM apparently only develops during the second half of gravidity and can also affect younger women (78). DPLM in these cases are virtually always pregnancy/hormone-associated. If not accompanied by uterine LM, DPLM has no impact on fertility and generally has no influence on the course of pregnancy and the development of the fetus. The corresponding nodules can grow dramatically as pregnancy progresses, a course that cannot even be halted by extensive tumor-reductive surgery in some cases. Another study reports a case in which a parasitic LM, that had developed after the patient had undergone morcellation, exhibited rapid growth during pregnancy (82). It is not clear whether gestation has any role to play in the development of metastasized DPLM. Whether a DPLM is pregnancy-associated, or constitutes metastasized DPLM incidentally diagnosed upon conservative surgery performed under the indication of LM, is determined by the further course. While the former generally spontaneously regresses after pregnancy, the latter does not or continues to progress (cf. Chapter 1, Vol. 1).

While most DPLM are asymptomatic, they can sometimes cause ambiguous abdominal complaints that in turn can affect a pregnancy. In extremely rare cases, DPLM can complicate gestation by causing an acute abdomen together with elevated CRP values and a leukocytosis (78).

Treating gestation-associated DPLM that are incidentally discovered, e.g. during a cesarean section, is not necessary. The masses and symptoms virtually always regress after delivery, even when courses have been dramatic during gestation. Some of the present masses should be R0 resected in order to histologically secure the diagnosis. Larger or grossly suspicious lesions should likewise be surgically removed leaving R0 resection margins so as to rule out STUMP or LMS. If resection during pregnancy is indicated due to mechanical, technical or other reasons, only those masses should be removed on which the indication for surgery is based. Otherwise, asymptomatic DPLM incidentally diagnosed during gestation can be subjected to observation to term.

For women who have already presented with a coincidence of pregnancy and DPLM in the past, it must be assumed that the DPLM will recur if they become pregnant again. There are no known prophylactic measures.

A case has been reported in which a DPLM developed and was subsequently surgically treated outside of gestation. The patient later conceived via in vitro fertilization and delivered a healthy child via cesarean section (16). Another study recounts two cases in which women with pre-existing, thus metastasized DPLM successfully delivered after in vitro fertilization (80).

Pregnancy-associated disseminated peritoneal leiomyomatosis only develops during gestation. It has no apparent impact on fertility or on the course of the pregnancy, and usually regresses spontaneously after gestation. Growth during gestation can cause abdominal complaints. Asymptomatic cases require no therapeutic treatment. Patients who become pregnant again need to reckon with recurrences, there are no known prophylactic measures. To be certain, large and macroscopically suspicious individual lesions should be R0 resected and subjected to histological analysis. It is not known whether metastasized peritoneal leiomyomatosis has an influence on reproduction or exhibits noticeable growth during pregnancy.

8.3 Intravenous (intravascular) leiomyomatosis

Up to the year 2000, there had been at total of 35 cases in which this rare disease coincided with pregnancy (47). This incidence allows the assumption that the impact of IVLM on patient's fertility is at least not greater than that associated with regular LM. In one case, an IVLM resected during gestation revealed pronounced edema and hemorrhages, but only very few mitoses (55). IVLM are very likely to grow and expand during pregnancy. Analogous to uterine LM, strong intrauterine and parauterine intravenous growth can cause miscarriage. Progressive intracardiac extension into the large veins can induce or amplify cardiopulmonary complaints (47). Unilateral "thick legs" are also suspicious. In the latter case, for certainty, the possible presence of thrombosis needs to be ruled out. Abdominal MRI is, therefore, indicated in unclear or ambiguous cases. Resecting the lesions during pregnancy is indicated when symptoms are severe or threatening. Depending on the patient's desire to bear a child and on gestational age, one can resort to "merely" removing the IVLM from the large veins in a palliative approach, and schedule hysterectomy for after pregnancy (52). Definitive surgery can be performed on the date of delivery or during a cesarean section when the child is viable (cf. Vol. 1, Chapter 1). No literature is currently available on this matter.

The impact of intravenous (intravascular) leiomyomatosis on patient fertility is apparently no greater than that associated with regular leiomyoma. Cardiopulmonary complaints can complicate gestation. In these cases, the tumor must be bilaterally or unilaterally resected, depending on the age of pregnancy.

8.4 Benign metastasizing leiomyomas

MLM do not have any influence on fertility and gestation per se. However, the presence of large pulmonary masses will likely cause respiratory problems with increasing gestational age. An interesting case has been reported of a pregnant woman with a uterus myomatosus who underwent a cesarean section due to severe pre-eclampsia. Surgery revealed numerous myomas with wide open veins. The patient developed dramatic pulmonary symptoms immediately after the operation, and imaging revealed an extensive MLM in the lung. Symptoms diminished under 150 mg MPA daily, but there was no remission. GnRH analogues were given after one week, and upon general recovery the patient underwent HE with BSO. While this treatment approach served to alleviate the symptoms, the combination of HT and BSO did not achieve a remission of the pulmonary lesions (56). In this case, the operation obviously must have caused dramatic hematogenous dissemination of leiomyomatous materials. Since HT achieved no objective remission in the pulmonary lesions, it cannot be ruled out that the symptoms might have regressed spontaneously, and that they might have in fact been associated with the pre-eclampsia. There has also been an interesting case of spontaneous remission during gestation (31).

Benign metastasizing leiomyomas generally have no impact or influence on fertility and gestation. However, pulmonary complications can result from tumor growth and should be reckoned with.

8.5 Leiomyoma and its variants

In principle, it can be assumed that the different variants of LM affect and influence fertility and gestation to the same degree as regular LM. Rapid growth needs to be reckoned with during pregnancy due to the changes in blood circulation and the elevated levels of progesterone exposure that occur during gestation in LM. ALM are known to cause pain during pregnancy, though to date, this feature has only been observed in patients with extragenital-extrapelvic ALM (28). ALM can potentially rupture during pregnancy, and the resulting bleeding can quickly become life-threatening. The possibility of rupture must be considered whenever patients with known ALM present with an acute abdomen. Myxoid LM are often encountered in connection with gestation, and usually exhibit rapid growth when the two coincide (37).

The main problem with this family of neoplasms is that they are virtually always diagnosed as such postoperatively. Imaging diagnostic procedures like sonography and/or MRI cannot serve to reliably discern them from sarcomas during pregnancy. However, when there is clinical doubt, MRI in combination with an assessment of LDH values can be helpful in assessing whether a lesion is malignant or benign (cf. Vol. 1, Chapters 1, 2 and 6).

Due to the mitogenic effect of progesterone, mitotically active LM are often associated with a pregnancy or an otherwise caused exposure to progestins (15). Progestins are also capable of provoking changes in myxoid LM. The gestation-associated elevation in MI levels found in variants of LM (CLM, mitotically active, epithelioid, myxoid, apoplectic LM and LM with bizarre nuclei) resected during pregnancy or during a cesarean section, make differentiation from an LMS or a STUMP considerably more difficult.

Pregnancy apparently has no influence on the prognosis for the different LM variants. No recurrences were found in three women who had undergone ME on bizarre LM and who subsequently conceived and delivered, two via spontaneous delivery and one via elective cesarean section (50, 81). In one case, no residual disease was found in a patient who successfully delivered a child via cesarean section after resection of a superficial cotyledonoid LM (67). A further publication reports an account in which a superficial cotyledonoid LM was resected in the 14th week of gestation. The uterus was found to be tumor-free during cesarean section performed to term (53).

ME is a possible option for patients with variants of LM who urgently wish to preserve their fertility (7, 68). However, due to the special growth pattern that cotyledonoid LM exhibit, recurrence must be reckoned with when conservative surgery is opted for and R1 resection margins are achieved. CLM, in particular such with chromosomal p1 deletions, and LM with diffuse p16 and p53 expression must be treated analogous to STUMP (cf. Vol. 1, Chapter 1). Likewise, tumor injury/perforation and R1/2 resections should be avoided.

The different variants of leiomyoma do not differ from regular Leiomyoma in terms of their influence on fertility and pregnancy. They can, however, grow rapidly and become painful. MRI in combination with LDH value measurement can be helpful when there are clinical doubts regarding the aggressiveness of the tumor. Pregnancy has no influence on prognosis for this group of neoplasms.

Histologically differentiating STUMP or leiomyosarcoma from leiomyoma resected during pregnancy, and especially from its variants, can be challenging. Uterus-sparing surgery is possible when patients wish to preserve their fertility, as long as the tumor is not injured or perforated.

8.6 Smooth muscle tumors of uncertain malignant potential

The STUMP tumor family is discussed at length in the chapter on smooth muscle tumors, their variants and smooth muscle tumors with uncertain malignant potential (Vol. 1, Chapter 1). Such tumors usually only come to be discussed in the context of fertility and gestation when they are discovered incidentally after patients have undergone conservative surgery under the indication of LM in order to preserve their fertility. STUMP do not appear to have a noticeable influence on pregnancy or fertility, regardless of whether they remain in situ or if they have been treated with organ-sparing surgery. There are reports of cases in which STUMP patients had multiple pregnancies after having undergone one or even two TE (13, 50). STUMP and regular LM are very similar in terms of their clinical behavior, localization and growth, making it reasonable to expect that they will have largely the same effects on gestation and fertility.

Determining whether smooth muscle tumors in pregnant patients are malignant or benign is exacerbated by the fact that even regular LM can exhibit high cellularity, elevated MI, necroses and myxoid change in the context of gestation. Moreover, deciding whether a smooth muscle tumor still constitutes a STUMP or whether it should already be classified as LMS is particularly difficult when the MI is near the threshold/cut-off point and the type of necrosis is unclear. Please refer to the chapter on STUMP for more detailed information (Vol. 1, Chapter 1). In this regard, in one case study (92), a tumor was detected and extirpated during a cesarean section. The lesion was classified as LMS, and the case took a positive course. However, critical assessment of the case suggests that the tumor was in fact a STUMP.

While there are reports of pregnancies that took a successful course (13, 50), complications can still arise and courses can be unusual. In one case of a woman with coinciding gestation and STUMP, pregnancy had to be ended via preterm birth, probably due to a chorioamnionitis (14). There are also accounts of rapid tumor growth during pregnancy (50). In one DKSM consultancy case, an LM that had already been suspicious in sonography increased 3-fold in surface from 1 year before pregnancy to the 36th week of gestation, and 7-fold by the time pregnancy ended (41). The tumor had a diameter of 7 cm and was resected during a cesarean section after an otherwise uneventful pregnancy. The tumor constituted a labor obstruction. Histological analysis revealed only minimal TCN, 5 M/10 HPF and focally disseminated significant cellular atypia. The tumor was classified as a STUMP in the gestational context, though outside of that context it would more likely have been classified as an LMS (Fig. 8.6.1 (A)–(C)). What was noticeable about this tumor was that it was negative for ER but had strong PGR expression. Its rapid growth was most likely progesterone associated, not least because progesterone is said to influence LM growth (34, 40).

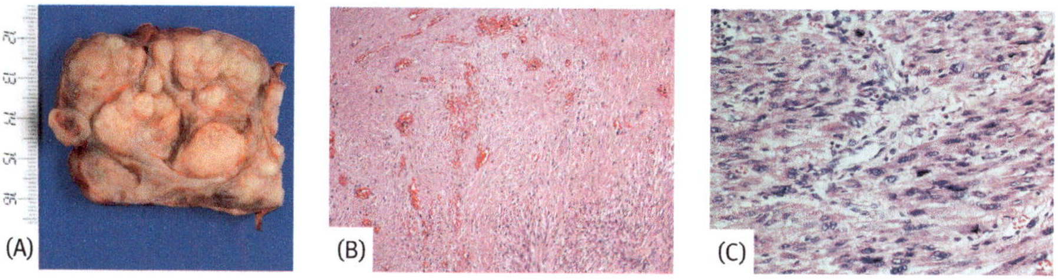

Fig. 8.6.1: (A) STUMP that had grown rapidly during pregnancy, macroscopic findings; (B) described tumor cell necroses were clearly discernible under the microscope, but did not fulfill the criteria necessary to be classified as tumor cell necroses in leiomyosarcoma; (C) the microscopic features exemplified in (B), together with significant atypia and ample mitotic activity, create a histological picture strongly reminiscent of LMS. Follow-up is still ongoing, but the patient did not relapse within the first year.

In principle, patients who wish to preserve their fertility can undergo organ-sparing surgery (13, 50). However, they must be informed, not only that it is not uncommon for STUMP to recur after conservative surgical procedures, but also that they can recur as LMS (for details see Vol. 1, Chapter 1). Therefore, indications for organ-preserving surgical procedures need to be based on strict criteria, and patients must be unequivocally informed of the increased risk of recurrence.

A case has been reported in which a patient became pregnant following removal of a STUMP via TE. At the time of the later cesarean section, a large uterine fibroid was again present. The patient underwent HE one year later, revealing numerous LM, but no STUMP (13). One literature review (13) also covered cases of women with STUMP who underwent TE, followed by successful pregnancy and birth of a living child. Among them, not one recurrence or de novo STUMP was observed. The same applies to the two cases in said review in which TE was performed during gestation.

While the courses witnessed after having performed TE on STUMP have thus far been promising ones, the goal should nonetheless be to become pregnant as shortly after surgery as possible. THE should then be undergone as soon as the patient's desire to have children has been satisfied. Where the desire to have children is not "acute", follow-up LSC should be performed within 3–6 mo (see Vol. 1, Chapters 1 and 6) (60, 74). There are no known prophylactic measures for preventing relapse.

LM and STUMP can also arise in the region of the vulva, vagina and ovaries during gestation. The myxoid variants, in particular, exhibit rapid growth during pregnancy

(58, 83). Overall, it is typical for vulvar LM and STUMP in pregnant women to exhibit extensive myxoid differentiation, while significant cellular atypia and an elevated MI are not found to be present (83).

Morcellation is associated with potentially elevated risks of recurrence and metastasis, and should thus never be opted for in any form in STUMP patients. The main problem in this regard is that STUMP are usually incidentally diagnosed as such post-surgery, and that lesions could in fact also be LMS. Analogous to the uterine neoplasms, DD are exacerbated by the fact that the MI is often elevated in smooth muscle tumors during gestation. MRI and color Doppler sonography should be performed when diagnosis is uncertain. Transcervical punch biopsy can be considered if diagnostic uncertainty persists and the intervention is technically feasible (cf. Vol. 1, Chapters 2 and 6). The challenges and pitfalls pertaining to punch biopsy are referred to in the chapters on STUMP, LMS and prevention of inadequate surgery (Vol. 1, Chapters 1, 2 and 6).

R0 resection is sufficient for vulvar and vaginal LM and STUMP, and can be performed during pregnancy. Follow-up treatment is not necessary.

Ovarian smooth muscle tumors in pregnant women usually also present with rapid growth, high cellularity, elevated mitotic activity and extensive hyaline necrosis. Consequently, diagnostically differentiating between LM and STUMP in pregnant patients can be challenging.

STUMP apparently have no influence or impact on fertility or gestation per se. It is highly unlikely that pregnancy will impact negatively on patient prognosis, but it does make discerning STUMP from regular leiomyoma and leiomyosarcoma considerably more difficult. Undergoing organ-sparing surgery is associated with an increased risk of recurrence, but is an option for patients who still desire to have children, so long as they are comprehensively informed. Patients should come in for endoscopic follow-up with 3–6 months of conservative surgery. Such patients should seek to become pregnant without undue delay. Total hysterectomy should be performed as soon as possible once the patient's desire to have children has been fulfilled.

8.7 Leiomyosarcoma

Women who develop an LMS at a more advanced age apparently do not suffer adverse effects on their fertility. Accordingly, only about 11 % of women with an LMS are nulliparous (1). When adjusted for patient age and stage of disease, the number of previous pregnancies has no influence on prognosis for LMS patients (1). Even pre-existing and recurrent LMS do not seem to have any bearing on fertility and the course of gestation (36). The same applies to retroperitoneal LMS and LMS of other sites, for example the vagina and the vulva (6, 19, 85).

Uterine and extrauterine LMS can produce HCG and thus generate the wrong impression that the patient is pregnant (46).

It has not yet been clarified whether or not gestation has an influence on LMS in terms of growth and prognosis. Since LMS are largely HR positive, one could assume that pregnancy would serve to accelerate growth of present LMS or facilitate the recurrence of LMS that have been subjected to conservative surgery prior. After all, progesterone does have a mitogenic effect on myogenic cells (40). However, PGR expression is typically only low or entirely absent in LMS (cf. Vol. 1, Chapter 2). The positive prognosis with which HR positive LMS as well as LMS in premenopausal women are associated rather suggests that pregnancy is unlikely to stimulate disease. With the exception of two observed patient deaths (54), there is at least no evidence to suggest that pregnancy has an unfavorable impact on prognosis.

There are accounts of 9 coincidences of gestation and LMS, in 4 of which the pregnancy was carried out. In one case that took a fatal course, the recurrent tumor was discovered during a cesarean section. All tumors had been R0 resected, i.e. the resection margins were microscopically disease-free. More closely studying the sources (48, 68) reveals that the majority of these tumors had in fact been STUMP. These findings must, therefore, be regarded critically and should not simply be taken at face value.

If clinical examination and medical imaging reveal a justifiable suspicion of an LMS in a pregnant patient, diagnostics can be expanded to include transcervical punch or fine needle biopsies if technically feasible (cf. Vol. 1, Chapters 2 and 6).

Organ-sparing operations and intraoperative tumor injuries and/or perforations significantly worsen the prognosis. Therefore, any form of conservative intervention must be abstained from, even if the patient still desires to bear children. If such course of action is opted for nonetheless, the patient must be unequivocally informed of the elevated risk that such procedures are associated with in terms of DFS and OS. Endoscopic follow-up should occur within 3–6 months of such surgeries (60, 74). Patients in these cases should seek to become pregnant as quickly as possible and definitive surgery should be performed as soon as the patient has fulfilled her desire to have children. Details pertaining to diagnostics and organ-sparing surgery are discussed at length in the chapter on LMS (Vol. 1, Chapter 2). In general, when considering pregnancy, patients who have undergone conservative operations should bear in mind that LMS have an extraordinarily poor prognosis.

It is unclear whether the discovery of a uterine LMS during gestation mandatorily requires that pregnancy be ended immediately, not least because OS does not depend on whether a uterine LMS is diagnosed early or late. Given the very poor prognosis, if the child is not yet viable, terminating pregnancy and simultaneously subjecting the LMS to adequate surgical treatment should be given serious consideration. No experiences or data have yet been published relating to the administration of neoadjuvant CHT in the 2nd or 3rd gestational trimester. Neoadjuvant CHT generally achieves low response rates in LMS and therefore constitutes a risk that is far from insignificant.

Pre-existing, even recurrent extrauterine LMS apparently have no influence on fertility and the course of pregnancy. The same applies to vaginal, vulvar and retroperitoneal LMS. In general, extrauterine genital sarcomas can, however, develop into an obstruction for labor. Vulvar LMS can also be extirpated during gestation. Meticulous effort must be taken to achieve wide R0 resection margins so as to spare the patient postoperative RT. In principle, vaginal LMS can also be subjected to surgery during pregnancy, if their size makes such surgery technically possible. Otherwise, it must be considered in each case individually whether pregnancy should be ended and the tumor simultaneously resected (cf. Vol. 1, Chapter 2).

Only two accounts of vaginal LMS in pregnant women have been published. Diagnostics and therapy largely correspond to those of vaginal LMS in non-gestational patients (6, 54).

On the basis of current knowledge, performing unilateral ovarectomy can suffice in cases of patients with unilateral ovarian LMS who desire to preserve their fertility. In principle, the same applies to ovarectomies in cases of pregnant women. In any case, the poor prognosis with which such tumors are associated must always be borne in mind. LMS localized in the vulva have the most promising starting point. Details are presented in the context of extrauterine LMS (cf. Vol. 1, Chapter 2).

Leiomyosarcoma apparently have no influence on fertility and gravidity. It is highly unlikely that pregnancy will impact negatively on prognosis. Subjecting Leiomyosarcoma patients who wish to bear children to organ-sparing surgery is associated with a poorer progression free interval and poorer overall survival. The poor overall disease-specific prognosis already serves to contraindicate conservative surgical interventions. When they are nonetheless opted for, patients must be unequivocally and comprehensively informed of the risks involved. Laparoscopic follow-up should be scheduled within three months of undergoing conservative surgery. Moreover, patients should seek to become pregnant without considerable undue delay. Once the desire to bear children has been fulfilled, total hysterectomy should be performed as quickly as possible. Pregnancies in which the child would not be viable should be aborted and the tumor subjected to adequate surgery.

8.8 Endometrial stromal nodules and uterine tumors with sex cord-like elements type I and II (ESTSCLE and UTROSCT)

The data situation is too weak to allow conclusions to be drawn in terms of whether ESN affect fertility or gestation. Notwithstanding, it can be assumed that ESN will have a similar influence to LM, as these two types of neoplasm have numerous features in common in terms of clinical behavior, localization and growth.

Bearing in mind that ESN exhibit a strong expression of ER and PGR almost without exception, it is at least thinkable that pregnancy will have an impact on the growth of such tumors, or might promote transformation into an LG-ESS. Elevated mitotic rates, constituting an expression of increased proliferation, have been reported during pregnancy (38). However, ESN in nonpregnant women have also been described as having this feature. The observed decidualization of ESN is most likely effected by gestation. In one case, sonography revealed a 5 cm large ESN situated at the interface between the placenta and the decidua in the 28th week of pregnancy. At the time of normal term delivery, the tumor was found to be embedded within the placenta (38).

Pregnant patients with ESN who urgently desire to bear the child and to preserve their fertility can undergo organ-sparing surgery. More information to this end is provided in the chapter on ESN under surgical therapy (cf. Vol. 1, Chapter 3). Since diagnostically differentiating ESN from LG-ESS poses such a challenge, patients with ESN should undergo laparoscopic follow-up within 3–6 months, if they have been subjected to morcellation or conservative operations.

In one DKSM consultation case, a patient whose ESN had been extirpated became pregnant soon after surgery. Pregnancy took an uneventful course and culminated in the birth of a healthy child. Multiple peritoneal and uterine biopsies revealed no findings suggestive of ESN or LG-ESS, even though the tumor – not known to be ESN at the time of primary diagnosis – had been intraperitoneally punctured during primary surgery (cf. Vol. 1, Chapter 3) (3).

Conservative surgery leaving R0 resection margins can be considered for patients with uterine tumors with sex cord-like elements (cf. Vol. 1, Chapter 3) who wish to bear children (8, 9, 25, 30), but should only be opted for in exceptional cases. Since such procedures are generally associated with an elevated risk of recurrence, they should only be performed when the following criteria are fulfilled: not ESTSCLE, no LVI, no distant metastasis, tumor < 10 cm (9).

In one case, a patient who underwent enucleation subsequently successfully carried out a regular pregnancy, even though the tumor had pushing invasive margins (30). In another case, a patient was diagnosed with a metastasized ESTECLE in the 35th week of gestation. The peritoneal masses were subjected to maximal cytoreductive surgery during cesarean section. However, the patient had also developed pulmonary metastases. Neither CHT using ifosfamide plus carboplatin, nor a combination of cyclophosphamide, vincristine, doxorubicin plus dacarbazine effected a remission. The patient died 9 mo after surgery (20).

Endometrial stromal nodules apparently have no influence on patient fertility. The situation corresponds to that of leiomyoma or endometrial stromal sarcomas in this context. Pregnancy could promote their growth. Organ-sparing surgery is possible if patients desire to preserve fertility. Conservative procedures should not be performed on patients with uterine tumors with sex cord-like elements due to the elevated risk of recurrence.

8.9 Low-grade endometrial stromal sarcoma

Fertility and gestation usually only really become an issue when an LG-ESS is incidentally diagnosed in patients who desire to preserve their fertility and thus undergo conservative surgery under the indication of LM. Neither existing LG-ESS, nor those that have been subjected to organ-sparing surgery, appear to have a noticeable influence on fertility or pregnancy (4, 17, 21, 42, 45, 59, 87, 90, 95). In one case, cesarean section revealed a retroplacental LG-ESS within the decidua. The tumor had had no impact on gestation (40). Since LG-ESS and LM share numerous commonalities in terms of their clinical behavior, localization and growth (cf. Vol. 1, Chapter 4), it can be expected that their influence and impact on gestation is also similar. No accounts of transplacental passage of uterine sarcoma have yet been published (54).

The few available reports pertaining to the course of LG-ESS following pregnancy, with and without prior surgical interventions, are contradictory and ambiguous. In one case, a patient underwent conservative surgery and subsequent CHT on a tumor classified at the time as high-grade ESS. Following treatment, she conceived naturally and subsequently delivered a healthy child. The patient did not relapse within the 5-year follow-up period (90). However, the histological findings and the evaluation thereof were questionable overall. In another instance (17), a 16-year-old patient with LG-ESS (pre-2014 nomenclature) underwent an organ-sparing resection. She conceived after 8 years of adjuvant MGA therapy and carried out the pregnancy. Her further course is not known. The presented microscopic findings do not serve to reliably rule out whether the patient had in fact had primary ESN. A further publication recounts the case of a woman who conceived rapidly after hysteroscopic resection of an LG-ESS, and who duly delivered her child. Extensive peritoneal recurrence was diagnosed in the immediate postpartum period and subsequently surgically resected. The patient was treated with AI upon removal of a further recurrence (42). In a similar case, a patient with LG-ESS opted for primary conservative surgery with 16 mo of subsequent progestin treatment. She subsequently conceived and gave birth to premature twins via cesarean section in the 32nd week of gestation. Postpartum follow-up revealed that the patient had developed recurrences (70). A further case study reports a lethal course within 4 mo of having undergone a cesarean section with simultaneous resection of an LG-ESS (87). A further publication recounts a case in which stage III LG-ESS was revealed in a patient who presented with persistent postpartum bleeding (45).

Since LG-ESS are generally HR positive and respond well to palliative HT, in light of the case studies at hand, it is justifiable to assume that pregnancy can accelerate or induce growth in present LG-ESS or those that have been subjected to conservative surgery prior. When technically feasible, transcervical punch biopsy can be performed during pregnancy, if a lesion's clinical behavior and imaging diagnostic features create a reasonable suspicion of LG-ESS. The problems and challenges associated with this procedure are discussed in the chapters on LMS, LG-ESS and prevention of inadeqate surgery (cf. Vol. 1, Chapters 2, 4 and 6). Besides the possibility of terminating pregnancy and performing an HE, LG-ESS can also first be enucleated. Since this procedure is associated with a very high risk of recurrence, it could be sensible to end pregnancy via cesarean section once the child is viable, and to perform simultaneous definitive surgery. The lack of reliable data makes it imperative that the potential risks are precisely discussed with the patient beforehand. Due to the fact that tumors subjected to conservative surgery have been observed to recur after pregnancy, to be certain, administering postpartum progestin therapy should be given serious consideration. Taken together, the available data do suggest that such course of action should at least be considered.

Due to the aforementioned factors and to the fact that undergoing inadequate surgery serves to shorten RFI considerably, conservative operations should not be resorted to "merely" to fulfill the patient's desire to preserve their fertility (cf. Vol. 1, Chapter 4). On the other hand, effects on OS have yet to be observed. Therefore, despite reports of several cases in which outcomes were favorable, conservative surgery should only be considered exceptionally for LG-ESS patients, and only after they have been comprehensibly informed of the potential risks involved (77). Resection must reliably occur entirely in disease-free tissue (R0 margins). Extensive LVI must be deemed a contraindication. Likewise, conservative surgery is contraindicated if the patient is already suffering other fertility disorders. Patients should undergo follow-up LSC within 3–6 mo of surgery before considering conception (74). Otherwise, one runs the risk that recurrence could already (potentially avoidably) be present at the onset of pregnancy. Since an R1 or RX situation must be presumed following conservative surgery in many cases, administering immediately postoperative adjuvant HT with progestins should be considered as a means for reducing the risk of recurrence. One case report recounts positive experiences being made by administering postoperative progestin therapy to a patient who underwent prior resection of an LG-ESS and later became pregnant (21). The literature offers no usable information or recommendations in terms of what duration such adjuvant HT should be administered for in this context, though a two-year timeframe seems appropriate. Giving patients adjuvant HT is also in line with the current NCCN recommendations (57). However, it has yet to be reliably proven that such therapy is effective in preventing pregnancy-associated recurrence. One reported case exemplifies that following up conservative operations with HT need not necessarily always be enough to protect patients from developing recurrences during gestation (70). THE should be performed as soon as the patient has fulfilled her desire to bear children (4).

Vulvar and vaginal LG-ESS should be surgically R0 resected while pregnancy is still ongoing so as to prevent that the gestation context potentially accelerates tumor growth. For LG-ESS in the ovary, performing an ovarectomy can be classified as adequate surgery, also during pregnancy.

Low-grade endometrial stromal sarcomas apparently have no influence on fertility and/or gestation per se. Pregnancy will most likely influence the prognosis unfavorably. Organ-sparing surgery opted for on grounds of a patient's desire to preserve fertility is associated with a higher risk of recurrence that is likely exacerbated by the pregnancy context. Endoscopic follow-up should occur within 3–6 months of conservative surgery. It seems sensible to seriously consider undergoing adjuvant hormone therapy prior to conceiving. Total hysterectomy should follow as soon as the patient has fulfilled her desire to bear children. Whether undergoing temporary postpartum hormone therapy, with a view to preventing recurrence, is sensible, has yet to be reliably proven, though it should be at least considered.

8.10 High-grade endometrial stromal sarcomas and undifferentiated uterine sarcomas

Virtually no data are available that relate to the influence of HG-ESS and UUS on fertility and gestation, nor that concern the impact of pregnancy on these types of neoplasms. This state of affairs is a consequence of both the generally low incidences of such tumors and the fact that they predominantly arise in postmenopausal women. UUS were recently first included in the current WHO Classification (62), but absolutely no data are available on these neoplasms in the context of fertility and pregnancy. In one case, an HG-ESS presented as an endocervical polyp in the 25th week of pregnancy. Pregnancy took an uneventful, regular course after resection. Gestation was ended in the 34th week of pregnancy via cesarean section combined with HE and LNE, and culminated in the delivery of a healthy child (72).

One HG-ESS discovered in the 15th week of gestation already exhibited wide intraperitoneal spread (2). Pregnancy was terminated via TAH, and the patient died within 6 weeks. Whether or not the tumor had in fact originated in the uterus, however, remained unclear. HG-ESS can also be HR positive (44). In these cases, as for LG-ESS, it must be reckoned with that pregnancy will have an unfavorable impact on the tumor (in all of the aforementioned cases, the nomenclature prior to 2014 was used).

Since HG-ESS and UUS are known to grow very rapidly, it must be assumed that an incurable condition will develop during pregnancy if intervention is not immediate. In HG-ESS that are HR positive, pregnancy is even likely to stimulate tumor growth even further. Against this backdrop, the sensible option is to end the pregnancy without delay, also via abortion or premature birth, whenever these tumors are diagnosed, and to immediately undertake adequate surgery. While administering systemic (neoadjuvant) therapy until the child is viable might seem like a sensible option, due to the poor rates with which CHT achieves a response, and the fact that responses are only very short, such course of action would constitute an unjustifiable risk. In a similar vein, for HG-ESS and UUS, any form of uterus-sparing surgery is strongly contraindicated, even when technically feasible. Overall, it appears unlikely that pregnancy per se has an unfavorable influence on the prognosis for HR negative HG-ESS and UUS.

Barely any usable data are available pertaining to the relationship between fertility and gestation on the one hand, and high-grade endometrial stromal sarcomas and undifferentiated uterine sarcomas on the other. Due to the extremely poor prognosis with which these neoplasms are generally associated, pregnancy should be terminated by whatever means are appropriate in the individual case, and the tumor should be subjected to adequate definitive surgery in the same sitting.

8.11 Angiosarcoma

There is nothing in the literature about uterine, vulvar and vaginal ANS in the context of fertility and gravidity. This is likely to be connected to the fact that uterine ANS predominantly arise in postmenopausal women. In contrast, the majority of ovarian ANS patients are premenopausal. However, barely any cases of ovarian ANS in pregnant women are known. In one case, a 28-year-old woman presented with ovarian ANS and underwent unilateral ovarectomy. She relapsed within 15 mo. The recurrent tumor had infiltrated the pelvic colon, the rectum and the abdominal wall. The patient retained her uterus and remaining ovary by undergoing maximal cytoreductive surgery and subsequent CHT using doxorubicin and ifosfamide. After two years of hormonal contraception, the patient became pregnant and later delivered a healthy child. She suffered no further relapse (32). In a further case, CT revealed a pelvic mass in a patient who was three months pregnant and who had undergone surgery on a primary ANS of the mammary two years prior. Cesarean section in the 36th week of gestation, in the course of which a healthy child was delivered, revealed a well-capsulated ANS metastasis to the ovary. The ovary was resected, the uterus and the other adnexa were preserved (86).

According to the literature, ANS in the ovaries as well as those in other organs apparently have no influence on fertility or on the intrauterine development of the child. There have been no accounts of metastasis to the placenta. The aforementioned case (86) as well as accounts of ANS in other sites like the mammary, the skull and the chest (23, 69, 71), are at least suggestive of the possibility that pregnancy can impact negatively on the course of ANS, or can promote their growth. Given the fact that ANS are generally already associated with a poor prognosis, patients should rather be dissuaded from conceiving.

Angiosarcomas and pregnancy only rarely coincide. Such neoplasms have no apparent impact on fertility or on the adequate development of unborn children. Gestation could possibly have an unfavorable influence on the prognosis of angiosarcomas in all localizations.

8.12 Liposarcoma

It is not known whether or not uterine LS have any influence on fertility. Lipogenic tumors are easy to recognize as such in sonography and MRI. Transcervical or fine needle aspiration biopsy can be performed. The problems and challenges that can arise in this context are described in the chapter on LS (Chapter 2).

Exceptionally, uterus-sparing tumor extirpation can be considered for patients with uterine LS who wish to preserve their fertility. This decision ultimately depends on the tumor's degree of malignancy or its dedifferentiation. Such an approach would most likely be conceivable for well-differentiated LS, though there have been no reports of this type of neoplasm having arisen in the uterus to date. For all other variants, conservative surgery must be regarded as inadequate and thus contraindicated, due to their strong potential for recurrence and metastasis. In direct comparison, that potential is lower in dedifferentiated and myxoid round cell LS, and highest in pleomorphic LS (cf. Chapter 2). Even patients with well-differentiated LS must be insistently and comprehensively informed of the high risk of recurrence.

Uterus-sparing operations must thus always be regarded critically, especially if it cannot be guaranteed beyond doubt that the resection margins will be disease-free. In once DKSM consultancy case (41), a 23-year-old patient who underwent R0 resection of a uterine dedifferentiated LS did not relapse during the 4-year follow-up period. Analogous to the other types of uterine sarcoma, an endoscopic follow-up examination should be considered within 3–6 months. Uterine sonography should likewise be regarded as an essential element of oncologic follow-up.

Within the group of LS, retroperitoneal LS appear to coincide most frequently with pregnancy. Up until 2014, the literature provided accounts of 67 pregnancies that coincided with retroperitoneal LS (35, 49, 61, 66, 84, 88). Even entirely resected, extremely large pelvic-retroperitoneal LS do not appear to have any impact on gestation or fertility (49, 79). In one case in which a huge dedifferentiated LS was discovered at 29 weeks gestation, the patient had previously already had five miscarriages (61). In a case involving a pregnant patient with simultaneous pleomorphic LS, fetal development was normal, though delivery was premature (84). It appears unlikely that premature delivery stood in connection to the LS. Roughly 25 % of the 67 cases of LS described in the literature significantly progressed either during or immediately after gestation and took a lethal course. Those cases included patients who were operated on either before, during or after pregnancy. CHT and/or RT failed to impact on the further course. In one case, a well-differentiated (low-grade) purely myxoid LS was radically excised from a pregnant patient at 36 weeks' gestation at the time of cesarean delivery. The resection margins were not disease-free (not R0), and the tumor recurred as a poorly differentiated (high-grade) myxoid/round cell LS. The patient eventually died of the disease. Pregnancy might possibly have an unfavorable influence on LS in terms of prognosis.

Overall, completely resecting retroperitoneal LS while gestation is still ongoing seems to be a sensible option (65). In one case, a pleomorphic LS in a pregnant patient was wrongly classified as pedunculated myoma (84). Despite CHT, the case took a dramatic further course. In cases of well-differentiated LS, definitive surgery can be performed during cesarean section once the child's lungs have matured (88).

MRI (see also imaging, Chapter 2) and FDG-PET-CT are highly reliable means for verifying/securing a diagnosis of well-differentiated LS (75). Notwithstanding, the diagnosis should be confirmed via punch biopsy. On the basis of what is known today, subject to strict indication criteria, FDG-PET-CT can be performed as of the second trimester (93, 94). Overall, LS do not appear to impact negatively on the child's development in any way.

It is not known whether uterine liposarcomas have any influence on fertility and pregnancy. Arising space constraints could necessitate or facilitate a premature delivery. Uterus-sparing operations, as means of fertility preservation, should only be performed upon highly critical consideration. Where possible, extrauterine LS should be surgically excised leaving clean R0 resection margins while the patient is still pregnant. Until further data are available, patients whose uterine, genital or retroperitoneal tumors have been resected, but without achieving R0 resection margins, should rather be dissuaded from becoming pregnant. The question whether gestation has a negative impact on the prognosis for liposarcomas remains an open one, but it might possibly have an unfavorable influence.

8.13 Rhabdomyosarcoma

Only four cases of RMS coinciding with gestation have been reported. Patients were aged between 18 and 29 years (54). One patient with botryoid RMS was lost within 12 months. In the remaining three cases, follow-up lasted for 12–54 months. Embryonal/botryoid RMS generally have a relatively promising prognosis (cf. Chapter 3). The tumors were all localized in the upper two-thirds of the vagina, were discovered incidentally during obstetric examination, and were primarily recognized and diagnosed as such. Patients became symptomatic with bleeding during the last third of gestation. Three RMS patients were operated on during the third trimester and two underwent surgery postpartum. In one case, considerable tumor growth made a cesarean section necessary. One patient received CHT, another underwent both CHT and additional ERT. The majority of the sources covered in the corresponding literature review (54) are more than 20 years old.

Overall, the RMS did not appear to have had any impact on patient fertility or gestation (54). A recent publication recounts a case in which a large retroperitoneal spindle cell ERMS was incidentally discovered immediately after spontaneous vaginal delivery of a healthy child (91). The tumor had had no discernible influence on the pregnancy.

ERMS usually clinically present as polypoid tumors growing into the vagina. Diagnosis is usually reached via biopsy. No cases of primary metastatic disease have been reported, most likely because ERMS generally have a rather favorable prognosis. The review at hand, as well as another case study, yielded no findings which would suggest that pregnancy has an unfavorable influence of the prognosis of patients with ERMS and ARMS (54, 76, 91). RMS fall within the domains of pediatric oncology and hemato-oncology. Such neoplasms generally require a multimodal therapeutic strategy that needs to be interdisciplinarily discussed among representatives from the corresponding disciplines as well as radiologists. The same applies to RMS that coincide with gestation. Nowadays, multimodal therapeutic models achieve cure rates of over 90 %. A case has recently been reported in which a pregnant patient (27th week of gestation) with extrauterine ARMS was successfully treated with CHT. Treatment had no apparent influence on the fetus (76). A healthy child was delivered by cesarean section, and the mother did not relapse within the 2-year follow-up period.

Coincidences of genital rhabdomyosarcoma and pregnancy are the exception. Rhabdomyosarcomas do not have a negative impact on fertility or fetal development. Pregnancy has no apparent influence on the prognosis for this neoplasm.

8.14 PEComa

No cases have yet been observed in which pregnancy and PEComa coincided. Accordingly, it is unclear whether pregnancy impacts negatively on the clinical course or prognosis of such tumors. Women who develop a PEComa later do not appear to suffer any limitations or detrimental effects in terms of their fertility. It is also unknown whether PEComas are epidemiologically associated with prior pregnancies. It is not uncommon for benign, semi-malignant and malignant PEComas to occur in children and women under the age of 30, i.e. in girls and women who potentially still have a desire to bear children (11, 15, 63, 89). In terms of conservative surgery, the same rules apply as for STUMP and LMS. Reference can be made to the chapter on PEComas (cf. Chapter 4) in this regard. It is also unknown whether pregnancy impacts negatively on the prognosis for PEComas that have been subjected to conservative surgery prior to gestation.

No publications have yet been devoted to the issue of fertility/gestation and PEComas. Regarding conservative operations and the desire to preserve fertility, reference can be made to the data and information pertaining to leiomyosarcoma and STUMP.

8.15 Adenofibroma

In one case in which a patient had had a positive pregnancy test, a cystic tubal tumor containing embryo-like solid components was mistaken for a tubal pregnancy. Salpingectomy revealed the solid mass to be AF. The embryo was later found in the uterus, and pregnancy culminated in the birth of a healthy child (24).

Literature covering possible associations between adenofibromas and gestation is virtually nonexistent.

8.16 Adenosarcoma

Due to a lack of data, it is not known whether AS that have been treated with conservative surgery prior to gestation have any influence on fertility, or whether pregnancy has a negative impact on the prognosis of such tumors. Given that AS and stromal sarcomas exhibit largely identical behavior (73), reference can be made to the uterine stromal sarcomas in the context of these issues as well. In particular, the data and information pertaining to LG-ESS can also be largely applied to AS without OS, and with positive HR.

Local excision can be an option for patients with favorably localized AS without SO, who urgently desire fertility-preserving treatment (29, 51). Resection must leave disease-free (RO) margins. No recurrences were observed in one patient who underwent curettage and two patients who underwent SHE (7). Among 8 adolescents with cervical AS who underwent organ-sparing surgery, 5 developed recurrences (12, 22). Pedunculated tumors confined to the endometrium are best suited for a conservative surgical strategy, assuming RO resection margins are achieved in the process (29). In general, organ-sparing surgical interventions must nonetheless be classified as inadequate operations, not least because (analogous to LG-ESS) leaving the ovaries in situ in patients with HR positive AS can potentially foster recurrence. Among the cases covered in one publication, retaining the adnexa was not associated with recurrence during the follow-up period (51). Long-term data have yet to be published, however. Patients in this context need to be comprehensively informed of the generally elevated risk of recurrence that arises when sarcomas are treated conservatively. Furthermore, it is particularly important that patients in these cases undergo accurate follow-up examinations using sonography and MRI, when necessary. Analogous to the other uterine sarcomas, patients should undergo follow-up LSC within 3 to 6 months of conservative surgery (cf. Chapter 6 and Vol. 1, Chapter 4). The very poor prognosis generally associated with AS with SO forbids any and all forms of conservative surgery. Pregnancy-related data have not been published to date.

No data are available that pertain to the influence of AS that have been subjected to conservative surgical therapy prior to gestation on fertility. Nor can any reliable statements be made as to whether gestation impacts negatively on the prognosis for such tumors. Regarding organ-sparing operations and the desire to preserve fertility, reference can be made to the stromal sarcomas.

8.17 Carcinosarcoma

Analogous to EC, in some cases, UCS have been found to be associated with nulliparity (33). According to one publication, nulliparous women more frequently present with advanced CS at the time of primary diagnosis (1), while in another study, parity did not influence overall survival (10). There have been no publications over the last 50 years that describe the simultaneous occurrence of gestation and UCS, most likely because such tumors predominantly arise in postmenopausal women. If a CS is diagnosed at an early age of gestation, the very poor overall prognosis with which CS are associated serves as an urgent indication for terminating the pregnancy and performing definitive surgery. This generally applies to all genital CS.

No accounts of carcinosarcomas in pregnant patients have yet been described in the literature. When carcinosarcoma and gestation do coincide, treatment must be administered swiftly and consistently.

References

(1) Albrektsen G, Heuch I, Wik E, Salvesen HB. Prognostic impact of parity in 493 uterine sarcoma patients. Int. J. Gynecol Cancer 2009; 19: 1062–107

(2) Amant F, Van Calsteren K, Debiec-Rychter M, Heyns L, De Beeck KO, Sagaert X, Bollen B, Vergote I. High-grade endometrial stromal sarcoma presenting in a 28-year-old woman during pregnancy: A case report. J Med Case Reports 2010; 4: 243

(3) Andergassen U. Ein Fall von regelhaftem Schwangerschaftsverlauf nach organerhaltender Operation eines endometrialen Stromaknotens. Pers. Mitteilung 2014

(4) Bai H, Yang J, Cao D, Huang H, Xiang Y, Wu M, Cui Q, Chen J, Lang J, Shen K. Ovary and uterus-sparing procedures for low-grade endometrial stromal sarcoma: a retrospective study of 153 cases.Gynecol Oncol 2014; 132: 654–560

(5) Behranwala KA, Latifaj B, Blake P, Barton DP, Shepherd JH, Thomas JM. Vulvar soft tissue tumors. Int J Gynecol Cancer 2004; 14: 94–99

(6) Behzatoğlu K, Bahadir B, Inhan G, Altuğ M. Primary vaginal leiomyosarcoma in pregnancy. Gynecol Oncol 2003; 91: 627–629

(7) Bernard B, Clarke BA, Malowany JI, McAlpine J, Lee CH, Atenafu EG, Ferguson S, Mackay H. Uterine adenosarcomas: A dual-institution update on staging, prognosis and survival. Gynecol Oncol 2013; 131: 634–639

(8) Berretta R, Patrelli TS, Fadda GM, Merisio C, Gramellini D, Nardelli GB. Uterine tumors resembling ovarian sex cord tumors: A case report of conservative management in young women. Int J Gynecol Cancer 2009; 19: 808–810

(9) Blake EA, Sheridan TB, Wang KL, Takiuchi T, Kodama M, Sawada K, Matsuo K. Clinical characteristics and outcomes of uterine tumors resembling ovarian sex-cord tumors 13UTROSCT): A systematic review of literature. Eur J Obstet Gynecol Reprod Biol 2014; 181: 163–170

(10) Bodner-Adler B, Bodner K, Obermair A, Czerwenka K, Petru E, Leodolter S, Mayerhofer K. Prognostic parameters in carcinosarcomas of the uterus: A clinico-pathologic study. Anticancer Res 2001; 21: 3069–3074

(11) Bunch K, Sunde J. Fertility sparing treatment of a malignant uterine perivascular epithelioid cell tumor: A case report. Gynecol Oncol Case Rep 2014; 8: 14–16

(12) Buyukkurt S, Guzel AB, Gumurdulu D, Vardar MA, Zeren H, Sucu M. Mullerian adenosarcoma of the uterine cervix in an adolescent girl. J Pediatr Adolesc Gynecol 2010; 23: e13–55.

(13) Campbell JE, Knudtson JE, Valente PT, Robinson RD, Kost ER. Successful pregnancy following myomectomy for uterine smooth muscle tumor of uncertain malignant potential: A case report and review of the literature. Gynecol Oncol Rep 2016; 15: 1–3

(14) Clauss S, Höller S, Hegi L, Blum R, Hösli I. ["STUMP" (smooth muscle tumour of uncertain malignant potential), a tumour of the uterus in pregnancy—a diagnostic and therapeutic challenge]. Z Geburtshilfe Neonatol 2010; 214: 74–77
(15) Clement PB, Young RH. Atlas of Gynaecologic Surgical Pathology. Elsevier Saunders 2014
(16) De Angelis SL, Harris RR, Maiman MA, Knochenhauer ES. Live birth of a normal mature healthy baby by in vitro fertilization-embryo transfer (IVF-ET) after an exploratory laparotomy and multiple myomectomy for leiomyomatosis peritonealis disseminata. Fertil Steril 2009; 91: 1956–1957
(17) Delaney AA, Gubbels AL, Remmenga S, Tomich P, Molpus K. Successful pregnancy after fertility-sparing local resection and uterine reconstruction for low-grade endometrial stromal sarcoma. Obstet Gynecol 2012; 120: 486–489
(18) De Vivo A, Mancuso A, Giacobbe A, Savasta LM, De Dominici R, Dugo N, Dugo C, Vaiarelli A. Uterine myomas during pregnancy: A longitudinal sonographic study. Ultrasound Obstet Gynecol 2011; 37: 361–355
(19) Di Gilio AR, Cormio G, Resta L, Carriero C, Loizzi V, Parisi AM, Selvaggi L. Rapid growth of myxoid leiomyosarcoma of the vulva during pregnancy: A case report. Int J Gynecol Cancer 2004; 14: 172–175
(20) Di Vagno G, Cormio G, Resta L, Colucci GA, Provenzano L, Selvaggi L. Uterine tumour resembling an ovarian sex-cord tumour presenting with spontaneous haemoperitoneum in pregnancy. Aust N Z J Obstet Gynaecol 1996; 36:213–215
(21) Dong R, Pang Y, Mao H, Yang N, Liu P. Successful pregnancy following conservative management of low-grade endometrial stromal sarcoma: A case report. Oncol Lett 2014; 7: 1039–1042
(22) Fleming NA, Hopkins L, de Nanassy J, Senterman M, Black AY. Mullerian adenosarcoma of the cervix in a 10-year-old girl: case report and review of the literature. J Pediatr Adolesc Gynecol 2009; 22: e45–51.
(23) Fujita T, Taira N, Ogasawara Y, Omori M, Doihara H. Bilateral angiosarcoma of the breast detected by magnetic resonance imaging during pregnancy. Int J Clin Oncol 2009; 14: 560–563
(24) Fukushima A, Shoji T, Tanaka S, Sugiyama T. A case of fallopian tube adenofibroma: difficulties associated with differentiation from ectopic pregnancy. Clin Med Insights Case Rep. 2014 Nov 27;7:135–137. DOI: 10.4137/CCRep.S18859
(25) Garuti G, Gonfiantini C, Mirra M, Galli C, Luerti M. Uterine tumor resembling ovarian sex cord tumors treated by resectoscopic surgery. J Minim Invasive Gynecol 2009; 16: 236–240
(26) Gojnic M, Likic I, Pervulov M, Petkovic S, Fazlagic A, Vasiljevic B. The significance of Doppler flow in early detection of uterine sarcoma in older primigravida pregnancies. Eur J Gynaecol Oncol 2005; 26: 291–2933
(27) Goto A. Takeuchi S. Sugimura K. Maruo T. Usefulness of Gd-DTPA contrast-enhanced dynamic MRI and serum determination of LDH and its isozymes in the differential diagnosis of leiomyosarcoma from degenerated leiomyoma of the uterus. Int J Gynecol Cancer 2002; 12: 354–361
(28) Hachisuga T. Hashimoto H. Enjoji M. Angioleiomyoma. A clinicopathologic reappraisal of 562 cases. Cancer 1984; 54: 126–130
(29) Han XY, Xiang Y, Guo LN, Shen K, Wan XR, Huang HF, Pan LY. Clinicopathological analysis of mullerian adenosarcoma of the uterus. Chin Med J (Engl) 2010; 123: 756–759
(30) Hillard JB, Malpica A, Ramirez PT. Conservative management of a uterine tumor resembling an ovarian sex cord-stromal tumor. Gynecol Oncol 2004; 92: 347–352
(31) Horstmann JP, Pietra GG, Harman JA. Spontaneous regression of pulmonary leiomyomas during pregnancy. Cancer 1977; 39: 314 –321
(32) Jha S, Chan KK, Poole CJ, Rollason TP. Pregnancy following recurrent angiosarcoma of the ovary—a case report and review of literature. Gynecol Oncol 2005; 97: 935–937

(33) Inthasorn P, Carte J, Valmadr S. Beale P. Russel P. Dalrymple C. Analysis of clinicopathologic factors in malignant mixed Müllerian tumors of the uterine corpus. Int J Gynecol Cancer 2002, 12: 348–353
(34) Ishikawa H, Ishi K, Serna VA, Kakazu R, Bulun SE, Kurita T. Progesterone is essential for maintenance and growth of uterine leiomyoma. Endocrinology 2010; 151: 2433–2442
(35) Jeng CJ, Tzen CY, Huang WC, Yang YC, Shen J, Tzeng CR. Recurrent retroperitoneal myxoid liposarcoma during pregnancy: A case report and literature review. Int J Gynecol Cancer 2005; 15: 1235–1238
(36) Kagami S, Kashimura M, Toki N, Katuhata Y. Myxoid leiomyosarcoma of the uterus with subsequent pregnancy and delivery. Gynecol Oncol 2002; 85: 538–542
(37) Kamra HT, Dantkale SS, Birla K, Sakinlawar PW, Narkhede RR. Myxoid leiomyoma of cervix. J Clin Diagn Res 2013; 7: 2956–2957
(38) Karpf EF, Poetsch B, Langner C, Nogales FF, Regauer S. Endometrial stromal nodule embedded into term placenta. Acta Pathol Microbiol Immunol Scand 2007; 115: 1302–1305
(39) Katsanis WA, O'Connor DM, Gibb RK, Bendon RW. Endometrial stromal sarcoma involving the placenta. Ann Diagn Pathol 1998; 2: 301–305
(40) Kim JJ, Kurita T, Bulun SE. Progesterone action in endometrial cancer, endometriosis, uterine fibroids, and breast cancer. Endocr Rev 2013; 34: 130–162.
(41) Köhler G, Belau, A, Dennis K, Evert K, Evert M, Hesse J, Hegenscheid K, Köller M, Krichbaum J, Kühnast M, Lehnhoff H, Lehr A, Linke L, Marcinek A, Müller S, Riechmann C, Schalitz S, Simon J, Spring P, Schädler, J, Ständer C, Trojnarska D, Wilcke S, Witte N, Zygmunt M; Deutsches klinisches Kompetenzzentrum für genitale Sarkome und Mischtumoren an der Universitätsmedizin Greifswald (DKSM) und Kooperationspartner VAAO Deutschland und FK Frankfurt/Sachsenhausen. Datenbank und Promotions- und Forschungsgruppe genitale Sarkome, Greifswald 2016, http://www.medizin.uni-greifswald.de/gyn/dksm/
(42) Koskas M, Morice P, Yazbeck C, Duvillard P, Walker F, Madelenat P. Conservative management of low-grade endometrial stromal sarcoma followed by pregnancy and severe recurrence. Anticancer Res 2009; 29: 4147–4150
(43) Laughlin SK, Baird DD, Savitz DA, Herring AH, Hartmann KE. Prevalence of uterine leiomyomas in the first trimester of pregnancy: An ultrasound-screening study. Obstet Gynecol 2009; 113: 630–635
(44) Lee CH, Mariño-Enriquez A, Ou W, Zhu M, Ali RH, Chiang S, Amant F, Gilks CB, van de Rijn M, Oliva E, Debiec-Rychter M, Dal Cin P, Fletcher JA, Nucci MR. The clinicopathologic features of YWHAE-FAM22 endometrial stromal sarcomas: A histologically high-grade and clinically aggressive tumor. Am J Surg Pathol 2012; 36: 641–653
(45) Leunen K, Amant F, Debiec-Rychter M, Croes R, Hagemeijer A, Schoenmakers EF, Vergote I. Endometrial stromal sarcoma presenting as postpartum haemorrhage: report of a case with a sole t(10;17)(q22;p13) translocation. Gynecol Oncol 2003; 9: 265–271
(46) Liang S, Stone G, Chalas E, Pearl M, Callan F, Zheng W. A high-grade uterine leiomyosarcoma with human chorionic gonadotropin production. Int J Gynecol Pathol 2006; 25: 257–261
(47) Ling FT, David TE, Merchant N, Yu E, Butany JW. Intracardiac extension of intravenous leiomyomatosis in a pregnant woman: A case report and review of the literature. Can J Cardiol 2000; 16: 73–79
(48) Lissoni A, Cormio G, Bonazzi C, Perego P, Lomonocio S, Gabriele A, Bratina G. Fertility sparing surgery in uterine leiomyosarcoma. Gynecol Oncol 1998; 70: 348–350
(49) Lopes RI, Machado M, Paz C, Santos AC, Rezende WW. Successful outcome of a surgically treated giant retroperitoneal liposarcoma during pregnancy. Arch Gynecol Obstet 2009; 280: 1067–1069

(50) Ly A, Mills AM, McKenney JK, Balzer BL, Kempson RL, Hendrickson MR, Longacre TA. Atypical leiomyomas of the uterus: A clinicopathologic study of 51 cases. Am J Surg Pathol. 2013; 37:643–649

(51) Manoharan M, Azmi MA, Soosay G, Mould T, Weekes AR. Mullerian adenosarcoma of uterine cervix: report of three cases and review of literature. Gynecol Oncol 2007; 105: 256–260

(52) Marom D, Pitlik S, Sagie A, Ovadia Y, Bishara J. Intravenous leiomyomatosis with cardiac involvement in a pregnant woman. Am J Obstet Gynecol 1998; 178: 620–621

(53) Mathew M1, Gowri V, Al Hamdani A, Machado L, Rao K, Shabnam S. Cotyledonoid leiomyoma in pregnancy. Obstet Gynecol 2007; 109: 509–511

(54) Matsuo K, Eno ML, Im DD, Rosenshein NB. Pregnancy and genital sarcoma: A systematic review of the literature. Am J Perinatol 2009; 26: 507–518

(55) Miller JN Jr. Pregnancy complicated by intravenous leiomyomatosis. Am J Obstet Gynecol 1975; 22: 485–489

(56) Nardo LG, Iyer L, Reginald PW. Benign pulmonary metastasizing leiomyomatosis in pregnancy: A rare complication after cesarean section. Acta Obstet Gynecol Scand 2003; 82: 770–772

(57) National Comprehensive Cancer Network: NCCN Practice Guidelines in Oncology – V.2.2016, Uterine neoplasms. www.nccn.org

(58) Nielsen GP, Rosenberg AE, Koerner FC, Young RH, Scully RE. Smooth-muscle tumors of the vulva. A clinicopathological study of 25 cases and review of the literature. Am J Surg Pathol. 1996; 20:779–793

(59) Noventa M, Gizzo S, Conte L, Dalla Toffola A, Litta P, Saccardi C. Fertility sparing surgery in young women affected by endometrial stromal sarcoma: An oncologic dilemma or a reliable option? Review of literature starting from a peculiar case. Onco Targets Ther 2014; 8: 29–35

(60) Oduyebo T, Rauh-Hain AJ, Meserve EE, Seidman MA, Hinchcliff E, George S, Quade B, Nucci MR, Del Carmen MG, Muto MG. The value of re-exploration in patients with inadvertently morcellated uterine sarcoma. Gynecol Oncol 2014; 132: 360–365

(61) Oh SE, Kim HJ, Choi SJ, Oh SY, Roh CR, Kim JH. A case of huge retroperitoneal liposarcoma in pregnancy. Obstet Gynecol Sci 2014; 57: 236–239

(62) Oliva E, Caracangiu ML, Carinelli SG, Ip P, Loening T, Longacre TA, Nucci MR, Prat J, Zaloudek CJ. Mesenchymal tumors. In: Kurman RJ, Carcangiu ML, Herrington CS, Young RH (eds). WHO classification of tumors of female reproductive organs. 4th edn. IARC: Lyon 2014, pp. 135–152

(63) Ong LY, Hwang WS, Wong A, Chan MY, Chui CH. Perivascular epithelioid cell tumour of the vagina in an 8 year old girl. J Pediatr Surg 2007; 42: 564–566

(64) Rai H, Odunsi K, Kesterson J, Morrison C, Chan A, Mhawech-Fauceglia P. Epithelioid sarcoma of the vulva in a 17-year-old pregnant woman. Appl Immunohistochem Mol Morphol 2009; 17:270–273

(65) Roscher W. Fatal intrapartum hemorrhage in primary tubal sarcoma in a multigravida. Zentralbl Gynakol 1956; 78: 1063–1070

(66) Rousková L, Melichar B, Nikolov DH, Cerman J Jr, Havel E, Megancová J, Urminská H, Jandík P. Fulminant course of metastatic liposarcoma after delivery—case report. Eur J Gynaecol Oncol. 2007; 28: 67–68

(67) Saeki H, Suzuki C, Yamasaki S, Hashizume A, Izumi H, Suzuki F, Ishi K, Nojima M, Hino O. Cotyledonoid dissecting leiomyoma of the uterus: report of two cases. Arch Gynecol Obstet. 2015; 291: 357–361

(68) Salman MC, Guler OT, Kucukali T, Karaman N, Ayhan A. Fertility-saving surgery for low-grade uterine leiomyosarcoma with subsequent pregnancy. Int J Gynaecol Obstet 2007; 98: 160–161

(69) Samadian M, Rakhshan M, Haddadian K, Rezaei O, Zamani SA, Khormaee F. Angiosarcoma of skull in a pregnant woman: case report and review of the literature. Turk Neurosurg 2012; 22:113–115

(70) Sánchez-Ferrer ML, Machado-Linde F, Ferri-Ñíguez B, Sánchez-Ferrer M, Parrilla-Paricio JJ. Reproductive outcome after uterine-sparing surgery for endometrial stromal sarcoma. Gynecol Oncol Case Rep 2012; 3: 4–6
(71) Saraiva F, Antunes M, Providência LA. Cardiac angiosarcoma in a pregnant woman: A case report and review of the literature. Acta Cardiol 2012; 67: 727–731
(72) Schiavone MB, Smok D, Wright TC, Wright JD. High-grade uterine sarcoma during pregnancy. Gynecol Oncol 2011; 123: 424–425
(73) Seidman JD, Chauhan S. Evaluation of the relationship between adenosarcoma and carcinosarcoma and a hypothesis of the histogenesis of uterine sarcomas. Int J Gynecol Pathol. 2003; 22:75–82
(74) Seidman MA, Oduyebo T, Muto MG, Crum CP, Nucci MR, Quade BJ. Peritoneal dissemination complicating morcellation of uterine mesenchymal neoplasms. PLoS One. 2012; 7:e50058. DOI: 10.1371/journal.pone.0050058
(75) Sharma P, Kumar R, Singh H, Jeph S, Sharma JB, Jain SK, Sharma DN, Bal C, Malhotra A. Role of FDG PET-CT in detecting recurrence in patients with uterine sarcoma: comparison with conventional imaging. Nucl Med Commun 2012; 33: 185–190
(76) Siepermann M, Koscielniak E, Dantonello T, Klee D, Boos J, Krefeld B, Borkhardt A, Hoehn T, Asea A, Wessalowski R. Oral low-dose chemotherapy: successful treatment of an alveolar rhabdomyosarcoma during pregnancy. Pediatr Blood Cancer 2012; 58: 104–106.
(77) Stadsvold JL, Molpus KL, Baker JJ, Michael K, Remmenga SW. Conservative management of a myxoid endometrial stromal sarcoma in a 16-year old nulliparous woman. Gynecol Oncol 99 (2005) 243–245
(78) Summa B, Schem C, Weigel M, Strauss A, Jonat W, Maass N, Schäfer F, Bauerschlag DO. Leiomyomatosis peritonealis disseminata in a pregnant woman. Arch Gynecol Obstet 2010; 28: 1123–1127
(79) Susini T1, Taddei G, Massi D, Massi G. Giant pelvic retroperitoneal liposarcoma. Obstet Gynecol 2000; 95: 1002–1004
(80) Tanaka YO, Tsunoda H, Sugano M, Satoh T, Yagi H, Minami R, Shiigai M, Inadome Y, Yoshikawa H, Noguchi M, Minami M. MR and CT findings of leiomyomatosis peritonealis disseminata with emphasis on assisted reproductive technology as a risk factor. Br J Radiol 2009; 82: e44–7.
(81) Takeda A, Imoto S. Mori M, Nakamura H. Successful pregnancy outcome after laparoscopic-assisted excision of a bizarre leiomyoma: A case report. J Med Case Rep 2011; 5:344
(82) Takeda A, Imoto S, Mori M, Yamada J, Nakamura H. Rapid growth of parasitic myoma in early pregnancy: previously undescribed manifestation of a rare disorder after laparoscopic-assisted myomectomy. Eur J Obstet Gynecol Reprod Biol 2012; 162: 117–118
(83) Tavassoli FA, Norris HJ. Smooth muscle tumors of the vulva. Obstet Gynecol 1979; 53: 13–217
(84) Tebes S, Cardosi R, Hoffman M. Liposarcoma complicating pregnancy. Gynecol Oncol 2001; 83: 610–612
(85) Ulker V, Gungorduk K, Numanoglu C, Sahbaz A, Aslan O, Tekirdag AI, Gulkilik A. Complete surgical resection of retroperitoneal leiomyosarcoma in pregnancy: A case report. Arch Gynecol Obstet 2008; 277: 353–356
(86) Wang J, Fisher C, Thway K. Angiosarcoma of the breast with solitary metastasis to the ovary during pregnancy: An uncommon pattern of metastatic disease. Case Rep Oncol Med 2013; 2013:209610. DOI: 10.1155/2013/209610
(87) Woytoń J, Florjański J, Tomiałowicz M. [Stromal sarcoma in pregnancy – A case report]. Ginekol Pol 2002; 73: 400–403
(88) Yamamoto T, Marui T, Akisue T, Hitora T, Kawamoto T, Nagira K, Nakatani T, Yoshiya S, Kurosaka M. Management of liposarcoma occurring in pregnant women. Anticancer Res 2003; 23: 799–802

(89) Yamamoto E, Ino K, Sakurai M, Takigawa S, Iwase A, Kikkawa F. Fertility–sparing operation for recurrence of uterine cervical perivascular epithelioid cell tumor. Rare Tumors 2010; 2: e26
(90) Yan L, Tian Y, Fu Y, Zhao X. Successful pregnancy after fertility-preserving surgery for endometrial stromal sarcoma. Fertil Steril 2010; 93: 269.e1–3
(91) Yu L, Yang SJ. Spindle cell rhabdomyosarcoma of the retroperitoneum: An unusual case developed in a pregnant woman but obscured by pregnancy. Int J Clin Exp Pathol 2014; 7: 4904–4912
(92) Younis JS, Okon E, Anteby SO. Uterine leiomyosarcoma in pregnancy. Arch Gynecol Obstet 1990; 247: 155–160
(93) Zanotti-Fregonara P, Koroscil TM, Mantil J, Satter M. Radiation dose to the fetus from [(18)F]-FDG administration during the second trimester of pregnancy. Health Phys 2012; 102: 217–219.
(94) Zanotti-Fregonara P. Pregnancy should not rule out 18FDG PET/CT for women with cancer. Lancet 2012; 379:1948
(95) Zhan R, Wen H, Gao X, Yin L. Successful term pregnancy after laparoscopic surgery of low grade endometrial stromal sarcoma. Chinese Medical Journal 2014; 127: 391–392

Image references

Evert M, Evert K. Universitätsmedizin Greifswald, Institut für Pathologie, Greifswald.
Fig. 8.6.1 (A)–(C)

Index

Printed and bound by CPI Group (UK) Ltd, Croydon, CR0 4YY
13/09/2026
14960851-0003